AF510629

Veterinary Medicine: An Evidence-Based Approach

Veterinary Medicine: An Evidence-Based Approach

Editor: Gerardo Bailey

Callisto Reference

www.callistoreference.com

Callisto Reference,
118-35 Queens Blvd., Suite 400,
Forest Hills, NY 11375, USA

Visit us on the World Wide Web at:
www.callistoreference.com

© Callisto Reference, 2022

This book contains information obtained from authentic and highly regarded sources. Copyright for all individual chapters remain with the respective authors as indicated. All chapters are published with permission under the Creative Commons Attribution License or equivalent. A wide variety of references are listed. Permission and sources are indicated; for detailed attributions, please refer to the permissions page and list of contributors. Reasonable efforts have been made to publish reliable data and information, but the authors, editors and publisher cannot assume any responsibility for the validity of all materials or the consequences of their use.

ISBN: 978-1-64116-640-9 (Hardback)

Trademark Notice: Registered trademark of products or corporate names are used only for explanation and identification without intent to infringe.

Cataloging-in-Publication Data

Veterinary medicine : an evidence-based approach / edited by Gerardo Bailey.
p. cm.
Includes bibliographical references and index.
ISBN 978-1-64116-640-9
1. Veterinary medicine. 2. Animals--Diseases. 3. Animal health. I. Bailey, Gerardo.
SF745 .V48 2022
636.089--dc23

Table of Contents

Preface

This book has been a concerted effort by a group of academicians, researchers and scientists, who have contributed their research works for the realization of the book. This book has materialized in the wake of emerging advancements and innovations in this field. Therefore, the need of the hour was to compile all the required researches and disseminate the knowledge to a broad spectrum of people comprising of students, researchers and specialists of the field.

The branch of medicine which deals with the diagnosis, prevention and treatment of disease, disorder and injury in animals is known as veterinary medicine. It has a broad scope, ranging from domesticated animals to wild animals. It covers a wide spectrum of conditions which can affect different species. Professional care in veterinary medicine is mostly led by a veterinary physician. Other paraveterinary workers such as veterinary nurses and technicians can also provide professional veterinary care. The effectiveness of treatment in veterinary medicine is determined with the help of randomized controlled trials. Research in this domain is focused on wildlife and ecosystem health, human-animal interfaces and zoonotic diseases. This book brings forth some of the most innovative concepts and elucidates the unexplored aspects of veterinary medicine using an evidence based approach. It unravels the recent researches in this field. This book is appropriate for students seeking detailed information on veterinary medicine as well as for experts.

At the end of the preface, I would like to thank the authors for their brilliant chapters and the publisher for guiding us all-through the making of the book till its final stage. Also, I would like to thank my family for providing the support and encouragement throughout my academic career and research projects.

Editor

1

A comparison of the histopathologic pattern of the left atrium in canine dilated cardiomyopathy and chronic mitral valve disease

Izabela Janus[1*], Agnieszka Noszczyk-Nowak[2], Marcin Nowak[1], Rafał Ciaputa[1], Małgorzata Kandefer-Gola[1] and Urszula Pasławska[2]

Abstract

Background: Dilated cardiomyopathy (DCM) and chronic mitral valve disease (CMVD) in dogs are associated with heart chamber enlargement, also of the left atrium. DCM is often accompanied by rhythm disturbances (mainly atrial fibrillation or ventricular arrhythmias). In CMVD, arrhythmias are observed less frequently. It is still unclear whether left atrial enlargement in these diseases results from volume overload or if it is also connected with other factors (e.g. rhythm disturbances).

This study was conducted on the left atrial myocardial specimens from 31 dogs, including those from 16 dogs with clinically diagnosed DCM and 15 dogs with CMVD. After fixation and staining (using haematoxylin-eosin and Masson-Goldner trichrome stain), the specimens underwent evaluation. Parenchymal changes (fibrosis, fatty infiltration, and vessel narrowing), degenerative changes (loss of striation, changes in cardiomyocyte structure, and abnormal cell nuclei) and the presence of inflammatory infiltrates were assessed.

Results: More interstitial fibrosis (median 4 vs. 2.5 grid fields; $p < 0.05$) and less perivascular fibrosis (median score 1 vs. 2; $p < 0.05$) was observed in the DCM group compared to the CMVD group. Moreover, less distinct vessel narrowing was observed in the DCM group than in the CMVD group (median lumen area ratio 0.3 vs. 0.26 respectively; $p < 0.05$). Dogs with DCM showed more strongly defined degenerative changes than the CMVD dogs (median nuclei enlargement score 3 vs. 1, median loss of striation score 3 vs. 2 and median structural alterations score 3 vs. 2, respectively; $p < 0.05$).

Conclusion: The obtained results indicate a different nature of changes occurring in the left atrial myocardium of dogs with DCM compared to dogs with mitral valve disease, including differences in vessel narrowing, cardiomyocyte degeneration and in the distribution of connective tissue.

Keywords: Dilated cardiomyopathy, Mitral valve disease, Dog, Left atrium, Histopathology

Background

Dilated cardiomyopathy (DCM) is a polyetiological disease characterised by a dilation of heart chambers (mainly the left ventricle and left atrium) without other significant structural heart defects. In some cases, it is combined with myocardial failure [1, 2]. It is mostly encountered in large and giant breed dogs but it can also develop in dogs of other breeds (e.g. English and American cocker spaniels, poodles and Portuguese water dogs) [1–7]. During the development of DCM the radiographic, echocardiographic and post-mortem examinations reveal an enlargement of the left ventricle and left atrium or an enlargement of all the heart chambers [1, 2, 4, 5, 7]. The ventricular dilation in DCM alters the geometry of atrioventricular valves, which results in valvular insufficiency. Mitral regurgitation increases left atrial pressure that may

* Correspondence: izabela.janus87@gmail.com
[1]Division of Pathomorphology and Veterinary Forensics, Department of Pathology, Wroclaw University of Environmental and Life Sciences, Wroclaw 50375, Poland
Full list of author information is available at the end of the article

worsen the pathological remodelling of the left atrium and the left ventricle and independently stimulate the dilation of the heart chambers [8]. The disease is often accompanied by rhythm disturbances, mainly atrial fibrillation. However, there is no consent whether atrial fibrillation is the cause or result of atrial enlargement [9].

The histopathologic examination of the samples obtained from dogs with DCM demonstrates changes in the myocardial structure. There are two well-described forms of histopathologic lesions in the ventricular specimens of dogs with DCM: the attenuated wavy fibre type (AWF) and the fatty infiltration-degenerative (FID) type. Those lesions are mostly encountered in specimens from the left ventricle, but can also occur in the myocardium of the right ventricle and interventricular septum [1, 2, 4, 5, 8, 10]. Our previous study showed similar changes in atrial specimens from dogs with FID types of lesions in the ventricles. In dogs with the AWF type of ventricular lesions, the changes observed in atria can resemble either AWF or FID types of changes [11]. The attenuation of cardiomyocytes is a specific pathological feature of DCM. However, vacuolisation, extensive fibrosis and fatty infiltration may also occur in the ventricular walls during the course of that disease [1, 2, 4, 7]. Due to the fact that there is a similarity between the FID type of DCM and arrhythmogenic right ventricular cardiomyopathy, it is important to accurately characterise the disease based on the clinical and histopathological examinations [5].

The mechanism of changes occurring in the atrial myocardial structure in DCM is not well defined. It is suspected that the structural protein defects, impaired tissue oxygen supply and other factors may play a role in the development of the disease [1, 2]. It is not well understood whether the macroscopic and microscopic changes within the atria in dogs with DCM are a result of primary remodelling, the presence of arrhythmias, or a response of the cardiac tissue to functional disturbances, including volume overload (which also occurs in mitral valve disease).

Canine chronic mitral valve disease (CMVD) is the most common cardiovascular disease in dogs and the most frequent cause of congestive heart failure in those animals. The disease predominantly occurs in small breed dogs (e.g. Cavalier King Charles spaniels, Yorkshire terriers, dachshunds) and progresses with age [12–14]. The progressive dilation of the left ventricle and the left atrium in CMVD results from degenerative changes and an insufficiency of the mitral valve, leading to symptoms of heart failure [15]. Histopathologic changes within the ventricular walls include fibrosis and arteriosclerosis without or with slight myocyte atrophy [16, 17].

The purpose of the study was a histopathologic comparison of the left atrial wall specimens obtained from dogs with severe left atrial enlargement resulting from clinically diagnosed dilated cardiomyopathy (DCM) or chronic mitral valve disease (CMVD). To the authors' knowledge, there are no detailed studies comparing histopathologic changes occurring in the atria in those diseases.

Methods

Case selection

Thirty-one dogs aged from 4 to 19 years (23 males and 8 females) with either CMVD or DCM were included in the study. Dogs met the inclusion criteria if they had an enlarged left atrium according to an echocardiographic examination (left atrial (LA)-to-aortic root (Ao) diameter ratio; LA/Ao >1.7 [18]), which was confirmed in a post-mortem examination. Dogs were included in the DCM group if they had a dilated left ventricle and a decreased fractional shortening (FS < 20 %) noted during an echocardiographic examination [1, 2, 5] with normal or type 1 mitral valve lesions (according to Whitney [19]). Dogs were included in the CMVD group if they had preserved left ventricular systolic function (FS > 20 %, noted in the echocardiographic examination) with type 3 or 4 mitral valve lesions (according to Whitney [19]). At the time of death or euthanasia, all dogs presented with stage D heart failure (according to the ACVIM Consensus Statement [20]).

Ante-mortem examination

All animals underwent a clinical examination, echocardiography and electrocardiography, and were treated and re-examined every 6 months, until they died or were euthanized due to heart failure refractory to treatment. Only the LA/Ao ratio from the last examination of each dog served as an inclusion criterion.

The ECG was performed in right lateral recumbency using a 6-channel BTL SD08 device (BTL, UK) with I, II, III, aVL, aVR, aVF, and precordial (V1-V6) lead recordings. The echocardiographic examination was performed in standard views using the Aloka SSD 4000 and Aloka Alpha7 machines and included the assessment of the LA/Ao ratio, end-systolic and end-diastolic left ventricular measurements, ejection fractions and FS, blood velocity through the aortic and pulmonic valve, and the function of the atrioventricular valves. The relative left atrial size was estimated based on the LA/Ao. This parameter was determined using standard images acquired from a right short-axis view at the base of the heart. Estimates of left ventricular systolic function were obtained from the index of circumferential myocardial contraction and FS using the formula: FS[%] = ([LVIDd − LVIDs]/LVIDd) ×100, where LVIDd and LVIDs are the internal left ventricular dimensions at end-diastole and end-systole, respectively. Left ventricular dilation was estimated based on the comparison of chamber measurements (internal diameter and wall thickness) to standard breed-specific or body-weight specific values [21]. The function of the atrioventricular, pulmonary and aortic valves was examined using pulsed wave Doppler and color Doppler techniques.

Post-mortem examination

The results of the echocardiographic examination (left atrial and left ventricular enlargement) were confirmed during the post-mortem examination, where the type of mitral valve lesion was determined. Heart measurements were taken using a manual 150 mm Beerendonk caliper, measured to the nearest 1/20 mm. The measurements were taken in planes compatible with those used during the echocardiographic examination. Specimens from the left atrial wall were collected from each dog for further histopathologic analysis. They were fixed in 7 % buffered formalin, embedded in paraffin blocks, sectioned at 6 µm, stained using the standard haematoxylin-eosin (H&E) method and Masson-Goldner trichrome (for a better visualisation of connective tissue), and underwent a light microscopy evaluation. Photomicrographs of each studied specimen were subjected to computer-assisted image analysis, using a computer coupled to an optical Olympus BX53 microscope, equipped with a Color View IIIu digital Olympus camera (Olympus, Japan). A morphometric analysis was performed using Cell^A software (Olympus Soft Imaging Solution GmbH, Germany).

To accurately describe the histopathological changes in the atria, specimens were evaluated for the presence and severity of fibrosis, fatty infiltration, inflammatory infiltration, intra-myocardial arterial narrowing and degenerative changes in cardiomyocytes. The latter was expressed as the presence of abnormal cell nuclei (swollen nuclei with an altered structure surrounded by a "halo"), loss of striation, and other features of degeneration (e.g. swelling of the cardiomyocyte, blurring of the cell structure and alterations in staining).

The presence and severity of interstitial fibrosis and fatty infiltration were evaluated after superimposing a 16-field grid over the digital image and counting the number of fields that showed the presence of fatty infiltration or fibrosis (in 200× magnification, after Masson-Goldner trichrome staining), as proposed by Lobo et al. [7].

The severity of perivascular fibrosis was assessed using the following scoring system: 0, no fibrosis; 1, mild; 2, moderate; 3, severe fibrosis (in 100× magnification, after Mason-Goldner trichrome staining).

Inflammatory infiltrates were evaluated according to the number of inflammatory cells in a field at a 400× magnification (H&E staining).

Intra-myocardial arterial narrowing was assessed using the lumen area ratio (LAR; the luminal area of the vessel divided by the total vessel area, not including the adventitia), as proposed by Falk et al. [16] (at 200× magnification, after H&E staining).

Cardiomyocyte degenerative changes (abnormal cell nuclei, loss of striation and changes in cardiomyocyte structure) were assessed using the following scoring system: 0, none or involving <25 % of the myofibres; 1, involving 25–50 % of the myofibres; 2, involving 50–75 % of the myofibres; 3, involving >75 % of the myofibres (at 400× magnification, after H&E staining).

Each of the features was evaluated in 20 randomly chosen fields per slide (for fatty infiltrates, interstitial fibrosis, inflammatory infiltrates, and cardiomyocyte degenerative changes) or in at least 10 vessels per slide (for perivascular fibrosis and LAR), and a mean score was subsequently calculated for the slide.

Ethical consideration

According to the Polish law [22], standard diagnostic procedures and studies conducted on animal tissue do not require permission from the Ethical Board. Oral consent for the ante-mortem examination (electrocardiography and echocardiography) was obtained from all owners, as those examinations are used routinely to diagnose canine heart disease.

Statistical analysis

A statistical analysis was performed using StatisticaPL® software (StatSoft, Poland). The Shapiro-Wilk analysis was used to test the data normality. The Mann–Whitney *U* test (for data distributed non-normally) or Student's t test (for data distributed normally) were used to compare groups. The level of statistical significance was set at $P < 0.05$.

The results are shown as range and median values.

Results

The DCM group consisted of 16 dogs (9 Doberman pinschers, 4 German shepherds, 2 boxers, and 1 great Dane, aged 4–11 years, including 12 males and 4 females). Seven specimens from the left ventricle presented with an AWF type of lesion, while nine specimens had features of a FID type of lesion. The CMVD group comprised 15 dogs (10 mixed-breed dogs, 2 dachshunds, 1 Cairn terrier, 1 miniature pinscher, and 1 German pinscher, aged 8–19 years, including 11 males and 4 females) diagnosed with mitral valve disease combined with an enlarged left ventricle and left atrium (Table 1).

Dogs in the DCM group were significantly younger and heavier than those from the CMVD group, but there was no difference in the LA/Ao ratio between both groups (Table 1). All dogs in the DCM group and 26.7 % of dogs in the CMVD group had rhythm disturbances, as shown in Table 1.

The results of the histopathological analysis are shown in Table 2. The DCM group showed significantly more interstitial fibrosis, less perivascular fibrosis, a higher

Table 1 Population study and clinical findings in the examined groups

	DCM group $n = 16$	CMVD group $n = 15$	*p*-value
age (median; range) [years]	9 (4–11)	15 (8–19)	<0.001
weight (median; range) [kg]	31 (30–45)	11 (5–25)	<0.001
arrhythmia (*n*)	16	4[a]	
atrial fibrillation (*n*)	15	1	
ventricular tachycardia (*n*)	1	-	
atrial premature complexes (*n*)	-	2	
ventricular premature complexes (*n*)	-	2	
LA/Ao (mean ± SD)	3.14 ± 0.31	2.44 ± 0.71	0.08

LA/Ao left-atrial-to-aorta ratio, *SD* standard deviation
[a]one dog showing both single atrial premature complexes and ventricular premature complexes

LAR value, and no difference in fatty infiltration severity compared to the CMVD group (Figs. 1 and 2). Moreover, we noted a significantly more cardiomyocyte degenerative changes in the DCM group compared to the CMVD group (Figs. 1 and 2). They included the presence of abnormal cell nuclei, loss of striation and changes in the structure of the cardiomyocytes. No difference in the severity of inflammatory infiltrates was noted between both groups. The inflammatory infiltration consisted of single lymphocytes mainly localised subendocardially. The average number of inflammatory cells per field did not exceed 2 in any of the examined specimens.

Discussion

There have been numerous histopathological characterisations of canine DCM [1, 2, 4, 7]. However, changes occurring in the atrial tissue in the course of DCM remain poorly described. Similarly to our findings, Everett et al. [8] noted fibrosis and cardiomyocyte atrophy in specimens from the atria in Doberman pinschers with DCM. Those lesions were less extensive and less common than the lesions found in specimens from ventricles in the same animals.

According to Schaper et al. [23], normal cardiac tissue in failing hearts in humans is replaced by fibrosis. This is accompanied by changes within the cardiomyocyte nuclei (including nuclear enlargement). Sharov et al. [24] noted a disruption in the structure of cardiomyocytes with subsequent fibrosis in dogs with heart failure. The authors associated myocardial fibrosis with changes in the expression of structural proteins. We observed lesions in cardiomyocytes and interstitial tissue in both groups, which may reflect the response of the heart to volume overload, as described in the abovementioned studies. In our study, there was more interstitial fibrosis and nuclear enlargement in the DCM group.

When comparing ventricular specimens from dogs showing DCM and CMVD, Falk et al. [17] noticed that the majority of dogs with CMVD showed only a small degree of cardiomyocyte atrophy in the ventricular specimens or none at all. Such differences in the severity of cardiomyocyte degeneration were also observed in our study.

Studies on dogs with CMVD showed that animals developing congestive heart failure present with lower values of LAR as compared to controls, although this parameter is highly variable in each dog [16]. Falk et al. [17] showed that a decrease in LAR is directly associated with a decrease in fractional shortening in the left ventricle. This suggests the presence of alterations in intra-myocardial vessels in the course of heart dilation in CMVD. Although LAR is not a highly reliable parameter [17], its greater values observed in the DCM group in our study together with lower values of perivascular fibrosis may indicate that alterations in intra-mural vessels play a greater role in left atrial enlargement in CMVD than in DCM.

DCM in dogs is often connected with the occurrence of supraventricular and ventricular rhythm disturbances. Sustained arrhythmias in CMVD occur less frequently [1, 2, 5, 25, 26]. Noszczyk-Nowak et al. [27] and Crosara et al. [26] demonstrated a higher risk of developing supraventricular arrhythmias in dogs with an enlarged left atrium, although this phenomenon is not well understood. It has not been established whether arrhythmias, also found in dogs in pre-clinical stages of DCM, are a consequence of primary myocardial changes or if myocardial lesions result from long-lasting rhythm disturbances and secondary heart chamber dilation [5, 28].

Recent studies [28–30] emphasize the role of myocardial fibrosis in the development and progression of atrial fibrillation (AF) of different aetiology in humans. Platanov et al. [30] showed a significantly higher amount of

Table 2 Histopathological findings in the examined groups

	DCM group $n = 16$	CMVD group $n = 15$	*p*-value
interstitial fibrosis (median; range)	4 (1–7)	2.5 (1–5)	0.036
perivascular fibrosis (median; range)	1 (0–2)	2 (1–2)	0.006
fatty infiltration (median; range)	1 (0–10)	1 (0–6)	0.663
LAR (median; range)	0.3 (0.14–0.8)	0.26 (0.15–0.33)	0.041
abnormal cell nuclei (median; range)	3 (1–3)	1 (0–3)	0.008
loss of striation (median; range)	3 (1–3)	2 (0–3)	0.004
altered cardiomyocyte structure (median; range)	3 (2–3)	2 (0–3)	0.004
inflammatory infiltration (median; range)	0.36 (0–1.6)	0.35 (0–1.9)	0.796

LAR lumen area ratio

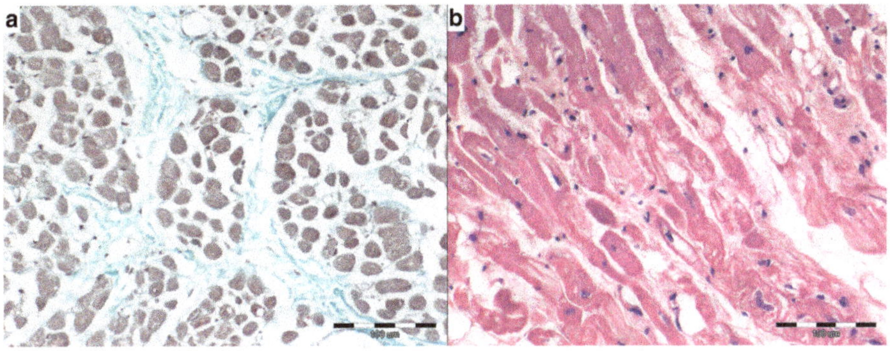

Fig. 1 Histopathologic pattern of atrial myocardium in DCM group. **a** interstitial fibrosis (Masson-Goldner trichrome), **b** myocardial degeneration presented by changes in cardiomyocyte structure, loss of striation and changes in cell staining (H&E)

connective tissue in heart specimens from patients with AF, compared to patients without atrial rhythm disturbances. Nattel and Harada [31] highlighted the possible role of fibrosis in cardiac conduction disturbances.

Frustaci et al. [32] noted changes in the atrial myocardial structure (inflammation, non-inflammatory cardiomyopathy or fibrosis) in patients with lone atrial fibrillation without coexisting heart chamber dilation (including atrial diameter). Moreover, Tuomainen et al. [33] noted significantly lower values of the left ventricular end-diastolic diameter, left ventricular end-diastolic volume and left ventricular end-systolic volume combined with a significantly higher value of the left atrial diameter in patients with chronic AF in DCM compared to patients with DCM and a sinus rhythm. Considering that all dogs with DCM in this study had an arrhythmia, it is impossible to determine whether the observed changes are a consequence of the primary myocardial disease or a consequence of the arrhythmia.

One of the limitations of our study was a lack of dogs with DCM without rhythm disturbances, which could be compared to dogs included in the study. Dogs with DCM often develop rhythm disturbances before the development of clinical symptoms. Further studies including dogs with DCM without arrhythmias may improve our knowledge of the pathogenesis of this disease.

Another limitation was an observed difference between body weight, age and breed distribution in both groups. This was a result of the different clinical courses of both diseases. DCM mostly occurs in young large-breed dogs, while CMVD mostly occurs in old small-breed dogs. To minimize those differences, we used an increased LA/Ao ratio as an inclusion criterion. There was no difference in the LA/Ao ratio between both groups. Therefore, we assumed that the comparison of atrial remodelling in both groups was justifiable.

The variety in the DCM group was a further limitation of the study. We included dogs with idiopathic DCM that developed arrhythmias in the course of the disease and dogs presenting with AF in the first examination. The latter dogs may have had tachycardia-induced cardiomyopathy. However, all the dogs in the DCM group did not respond well to treatment in late stages of the disease. They developed severe heart failure with left atrial enlargement, and presented with severe tachyarrhythmia at the time of death or prior to euthanasia. Hence, they were included in one group.

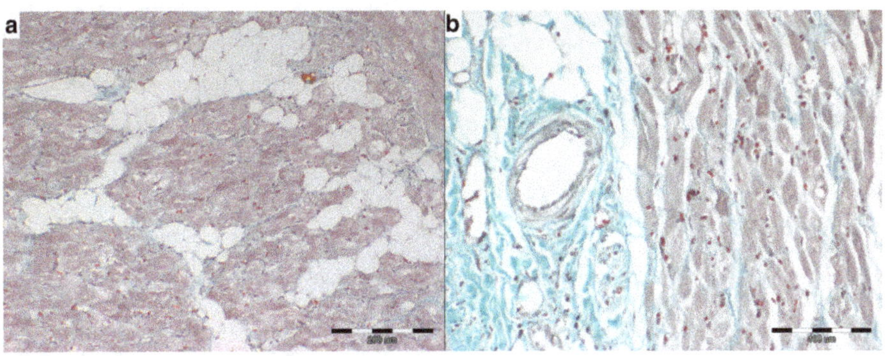

Fig. 2 Histopathologic pattern of atrial myocardium in CMVD group. **a** fatty infiltration with slight amount of interstitial fibrosis (Masson-Goldner trichrome), **b** perivascular fibrosis with slight amount of interstitial fibrosis (Masson-Goldner trichrome)

The last limitation was a lack of assessment of atrial pressure in the examined dogs prior to the histopathologic examination in order to exclude its influence on atrial remodelling. We attempted to minimise the possibility of other reasons for atrial enlargement (e.g. mitral stenosis) by performing an accurate ante-mortem and post-mortem examination.

Conclusion

Dogs with dilated cardiomyopathy show a different distribution of connective tissue, have less severe intra-myocardial arterial narrowing, and have more severe degenerative changes in the cardiomyocytes of the left atrium compared to dogs with chronic mitral valve disease. The changes noted in the atrial tissue from dogs in both groups resemble lesions noted in the ventricular tissue of dogs with the same diseases. Those differences may indicate that the atrial enlargement noted in DCM and CMVD has a different, disease-specific underlying mechanism and does not result only from volume overload.

Abbreviations

AF: atrial fibrillation; AWF: attenuated wavy fibres type; CMVD: chronic mitral valve disease; DCM: dilated cardiomyopathy; FID: fatty infiltration-degenerative type; FS: fractional shortening; H&E: haematoxylin-eosin stain; LA/Ao: left atrial-to-aortic root diameter ratio; LAR: lumen area ratio; LVIDd: end-diastolic left ventricular internal diameter; LVIDs: end-systolic left ventricular internal diameter.

Competing interests

The authors declare that they have no competing interests.

Authors' contributions

IJ prepared the manuscript and performed the histopathological examination, ANN performed the ante-mortem examination and treated the patients, MN supervised the post-mortem examination, RC performed the histopathological examination, MKG performed the histopathological examination, UP supervised the ante-mortem examination and treatment process. All authors read and approved the final manuscript.

Acknowledgements

We would like to thank the supporting staff of the Pathology Department of Wroclaw University of Environmental and Life Sciences for their experienced technical assistance.

Author details

[1]Division of Pathomorphology and Veterinary Forensics, Department of Pathology, Wroclaw University of Environmental and Life Sciences, Wroclaw 50375, Poland. [2]Department of Internal Medicine and Clinic of Diseases of Horses, Dogs and Cats Wroclaw University of Environmental and Life Sciences, Wroclaw 50366, Poland.

References

1. Tidholm A, Häggström J, Borgarelli M, Tarducci A. Canine idiopathic dilated cardiomyopathy. Part I: aetiology, clinical characteristics, epidemiology and pathology. Vet J. 2001;162(2):92–107.
2. Tidholm A, Jönsson L. Histologic characterization of canine dilated cardiomyopathy. Vet Pathol. 2005;42(1):1–8.
3. Alroy J, Rush JE, Freeman L, Amarendhra Kumar MS, Karuri A, Chase K, et al. Inherited infantile dilated cardiomyopathy in dogs: genetic, clinical, biochemical, and morphologic findings. Am J Med Genet. 2000;95(1):57–66.
4. Dambach DM, Lannon A, Sleeper MM, Buchanan J. Familial dilated cardiomyopathy of young Portuguese water dogs. J Vet Intern Med. 1999;13(1):65–71.
5. Dukes-McEwan J, Borgarelli M, Tidholm A, Vollmar AC, Häggström J, ESVC Taskforce for Canine Dilated Cardiomyopathy. Proposed guidelines for the diagnosis of canine idiopathic dilated cardiomyopathy. J Vet Cardiol. 2003;5(2):7–19.
6. Kittleson MD, Keene B, Pion PD, Loyer CG. Results of the Multicentre Spaniel Trial (MUST): taurine- and carnitine-responsive dilated cardiomyopathy in American cocker spaniels with decreased plasma taurine concentration. J Vet Intern Med. 1997;11(4):204–11.
7. Lobo L, Carvalheira J, Canada N, Bussadori C, Gomes JL, Faustino AM. Histologic characterization of dilated cardiomyopathy in Estrela mountain dogs. Vet Pathol. 2010;47(4):637–42.
8. Everett RM, McGann J, Wimberly HC, Althoff J. Dilated cardiomyopathy of Doberman Pinschers: retrospective histomorphologic evaluation of heart from 32 Cases. Vet Pathol. 1999;36(3):221–7.
9. Rossi L, Matturri L. Pathology of arrhythmias. In: Rossi L, Matturri L, editors. Clinicopathological approach to cardiac arrhythmias. A color atlas. Turin: Centro Scientifico Torinese Editore; 1990. p. 178–84.
10. Vollmar A, Fox PR, Meurs KM, Liu SK. Dilated cardiomyopathy in juvenile Doberman Pinschers. J Vet Cardiol. 2003;5(1):23–7.
11. Janus I, Nowak M, Madej JA. Pathomorphological changes of the myocardium in canine dilated cardiomyopathy (DCM). Bull Vet Inst Pulawy. 2015;59:135–42.
12. Borgarelli M, Buchanan JW. Historical review, epidemiology and natural history of degenerative mitral valve disease. J Vet Cardiol. 2012;14(1):93–101.
13. Borgarelli M, Häggström J. Canine degenerative myxomatous mitral valve disease: natural history, clinical presentation and therapy. Vet Clin North Am Small Anim Pract. 2010;40(4):651–63.
14. Fox PR. Pathology of myxomatous mitral valve disease in the dog. J Vet Cardiol. 2012;14(1):103–26.
15. Häggström J, Duelund Pedersen H, Kvart C. New insights into degenerative mitral valve disease in dogs. Vet Clin North Am Small Anim Pract. 2004;34(5):1209–26.
16. Falk T, Jönsson L, Olsen LH, Pedersen HD. Arteriosclerotic changes in the myocardium, lung, and kidney in dogs with chronic congestive heart failure and myxomatous mitral valve disease. Cardiovasc Pathol. 2006;15(4):185–93.
17. Falk T, Jönsson L, Olsen LH, Tarnow I, Pedersen HD. Associations between cardiac pathology and clinical, echocardiographic and electrocardiographic findings in dogs with chronic congestive heart failure. Vet J. 2010;185(1):68–74.
18. Borgarelli M, Savarino P, Crosara S, Santilli RA, Chiavegato D, Poggi M, et al. Survival characteristics and prognostic variables of dogs with mitral regurgitation attributable to myxomatous valve disease. J Vet Intern Med. 2008;22(1):120–8.
19. Whitney JC. Cardiovascular pathology. J Small Anim Pract. 1967;8(8):459–65.
20. Atkins C, Bonagura J, Ettinger S, Fox P, Gordon S, Häggström J, et al. Guidelines for the diagnosis and treatment of canine chronic valvular heart disease. J Vet Intern Med. 2009;23(6):1142–50.
21. Bonagura JD, O'Grady MR, Herrings DS. Echocardiography: principles of interpretation. Vet Clin North Am. 1985;15:1177–94.
22. The Polish Parliament: Act on the protection of animals used for scientific or educational purposes. http://orka.sejm.gov.pl/proc7.nsf/ustawy/2709_u.htm (2015). Accessed 15 July 2015.
23. Schaper J, Kostin S, Hein S, Elsässer A, Arnon E, Zimmermann R. Structural remodelling in heart failure. Exp Clin Cardiol. 2002;7(2–3):64–8.
24. Sharov VG, Kostin S, Todor A, Schaper J, Sabbah HN. Expression of cytoskeletal, linkage and extracellular proteins in failing dog myocardium. Heart Fail Rev. 2005;10(4):297–303.
25. Calvert CA, Jacobs GJ, Smith DD, Rathbun SL, Pickus CW. Association between results of ambulatory electrocardiography and development of cardiomyopathy during long-term follow-up of Doberman pinschers. J Am Vet Med Assoc. 2000;216(1):34–9.
26. Crosara S, Borgarelli M, Perego M, Häggström J, La Rosa G, Tarducci A, et al. Holter monitoring in 36 dogs with myxomatous mitral valve disease. Aust Vet J. 2010;88(10):386–92.
27. Noszczyk-Nowak A, Szałas A, Pasławska U, Nicpoń J. Comparison of P-wave dispersion in healthy dogs, dogs with chronic valvular disease and dogs with disturbances of supraventricular conduction. Acta Vet Scand. 2011;53:18.
28. Corradi D. Atrial fibrillation from the pathologist's perspective. Cardiovasc Pathol. 2014;23(2):71–84.

29. Akoum N, Marrouche N. Assessment and impact of cardiac fibrosis on atrial fibrillation. Curr Cardiol Rep. 2014;16(8):518.
30. Platonov PG, Mitrofanova LB, Orshanskaya V, Ho SY. Structural abnormalities in atrial walls are associated with presence and persistency of atrial fibrillation but not with age. J Am Coll Cardiol. 2011;58(21):2225–32.
31. Nattel S, Harada M. Atrial remodelling and atrial fibrillation. J Am Coll Cardiol. 2014;63(22):2335–45.
32. Frustaci A, Chimenti C, Bellocci F, Morgante E, Russo MA, Maseri A. Histological substrate of atrial biopsies in patients with lone atrial fibrillation. Circulation. 1997;96(4):1180–4.
33. Tuomainen PO, Magga J, Fedacko J, Kärkkäinen S, Miettinen K, Vanninen E, et al. Idiopathic dilated cardiomyopathy and chronic atrial fibrillation. Ciln Physiol Funct Imaging. 2014;34(2):133–7.

2

Comparison of angle, shape, and position of articular processes in Dobermans and Great Danes with and without cervical spondylomyelopathy

Marília de Albuquerque Bonelli[1,2], Ronaldo Casimiro da Costa[1*], Paula Martin-Vaquero[1,3] and Carolina Gonçalves Dias Lima[1]

Abstract

Background: Cervical spondylomyelopathy (CSM), also known as wobbler syndrome, affects mainly large and giant-breed dogs, causing compression of the cervical spinal cord and/or nerve roots. Structural and dynamic components seem to play a role in the development of CSM; however, pathogenesis is not yet fully understood. Physiologic and pathologic movements of the cervical spine depend on the morphology and morphometry of articular processes, as well as on intervertebral discs and vertebral column ligaments. Moreover, the characteristics of the articular processes affect motion and stability of the vertebral column. The goal of this study was to investigate the angle, shape, and position of the articular surfaces within the articular processes and compare them between Doberman Pinschers and Great Danes with and without cervical spondylomyelopathy.

Results: Magnetic resonance images were obtained for 60 dogs: 15 clinically normal Dobermans (Dob-N), 15 CSM-affected Dobermans (Dob-CSM), 15 clinically normal Great Danes (GD-N), and 15 CSM-affected Great Danes (GD-CSM). Angle, shape, and position (lateral distance) of the articular surfaces from the articular processes were analyzed from C_{2-3} to C_7-T_1. Results indicate that the mean angle was different between Dob-CSM and GD-CSM at C_{4-5}, C_{5-6}, and C_{6-7}, and between GD-N and GD-CSM at C_{6-7}. There were differences between Dob-N and GD-N, and between Dob-CSM and GD-CSM for the lateral distance at most locations, except C_{2-3}. Compared with Great Danes, Dobermans generally had a greater proportion of concave caudal surfaces at C_{4-5}, C_{5-6}, and C_{6-7}. Concave articular surfaces have been associated with greater axial rotation. This may explain the high proportion of disc-associated CSM in Dobermans compared to Great Danes. The differences between breeds suggest they may have different motion patterns in the caudal cervical vertebral column.

Conclusions: Considering that no differences in angle, shape, or position of the articular surfaces within the articular processes were found between normal and CSM-affected dogs, their relevance appears to have a secondary role in the pathogenesis of CSM.

Keywords: Articular facets, Cervical spine, Facet joint, Wobbler syndrome, Zygapophyseal joint

* Correspondence: dacosta.6@osu.edu
[1]Department of Veterinary Clinical Sciences, College of Veterinary Medicine, The Ohio State University, 601 Vernon Tharp St., Columbus, OH 43210, USA
Full list of author information is available at the end of the article

Background

Cervical spondylomyelopathy (CSM), commonly known as wobbler syndrome, is a disorder characterized by compression of the cervical spinal cord and/or nerve roots [1, 2] and can be divided into osseous-associated (OA-CSM) and disc-associated (DA-CSM), although overlap exists [1]. Structural changes of the cervical vertebral column, along with dynamic components, appear to be involved in the pathogenesis of CSM; however, the individual contribution of each is not yet fully understood [1, 2]. Dynamic lesions, where compression worsens as the amount of the space available within the vertebral canal increases or decreases depending on flexion and extension of the neck [1], are thought to be in part a consequence of the decrease in vertebral canal diameter during cervical extension [3].

Physiologic and pathologic movements of the cervical spine depend on the articular process joints which, along with the intervertebral discs and the vertebral column ligaments, facilitate the transfer of loads and guide and constrain the motion of the vertebrae [4]. Morphology, morphometry, and angle of the articular surfaces of the articular processes could affect the mechanical properties and patterns of motion of the articular process joints. As such, variations in articular process joint characteristics between breeds or vertebral levels could thus result in different motion patterns and be relevant to the pathogenesis of CSM [4–7]. A smaller horizontal angle, curved articular surfaces, and shorter distance from the center of the articular joint to the dorsal rim of the intervertebral disc have been associated with greater mobility [6, 7].

The objective of the present study was to investigate whether there are differences in the angle, shape, and position of the articular surfaces that form the articular processes between Doberman Pinscher and Great Dane dogs with and without CSM. Our primary hypothesis was that the articular surfaces would have a lower horizontal inclination angle, be more ventrally positioned, and with curved caudal articular surfaces in dogs with CSM. A second hypothesis was that there would be a significant difference between Dobermans and Great Danes, with Dobermans being supposed as having the aforementioned characteristics that would be considered related with greater mobility.

Methods

Magnetic resonance (MR) images of the cervical vertebral column of Doberman Pinscher and Great Dane dogs were retrospectively reviewed. All dogs had undergone thorough physical and neurological examinations. The MR studies consisted of at least sagittal and transverse T1- and T2-weighted images from C_2 to T_1, acquired using high-field magnets (1.5 T Magnetom Vision, Siemens; 3.0 T Achieva, Philips Healthcare), with a minimum of three transverse slices at each intervertebral disc level. The transverse images had been obtained parallel to the vertebral endplate. Slice thickness was 3 mm, with no interslice interval. For imaging, all dogs had received premedication with an opioid and a benzodiazepine or acepromazine and had been under general anesthesia using propofol and isoflurane and positioned in dorsal recumbency, with their cervical vertebral columns centered, extended and held in place with sandbags.

Dogs were included in the CSM-affected group if they had a confirmed diagnosis of CSM based on history, clinical signs, and presence of compatible magnetic resonance imaging (MRI) changes. Dogs were considered clinically normal based on absence of neurologic abnormalities at the time of the MRI scan and no history of neurologic disease. Dogs would have been excluded if they had unclear images of the articular surfaces, or MR image artifacts that interfered with visualization. All dogs were part of prospective studies carried out by the senior author [8–10].

T1-weighted images were used to obtain the measurements and perform the morphological analysis because they allowed clearer delimitation of the articular processes and their articular surfaces. All regions, from C_{2-3} to C_7-T_1, were studied. All analyses were performed by the same investigator (MAB), who was blinded to the clinical presentation of the dogs.

For measurements regarding the angle (Fig. 1) and lateral distance (Fig. 2) of the articular surfaces of the articular processes, the image with the clearest view of

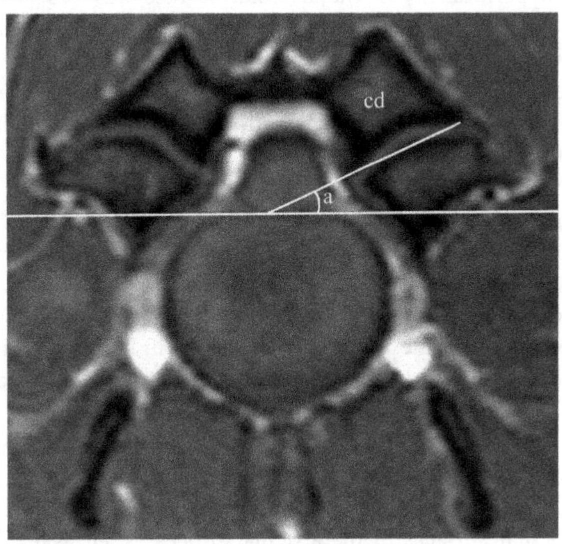

Fig. 1 Transverse T1-weighted magnetic resonance image from a CSM-affected Great Dane, demonstrating the measurement of the facet angle (**a**) of the *left* caudal articular process (cd)

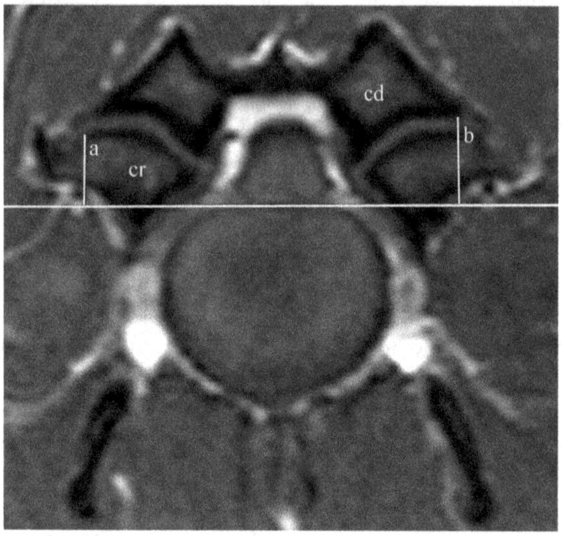

Fig. 2 Transverse T1-weighted magnetic resonance image from a clinically normal Doberman Pinscher, demonstrating the cranial lateral (**a**) and caudal lateral (**b**) distance points for the cranial (cr) and caudal (cd) articular processes

the articular surfaces for each articular process joint was selected. This was regularly the image that represented the middle of the articular joint. When two images were alike, the one closest to the cranial endplate of the caudal vertebra was selected. First, a vertical line was then drawn bisecting the spinous process and the intervertebral disc/vertebral body. Then, another line was drawn perpendicular to the first, with the most dorsal point of the floor of the vertebral canal as the reference line (Fig. 1). The articular surface of an articular process was considered to extend medially or laterally until a change in hyperintensity of the articular surface was observed. Both T1- and T2-weighted images were used to distinguish the articular surface from the hyperintense fat surrounding the articular process joint. All data were collected separately for left and right cranial and caudal articular surfaces/processes.

Angle of the articular surfaces

A line was drawn from the most lateral to the most medial point of the articular surface of each articular process, regardless of shape variations between these points. The angle was then determined in relation to the horizontal reference line (Fig. 1). This method was adapted from previous studies [6, 11, 12].

Shape of the articular surfaces

In order to establish the predominant shape of the articular surfaces of the articular processes, all available images for each articular process joint from C_{2-3} to C_7-T_1 were reviewed. To distinguish between shapes, a straight line was drawn from the medial to the lateral edge of the articular surface. Surfaces were classified as predominantly plane (less than 0.05 cm deviation), convex or concave (deviation greater than 0.05 cm to one side of the line), or sigmoid (deviations to both sides of the line) when that particular shape was present in the majority of images (Fig. 3). This classification was adapted from an osteological study [6]. Irregular shapes were also classified as sigmoid. Minor deviations in form (approximately less than 20% of the articular surface), were discarded to reduce the influence of the edges of the articular surfaces, where the surface sometimes followed the shape of the articular process.

Distance of the articular surfaces to the floor of the vertebral canal

As a reference to the position of the articular surfaces, the distance from the most lateral point of the articular surface of each respective articular process to the reference line was measured. While not representing the center of rotation for the joint, this point was selected as a representation of the position of the articular surface (referred to as distance) because it was the most easily identifiable edge of the articular surface for the cranial (Fig. 2, measurement a) and caudal (Fig. 2, measurement b) articular processes. The images used for these measurements were the same as the ones used to obtain angle measurements.

Statistical analysis

Quantile-quantile plots were used to check if the variables had a normal distribution. There were no large deviations from normal and no outliers, and the dataset was therefore treated as having a normal distribution.

Means for surface angle and distance, as well as proportions of surface shapes, were compared between clinically normal Dobermans (Dob-N) and CSM-affected Dobermans (Dob-CSM), between clinically normal Great Danes (GD-N) and CSM-affected Great Danes (GD-CSM), between Dob-N and GD-N, and between Dob-CSM and GD-CSM. Comparisons were also made between functional spinal units (FSU – pair of articulating vertebrae and intervertebral disc) within each of the four groups for left and right articular processes separately. Left and right measurements were also compared per FSU for each group, using a *t*-test.

For angle and distance, these comparisons were made using multivariate ANOVA with Tukey multiple comparisons, adjusted for the height of the vertebral bodies of the dogs (for distance). For shape, chi-square tests were used to determine if there were differences between the proportions of articular surface shapes across vertebral levels between all four groups. Measurements and shape classifications were repeated, using the same MRI scans, on three randomly selected dogs from each

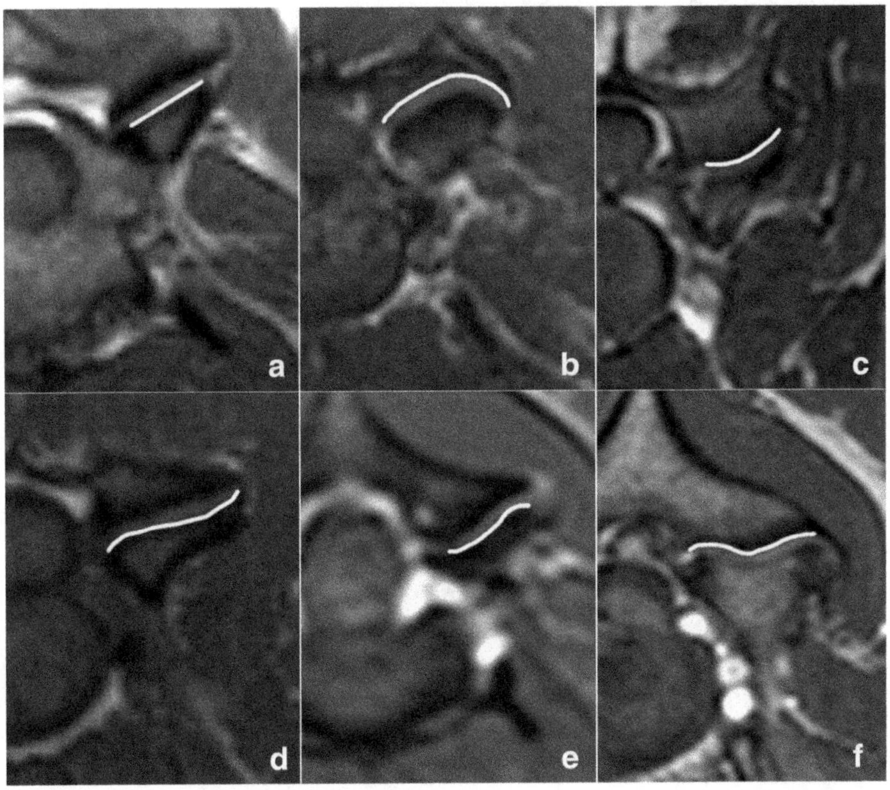

Fig. 3 Transverse T1-weighted magnetic resonance images illustrating the classification of the articular surface shapes: plane articular surface in a CSM-affected Doberman (**a**), concave caudal articular surface in a clinically normal Doberman (**b**), convex caudal articular surface in a clinically normal Great Dane (**c**), sigmoid cranial articular surface in a clinically normal Doberman (**d**) and in a clinically normal Great Dane (**e**). An irregular shape of the articular surface of a CSM-affected Great Dane, classified as sigmoid, is also shown (**f**). A *white line* has been drawn to highlight the shape of the articular surfaces

group ($n = 12$; 20%) to calculate intraobserver agreement (after one month) using intra-class correlation and interobserver agreement using inter-class correlation. Statistical analyses were performed by a professional statistician using SAS Version 9.4. Significance was set at $P < 0.05$.

Results

Sixty dogs were included: 30 Doberman Pinschers (15 CSM-affected and 15 clinically normal) and 30 Great Danes (15 CSM-affected and 15 clinically normal). The mean age for these dogs at the time of imaging was 6.3 years (3–12 years) for CSM-affected Dobermans; 4.3 years (2–8 years) for clinically normal Dobermans; 4 years (1–7.2 years) for CSM-affected Great Danes (mean age at onset 1.7 years); and 2.3 years (1–6.4 years) for clinically normal Great Danes.

Gender distribution for each group was: eight male and seven female CSM-affected Dobermans, eight female and seven male clinically normal Dobermans, 13 male and two female CSM-affected Great Danes, and eight male and seven female clinically normal Great Danes. Mean weight was 35 kg (26.3–50.8 kg) for CSM-affected Dobermans, 36.7 kg (26–52 kg) for clinically normal Dobermans, 57.8 kg (42–79.3 kg) for CSM-affected Great Danes, and 52.7 kg (40.5–73 kg) for clinically normal Great Danes.

The CSM-affected Dobermans had disc-associated CSM, with the main spinal cord compression at C_{6-7} (8), C_{5-6} (6), C_{4-5} (1). The main sites of spinal cord compression in the CSM-affected Great Danes, all of which had osseous-associated CSM, were C_{6-7} (8), C_{4-5} (3), C_{5-6} (2), C_{2-3} (1), and C_{3-4} (1). Seven CSM-affected Dobermans and thirteen CSM-affected Great Danes had multiple sites of compression, but the other compression sites were considered less clinically relevant.

Angle of the articular surfaces

In general, there were no differences in the angle of the articular surfaces between Dob-N and Dob-CSM or between GD-N and GD-CSM, except for C_{5-6} left cranial and C_{6-7} except for right caudal (greater for GD-CSM). When comparing breeds, there were differences between Dob-CSM and GD-CSM at C_{4-5}, C_{5-6}, C_{6-7} (greater for GD-CSM), but no differences between Dob-N and GD-N (Table 1).

Table 1 Mean angles ± standard error (and range) of the articular surfaces per group

Level	Dogs	Left Cranial Angle	Right Cranial Angle	Left Caudal Angle	Right Caudal Angle
C_{2-3}	Dob-N	26.56 ± 5.68 (5.2–37.7)	24.41 ± 7.11 (13.2–36.4)	28.35 ± 5.627 (7.6–39.2)	26.18 ± 8.156 (12.6–36.1)
	Dob-CSM	26.52 ± 5.68 (17.4–37.9)	22.68 ± 7.11 (14.9–31.5)	26.02 ± 5.62 (16.6–35)	25.54 ± 8.15 (12.9–31.9)
	GD-N	19.24 ± 5.68 (7.3–35.5)	23.18 ± 7.11 (3.5–38.3)	20.87 ± 5.62 (5.6–42.8)	23.83 ± 8.15 (0.2–41.1)
	GD-CSM	26.18 ± 5.68 (1.1–174.7)	36.43 ± 7.11 (0.3–170.7)	26.41 ± 5.62 (1.4–170.4)	46.24 ± 8.156 (2–171.9)
C_{3-4}	Dob-N	24.02 ± 5.33 (11.3–45)	21.24 ± 1.91 (12.6–36.6)	23.3 ± 2.18 (8.5–45.5)	21.98 ± 1.96 (11.7–38.5)
	Dob-CSM	20.2 ± 5.33 (10.2–28.3)	21.81 ± 1.91 (13.4–31.4)	19.37 ± 2.18 (8.3–28.8)	21.81 ± 1.96 (7.3–30.2)
	GD-N	24.02 ± 5.33 (8.4–29.1)	21.24 ± 1.91 (10.3–33.7)	23.3 ± 2.18 (9.9–30.6)	21.98 ± 1.96 (11.5–35)
	GD-CSM	34.1 ± 5.33 (8.3–174.3)	21.473 ± 1.91 (0.3–35.7)	23.3 ± 2.18 (1.3–45.1)	20.97 ± 1.96 (1.1–32.5)
C_{4-5}	Dob-N	23.52 ± 1.72 (10.5–37.9)	24.59 ± 1.74 (16.8–36.9)	21.50 ± 1.7 (7.5–37.9)	24.96 ± 1.75 (15.2–37.1)
	Dob-CSM	21.91 ± 1.72 [c] (14–30.1)	22.56 ± 1.74 [c] (8.5–39.7)	20.76 ± 1.7 [c] (11.4–30.5)	23.7 ± 1.759 [c] (10.6–43.9)
	GD-N	25.82 ± 1.72 (13.9–33.5)	26.69 ± 1.74 (16.7–32.3)	26.24 ± 1.7 (16.4–37.5)	26.72 ± 1.75 (21–32.8)
	GD-CSM	31.36 ± 1.72 [c] (19.3–42.5)	31.69 ± 1.74 [c] (14.5–40.7)	32.37 ± 1.7 [c] (22.2–43.7)	31.7 ± 1.75 [c] (18.4–39.3)
C_{5-6}	Dob-N	27.8 ± 1.87 (18.7–41.4)	26.52 ± 2.01 (19.1–37.7)	26 ± 2.11 (18.8–39.1)	26.73 ± 2.07 (16.4–37.1)
	Dob-CSM	23.62 ± 1.87 [c] (12.1–41.2)	21.77 ± 2.01 [c] (7.7–41.9)	22.93 ± 2.11 [c] (11.4–41.4)	21.47 ± 2.07 [c] (7.4–43.2)
	GD-N	25.4 ± 1.87 [a] (16.4–33.3)	27.28 ± 2.01 (9.9–39.9)	24.94 ± 2.11 (12.9–33.6)	28.1 ± 2.07 (13.5–39.5)
	GD-CSM	33.58 ± 1.87 [a, c] (22.8–48.5)	33.04 ± 2.01 [c] (21.3–45.8)	31.96 ± 2.11 [c] (16.2–46.2)	32.07 ± 2.07 [c] (18.6–47.3)
C_{6-7}	Dob-N	33.04 ± 2.05 (23.6–48.5)	32.42 ± 2.5 (22.1–45.4)	31.63 ± 2.43 (18.5–44.6)	31.92 ± 2.61 (21.2–43.2)
	Dob-CSM	29.36 ± 2.05 [c] (15.3–39.5)	30.02 ± 2.5 [c] (16.9–50.5)	27.4 ± 2.43 [c] (10.2–41.6)	28.11 ± 2.61 [c] (16.5–45.4)
	GD-N	29.1 ± 2.05 [a] (16.7–40.5)	30.45 ± 2.5 [a] (15.7–50.3)	27.44 ± 2.43 [a] (14.9–47.2)	31.56 ± 2.61 (13.4–50.8)
	GD-CSM	38.29 ± 2.05 [a, c] (21.8–64.4)	41.1 ± 2.5 [a, c] (22.9–73.4)	37.88 ± 2.43 [a, c] (19.5–66.5)	39.37 ± 2.61 [c] (18.5–78.6)
C_7-T_1	Dob-N	36.32 ± 2.79 (19.8–48.7)	33.24 ± 2.72 (24.5–39.8)	32.81 ± 3.04 (14.2–44.7)	30.86 ± 2.88 (17.7–39.5)
	Dob-CSM	36.92 ± 2.79 (21.4–56.3)	35 ± 2.72 (16.6–52.4)	37.84 ± 3.04 (16.9–60.3)	33.06 ± 2.88 (14.4–54.4)
	GD-N	36.15 ± 2.79 (26.5–57.4)	39.12 ± 2.72 (23.7–59.1)	33.32 ± 3.04 (18.4–51.2)	35.12 ± 2.88 (23.5–55.7)
	GD-CSM	43.83 ± 2.79 (24.6–79.8)	40.05 ± 2.72 (24.5–69.7)	41.69 ± 3.04 (21.2–79.4)	40.08 ± 2.88 (18.7–69.1)

Mean angles ± standard error adjusted for height of the vertebral bodies, with minimum and maximum values in parenthesis, for the cranial and caudal articular surfaces for clinically normal Doberman Pinschers (Dob-N) and Great Danes (GD-N) and Doberman Pinschers and Great Danes with cervical spondylomyelopathy (Dob-CSM, GD-CSM)
[a]Statistically significant difference between clinically normal and CSM-affected Great Danes ($P < 0.05$)
[b]Statistically significant difference between clinically normal Doberman Pinschers and clinically normal Great Danes ($P < 0.05$)
[c]Statistically significant difference between CSM-affected Doberman Pinschers and CSM-affected Great Danes ($P < 0.05$)

Among FSU, there was no significant difference between angles at C_{6-7} and C_7-T_1, which were greater than the other FSU in Dob-N. In Dob-CSM, the angle measurements were significantly greater for C_7-T_1 than for most other FSU, except for C_{6-7} cranial and caudal articular surfaces on the right side. Also, there were generally no significant differences in angles between FSU among Great Danes except for C_7-T_1 in GD-N, which was greater than the other FSU. When comparing sides, there was no significant difference in any of the groups, except for GD-N at cranial C_{2-3} and caudal C_{5-6} and C_{6-7}.

Angle measurements for the cranial and caudal articular surfaces are displayed in Additional files 1, 2, 3 and 4.

Shape of the articular surfaces

A predominant shape was recorded for all FSU except C_7-T_1, where the available transverse images did not consistently yield a predominant shape. There was a statistical difference in the proportion of shapes when comparing Dob-N with GD-N and Dob-CSM with GD-CSM, with an overall higher proportion of concave caudal processes in Dob-N (C_{4-5}, C_{5-6}, C_{6-7}) compared with GD-N, and Dob-CSM (C_{4-5} and C_{5-6}) compared with GD-CSM (Tables 2 and 3). Overall, there were no significant differences in the proportions of the four shapes between Dob-N and Dob-CSM or between GD-N and GD-CSM.

In general, when comparing FSU within a group, C_{3-4}, C_{4-5}, C_{5-6}, and C_{6-7} had a greater proportion of concave caudal and convex cranial surfaces, while C_{2-3} had comparatively more sigmoid and plane shapes. Interestingly, three CSM-affected Great Danes exhibited medially angled sigmoid caudal surfaces at C_{2-3} ($n = 2/15$) and C_{3-4} ($n = 1/15$).

Table 2 Shape distribution for cranial articular surfaces per group

Level	Dogs	Cc (RCr)	Cv (RCr)	P (RCr)	S (RCr)	Cc (LCr)	Cv (LCr)	P (LCr)	S (LCr)
C_{2-3}	Dob-N	10[b]	1	2	2[b]	10[b]	1	2	2[b]
	Dob-CSM	9[c]	2	4	0[c]	8[c]	2	5	0[c]
	GD-N	2[b]	0	2	11[b]	0[b]	0	2	13[b]
	GD-CSM	3[c]	1	1	10[c]	4[c]	3	1	7[c]
C_{3-4}	Dob-N	0	14	1	0	0	13	2	0
	Dob-CSM	0	15[c]	0[c]	0[c]	0	15[c]	0	0
	GD-N	2	7	2	4	2	8	2	3
	GD-CSM	0	5[c]	5[c]	5[c]	2	8[c]	2	3
C_{4-5}	Dob-N	1	12[b]	1[b]	1[b]	1	13[b]	0[b]	1[b]
	Dob-CSM	0	14	1	0	0	13	0	2
	GD-N	1	5[b]	5[b]	4[b]	0	4[b]	7[b]	4[b]
	GD-CSM	2	7	4	2	2	7	3	3
C_{5-6}	Dob-N	1[b]	12	0[b]	2	1[b]	1[b]	11[b]	2[b]
	Dob-CSM	1	12	0	2[c]	0	9	0	6
	GD-N	5[b]	4	3[b]	3	2[b]	3[b]	1[b]	9[b]
	GD-CSM	2	5	2	6[c]	2	4	2	7
C_{6-7}	Dob-N	0[b]	14[b]	1[b]	0	0[b]	14[b]	1[b]	0
	Dob-CSM	0	12	2	1	0	10	3	2
	GD-N	4[b]	6[b]	4[b]	1	3[b]	7[b]	4[b]	1
	GD-CSM	0	10	3	2	0	11	3	1

Shape distribution for the articular surface of the right (RCr) and left (LCr) cranial articular processes from C2-3 to C6-7 in clinically normal Doberman Pinschers (Dob-N) and Great Danes (GD-N) and Doberman Pinschers and Great Danes with cervical spondylomyelopathy (Dob-CSM, GD-CSM)

Cc concave, *Cv* convex, *P* plane, *S* sigmoid

[a]Statistically significant difference between clinically normal and CSM-affected Great Danes ($P < 0.05$)

[b]Statistically significant difference between clinically normal Doberman Pinschers and clinically normal Great Danes ($P < 0.05$)

[c]Statistically significant difference between CSM-affected Doberman Pinschers and CSM-affected Great Danes ($P < 0.05$)

Distance of the articular surfaces to the floor of the vertebral canal

There were no statistical differences between mean distance measurements for Dob-N and Dob-CSM or between GD-N and GD-CSM. There were significant differences in mean cranial and caudal lateral distance measurements between Dob-N and GD-N and between Dob-CSM and GD-CSM, with higher values for GD-N and GD-CSM (Table 4).

Among FSU, both groups of Dobermans usually had higher values for C_{2-3}, together with or followed by C_7-T_1, and then C_{3-4} through C_{6-7}, with no difference from C_{3-4} through C_{6-7} for cranial and caudal lateral distances. In GD-N, measurements at C_7-T_1 were generally higher, followed by (cranial) or equal to (caudal) those for C_{2-3}. In GD-CSM, C_7-T_1 values were higher for cranial and caudal lateral reference points, followed by C_{2-3}. Comparison between sides showed no significant difference overall.

Distance measurements for the cranial and caudal articular surfaces are available in Additional files 5, 6, 7 and 8.

Intraobserver and interobserver agreement

Intra-class correlations for measurements were generally greater than 0.95 for intraobserver agreement. The highest correlation was seen for the lateral distance for the left cranial articular process (0.9765) and the lowest for the right cranial articular surface angle (0.9090). Shape identifications were 80% consistent, with the least consistency observed for the cranial left articular surfaces (73%) and the highest for the caudal left (85%).

For interobserver agreement, inter-class correlations for measurements were 0.8 in average, with the highest correlation for the lateral distance of the left cranial articular process (0.9373) and the lowest for the right caudal articular surface angle (0.6). Interobserver shape identifications were 69% consistent, with the least consistency observed for the caudal right (62%) and the highest for the cranial left articular surface (75%).

Discussion

In this study, we investigated the angles, position (as given by lateral distance) and shapes of the articular surfaces of the cervical vertebral articular processes in

Table 3 Shape distribution for the caudal articular surfaces per group

Level	Dogs	Cc (RCd)	Cv (RCd)	P (RCd)	S (RCd)	Cc (LCd)	Cv (LCd)	P (LCd)	S (LCd)
C_{2-3}	Dob-N	2	6^b	3^b	4^b	2	5^b	5^b	3^b
	Dob-CSM	2	6^c	4^c	3^c	2	3^c	5^c	5^c
	GD-N	1	1^b	1^b	12^b	2	0^b	1^b	13^b
	GD-CSM	4	1^c	0^c	10^c	5	1^c	0^c	9^c
C_{3-4}	Dob-N	14	0	1	0	13	0	2	0
	Dob-CSM	15	0^c	0^c	0^c	15	0^c	0	0
	GD-N	8	0	4	3	9	0	4	2
	GD-CSM	6	0^c	4^c	5^c	11	1^c	1	2
C_{4-5}	Dob-N	13^b	0	1^b	1^b	13	0	1	1
	Dob-CSM	15^c	0	0^c	0	13	0	0	2
	GD-N	5^b	1	5^b	4^b	5	0	7	3
	GD-CSM	8^c	1	5^c	1	7	1	4	3
C_{5-6}	Dob-N	12^b	0^b	2	1	11^b	0	3	1^b
	Dob-CSM	14^c	0	0	1	12	0	0	3
	GD-N	4^b	4^b	3	4	4^b	0	2	9^b
	GD-CSM	6^c	1	3	5	6	2	2	5
C_{6-7}	Dob-N	15^b	0	0^b	0	15	0	0	0
	Dob-CSM	14	0	1	0	12	0	2	1
	GD-N	8^b	2	4^b	1	10	2	2	1
	GD-CSM	13	0	2	0	13	0	2	0

Shape distribution for the articular surface of the right (RCd) and left (LCd) caudal articular process from C2-3 to C6-7 in clinically normal Doberman Pinschers (Dob-N) and Great Danes (GD-N) and Doberman Pinschers and Great Danes with cervical spondylomyelopathy (Dob-CSM, GD-CSM)

Cc concave, *Cv* convex, *P* plane, *S* sigmoid

[a]Statistically significant difference between clinically normal and CSM-affected Great Danes ($P < 0.05$)

[b]Statistically significant difference between clinically normal Doberman Pinschers and clinically normal Great Danes ($P < 0.05$)

[c] Statistically significant difference between CSM-affected Doberman Pinschers and CSM-affected Great Danes ($P < 0.05$)

Dobermans and Great Danes with and without CSM. Such a thorough investigation of these characteristics and their relationships with CSM had not been previously performed.

Although our second hypothesis, that there would be a difference between breeds, was confirmed, our primary hypothesis, that there would be significant differences in articular surface shape, angle, and position between CSM and non-CSM-affected dogs, was not confirmed.

Overall, there were no significant differences in angle, lateral distance, or predominant shape of the articular surfaces between Dob-N and Dob-CSM or between GD-N and GD-CSM, suggesting that biomechanical differences between dogs with and without CSM are likely not related to these characteristics in these breeds. These findings also suggest that a difference in the overall size of the articular processes as a consequence of the osseous changes commonly seen in CSM-affected Great Danes [10, 13], may not result in a significant difference in position of the articular surface itself.

Overall, the shape of the articular surfaces was not associated with clinical disease in either breed. There was, however, a significant difference in shape patterns between breeds (comparing Dob-N to GD-N and Dob-CSM to GD-CSM). In general, Dobermans had a greater proportion of concave caudal surfaces, which has been associated with a greater capacity for axial rotation [6, 14]. The higher proportion of concave caudal surfaces may explain why Dobermans typically have disc-associated CSM, whereas this form of CSM is uncommon in Great Danes. The shape of the articular surfaces may be partially responsible for the higher torsional forces seen in the caudal cervical region [15], facilitating development of intervertebral disc degeneration and protrusion in this region.

Interestingly, we found three medially angled sigmoid caudal surfaces in GD-CSM. These were considered the result of osseous proliferation with severe deformation of the articular process, although it cannot be ruled out that they could be an anatomical variant. However, this would likely not be related to the change in orientation observed in humans [4, 5] which does not occur in dogs [6, 16]. Also, sigmoid surfaces were observed as being medially concave-laterally convex or medially convex-laterally concave, with both sometimes

Table 4 Mean ± standard error (and range) lateral distance of the articular surfaces per group

Level	Dogs	Left Cranial Lateral	Right Cranial Lateral	Left Caudal Lateral	Right Caudal Lateral
C_{2-3}	Dob-N	1.22 ± 0.05 (1.05–1.37)	1.2 ± 0.06 (1.03–1.47)	1.32 ± 0.05 (1.09–1.46)	1.31 ± 0.06 (1.2–1.51)
	Dob-CSM	1.2 ± 0.05 (0.99–1.42)	1.15 ± 0.06 (0.83–1.44)	1.31 ± 0.05 (1.11–1.56)	1.28 ± 0.06 (1.05–1.55)
	GD-N	1.18 ± 0.05 (0.97–1.62)	1.29 ± 0.06 (0.89–1.64)	1.31 ± 0.05 (1.09–1.59)	1.41 ± 0.06 (1.01–1.79)
	GD-CSM	1.2 ± 0.05 (0.74–1.63)	1.25 ± 0.05 (0.61–1.79)	1.32 ± 0.05 (0.68–1.78)	1.34 ± 0.06 (0.56–1.93)
C_{3-4}	Dob-N	0.81 ± 0.07 [b] (0.69–1.14)	0.81 ± 0.06 [b] (0.6–1.01)	0.94 ± 0.06 [b] (0.75–1.19)	0.95 ± 0.05 [b] (0.71–1.1)
	Dob-CSM	0.82 ± 0.07 (0.57–1.15)	0.86 ± 0.06 (0.66–1.07)	0.92 ± 0.06 [c] (0.69–1.31)	0.97 ± 0.05 [c] (0.76–1.17)
	GD-N	1.23 ± 0.07 [b] (0.81–1.52)	1.17 ± 0.06 [b] (0.77–1.5)	1.3 ± 0.06 [b] (0.94–1.62)	1.3 ± 0.06 [b] (0.93–1.63)
	GD-CSM	1 ± 0.07 (−0.04–1.52)	1.06 ± 0.06 (0.29–1.37)	1.24 ± 0.06 [c] (0.35–1.68)	1.2 ± 0.05 [c] (0.48–1.49)
C_{4-5}	Dob-N	0.81 ± 0.05 [b] (0.53–1.13)	0.81 ± 0.05 [b] (0.62–1.08)	0.92 ± 0.05 [b] (0.7–1.16)	0.94 ± 0.05 [b] (0.76–1.19)
	Dob-CSM	0.77 ± 0.05 [c] (0.52–0.99)	0.73 ± 0.05 (0.5–0.95) [c]	0.87 ± 0.05 [c] (0.6–1.07)	0.86 ± 0.05 [c] (0.61–1.06)
	GD-N	1.19 ± 0.05 [b] (0.85–1.44)	1.18 ± 0.05 [b] (0.83–1.49)	1.32 ± 0.05 [b] (1.07–1.71)	1.31 ± 0.05 [b] (1.06–1.62)
	GD-CSM	1.33 ± 0.05 [c] (0.81–1.81)	1.3 ± 0.05 [c] (0.7–1.72)	1.47 ± 0.05 [c] (0.98–2.09)	1.41 ± 0.05 [c] (0.89–1.89)
C_{5-6}	Dob-N	0.83 ± 0.06 [b] (0.43–1.26)	0.83 ± 0.06 [b] (0.55–1.14)	0.94 ± 0.05 [b] (0.59–1.31)	0.93 ± 0.06 [b] (0.7–1.18)
	Dob-CSM	0.71 ± 0.06 [c] (0.36–0.99)	0.69 ± 0.06 [c] (0.39–0.98)	0.82 ± 0.05 [c] (0.5–1.11)	0.81 ± 0.06 [c] (0.52–1.05)
	GD-N	1.3 ± 0.06 [b] (0.88–1.52)	1.34 ± 0.06 [b] (−0.51–0.22)	1.44 ± 0.06 [b] (1.06–1.68)	1.5 ± 0.06 [b] (1.03–2.11)
	GD-CSM	1.5 ± 0.06 [c] (0.92–1.99)	1.5 ± 0.06 [c] (1.02–1.86)	1.6 ± 0.06 [c] (1.02–2.09)	1.6 ± 0.06 [c] (1.11–1.97)
C_{6-7}	Dob-N	0.78 ± 0.04 [b] (0.55–0.91)	0.78 ± 0.05 [b] (0.6–1.03)	0.89 ± 0.04 [b] (0.69–1)	0.89 ± 0.05 [b] (0.7–1.12)
	Dob-CSM	0.79 ± 0.04 [c] (0.42–1.18)	0.82 ± 0.05 [c] (0.44–1.22)	0.91 ± 0.04 [c] (0.5–1.18)	0.92 ± 0.05 [c] (0.5–1.28)
	GD-N	1.18 ± 0.04 [b] (0.69–1.44)	1.23 ± 0.05 [b] (0.83–1.67)	1.34 ± 0.04 [b] (0.9–1.49)	1.38 ± 0.05 [b] (0.99–1.78)
	GD-CSM	1.36 ± 0.04 [c] (0.99–1.59)	1.38 ± 0.05 [c] (0.92–1.67)	1.47 ± 0.04 [c] (1.05–1.68)	1.53 ± 0.05 [c] (1.07–1.88)
C_7-T_1	Dob-N	1.02 ± 0.06 [b] (0.65–1.33)	1.05 ± 0.05 [b] (0.74–1.35)	1.1 ± 0.06 [b] (0.76–1.44)	1.15 ± 0.05 [b] (0.81–1.46)
	Dob-CSM	1.12 ± 0.06 [c] (0.88–1.39)	1.11 ± 0.05 [c] (0.9–1.43)	1.23 ± 0.06 [c] (0.96–1.45)	1.2 ± 0.05 [c] (0.98–1.56)
	GD-N	1.45 ± 0.06 [b] (1.26–1.81)	1.51 ± 0.05 [b] (1.27–1.84)	1.54 ± 0.06 [b] (1.36–1.89)	1.61 ± 0.05 [b] (1.42–1.92)
	GD-CSM	1.55 ± 0.06 [c] (1.1–2.12)	1.58 ± 0.05 [c] (1.07–2.12)	1.67 ± 0.06 [c] (1.22–2.21)	1.7 ± 0.05 [c] (1.27–2.19)

Mean ± standard error adjusted for height of the vertebral bodies, with minimum and maximum values in parenthesis for lateral distance of the articular surface of cranial and caudal articular processes, given as the distance to the floor of the vertebral canal (reference line), in clinically normal Doberman Pinschers (Dob-N) and Great Danes (GD-N) and Doberman Pinschers and Great Danes with cervical spondylomyelopathy (Dob-CSM, GD-CSM), in centimeters

[a]Statistically significant difference between clinically normal and CSM-affected Great Danes ($P < 0.05$)

[b]Statistically significant difference between clinically normal Doberman Pinschers and clinically normal Great Danes ($P < 0.05$)

[c]Statistically significant difference between CSM-affected Doberman Pinschers and CSM-affected Great Danes ($P < 0.05$)

present in the same dog, which had not been previously described [6].

Limitations of this study include a limited number of dogs per group. A greater number of subjects might have resulted in additional significant differences between clinically normal and CSM-affected dogs. Nonetheless, these numbers are consistent with previous comparative studies focusing on CSM [8, 17, 18]. A power analysis after completion of the study obtained a power of 75%. This power was considered adequate for this specific study.

The use of a single observer, though reducing variability, can be considered another limitation; however, intraobserver agreement indicated a high degree of reliability in the measurements and interobserver agreement was considered good for the majority of the measurements [19]. Although another limitation can be the selection of a single image of the articular surface for the measurements, which would not be representative of the variations within a joint, this permits standardization of the measurement method and is consistent with other studies that looked at articular surface angles [11, 12].

Other comparisons, such as between sites with and without spinal cord compression or between the sites immediately cranial or caudal to a site of spinal cord compression and sites that were not adjacent to a site of spinal cord compression, would have been interesting, however, there were not enough compression sites in CSM-affected Dobermans or sites without compression in CSM-affected Great Danes to make such comparisons worthwhile. Furthermore, joining all sites of compression regardless of location (C_{2-3}, C_{3-4}, C_{4-5}, C_{5-6}, C_{6-7}, C_7-T_1) would likely result in another type of error since most of the compression sites were in the caudal cervical vertebrae.

Conclusions

Differences in angle, shape, and position of the articular surfaces between Dobermans and Great Danes suggest that the movements of the caudal cervical region of the vertebral column may differ between these breeds. The higher proportion of concave articular surfaces in Dobermans may explain why this breed has a higher proportion of disc-associated CSM compared to Great Danes.

Considering that no differences in angle, shape or position of the articular processes were found between normal and CSM-affected Dobermans or Great Danes, their relevance to the development of CSM in these breeds appears to have a secondary role.

Additional files

Additional file 1: Angle of the cranial and caudal articular surfaces to the reference line for clinically normal Doberman Pinschers. Angle measurements for the articular surface of the right (R) and left (L) cranial and caudal articular processes in 15 clinically normal Doberman Pinschers (Dob-N).

Additional file 2: Angle of the cranial and caudal articular surfaces to the reference line for Doberman Pinschers with cervical spondylomyelopathy. Angle measurements for the articular surface of the right (R) and left (L) cranial and caudal articular processes in 15 Doberman Pinschers with cervical spondylomyelopathy (Dob-CSM).

Additional file 3: Angle of the cranial and caudal articular surfaces to the reference line for clinically normal Great Danes. Angle measurements for the articular surface of the right (R) and left (L) cranial and caudal articular processes in 15 clinically normal Great Danes (GD-N).

Additional file 4: Angle of the cranial and caudal articular surfaces to the reference line for Great Danes with cervical spondylomyelopathy. Angle measurements for the articular surface of the right (R) and left (L) cranial and caudal articular processes in 15 Great Danes with cervical spondylomyelopathy (GD-CSM).

Additional file 5: Distance from the lateral edge of the cranial and caudal articular surfaces to the reference line for clinically normal Doberman Pinschers. Distance (in centimeters) from the lateral edge of the articular surface of the right and left cranial and caudal articular processes to the reference line in 15 clinically normal Doberman Pinschers (Dob-N).

Additional file 6: Distance from the lateral edge of the cranial and caudal articular surfaces to the reference line in Doberman Pinschers with cervical spondylomyelopathy. Distance (in centimeters) from the lateral edge of the articular surface of the right and left cranial and caudal articular processes to the reference line in 15 Doberman Pinschers with cervical spondylomyelopathy (Dob-CSM).

Additional file 7: Distance from the lateral edge of the cranial and caudal articular surfaces to the reference line in clinically normal Great Danes. Distance (in centimeters) from the lateral edge of the articular surface of the right and left cranial and caudal articular processes to the reference line in 15 clinically normal Great Danes (GD-N).

Additional file 8: Distance from the lateral edge of the cranial and caudal articular surfaces to the reference line in Great Danes with cervical spondylomyelopathy. Distance (in centimeters) from the lateral edge of the articular surface of the right and left cranial and caudal articular processes to the reference line in 15 Great Danes with cervical spondylomyelopathy (GD-CSM).

Abbreviations

CSM: Cervical spondylomyelopathy; DA-CSM: Disc-associated cervical spondylomyelopathy; Dob-CSM: Cervical spondylomyelopathy-affected Doberman Pinschers; Dob-N: Clinically normal Doberman Pinschers; FSU: Functional spinal unit; GD-CSM: Cervical spondylomyelopathy-affected Great Danes; GD-N: Clinically normal Great Danes; MR: Magnetic resonance; MRI: Magnetic resonance imaging; OA-CSM: Osseous-associated cervical spondylomyelopathy

Acknowledgements

Dr. Bonelli received a scholarship grant from the Coordination for the Improvement of Higher Education Personnel (CAPES), Brazil. CAPES was not involved in any stage of this study. We would like to thank Dr. Steven Naber and Abhijoy Saha for their assistance with statistical analysis.

Funding

Not applicable.

Authors' contributions

MAB, RC_DC, and PMV participated in conception and design of the study. MAB and CGD performed the measurements and interpreted the results along with RC_DC. All authors contributed to, read, and approved the final version of the manuscript.

Competing interests

The authors declare that they have no competing interests.

Consent for publication

Not applicable.

Author details

[1]Department of Veterinary Clinical Sciences, College of Veterinary Medicine, The Ohio State University, 601 Vernon Tharp St., Columbus, OH 43210, USA. [2]Department of Veterinary Medicine, Federal Rural University of Pernambuco, R. Dom Manoel de Medeiros s/n, Recife, PE 52171-900, Brazil. [3]Ogilvy Healthworld, Avda. de Burgos 21, C. P. 28036 Madrid, Spain.

References

1. da Costa RC. Cervical spondylomyelopathy (wobbler syndrome) in dogs. Vet Clin North Am Small Anim Pract. 2010;40:881–913.
2. De Decker S, da Costa RC, Volk HA, Van Ham LM. Current insights and controversies in the pathogenesis and diagnosis of disc-associated cervical spondylomyelopathy in dogs. Vet Rec. 2012;171:531–7.
3. Ramos RM, da Costa RC, Oliveira AL, Kodigudla MK, Goel VK. Morphological changes of the caudal cervical intervertebral foramina due to flexion-extension and compression-traction movements in the canine cervical vertebral column. BMC Vet Res. 2015;11:184.
4. Jaumard NV, Welch WC, Winkelstein BA. Spinal facet joint biomechanics and mechanotransduction in normal, injury and degenerative conditions. J Biomech Eng. 2011;133:071010.
5. Pal GP, Routal RV, Saggu SK. The orientation of the articular facets of the zygapophyseal joints at the cervical and upper thoracic region. J Anat. 2001;198:431–41.
6. Breit S, Künzel W. Shape and orientation of articular facets of cervical vertebrae (C3-C7) in dogs denoting axial rotational ability: an osteological study. Eur J Morphol. 2002;40:43–51.
7. Benninger MI, Seiler GS, Robinson LE, Ferguson SJ, Bonél HM, Busato AR, et al. Effects of anatomic conformation on three-dimensional motion of the caudal lumbar and lumbosacral portions of the vertebral column of dogs. Am J Vet Res. 2006;67:43–50.
8. da Costa RC, Parent JM, Partlow G, Dobson H, Holmberg DL, Lamarre J. Morphologic and morphometric magnetic resonance imaging features of Doberman Pinschers with and without clinical signs of cervical spondylomyelopathy. Am J Vet Res. 2006;67:1601–12.

9. Foss K, da Costa RC, Rajala-Schuttz PJ, Allen MJ. Force plate gait analysis in Doberman Pinschers with and without cervical spondylomyelopathy. J Vet Intern Med. 2013;27:106–11.
10. Martin-Vaquero P, da Costa RC. Magnetic resonance imaging features of Great Danes with and without clinical signs of cervical spondylomyelopathy. J Am Vet Med Assoc. 2014;245:393–400.
11. Boden SD, Riew KD, Yamaguchi K, Branch TP, Schellinger D, Wiesel SW. Orientation of the lumbar facet joints: association with degenerative disc disease. J Bone Joint Surg Am. 1996;78:403–11.
12. Lee DY, Ahn Y, Lee SH. The influence of facet tropism on herniation of the lumbar disc in adolescents and adults. J Bone Joint Surg (Br). 2006;88:520–3.
13. Gutierrez-Quintana R, Penderis J. MRI features of cervical articular process degenerative joint disease in Great Dane dogs with cervical spondylomyelopathy. Vet Radiol Ultrasound. 2012;53:304–11.
14. Hofstetter M, Gédet P, Doherr M, Ferguson SJ, Forterre F. Biomechanical analysis of the three-dimensional motion pattern of the canine cervical spine segment C4-C5. Vet Surg. 2009;38:49–58.
15. Johnson JA, da Costa RC, Bhattacharya S, Goel V, Allen MJ. Kinematic motion patterns of the cranial and caudal canine cervical spine. Vet Surg. 2011;40:720–7.
16. Breit S, Künzel W. A morphometric investigation on breed-specific features affecting sagittal rotational and lateral bending mobility in the canine cervical spine (C3-C7). Anat Histol Embryol. 2004;33:244–50.
17. De Decker S, Gielen IM, Duchateau L, van Bree HJ, Waelbers T, Bavegems V, et al. Morphometric dimensions of the caudal cervical vertebral column in clinically normal Doberman Pinschers, English Foxhounds and Doberman Pinschers with clinical signs of disk-associated cervical spondylomyelopathy. Vet J. 2012;191:52–7.
18. Martin-Vaquero P, da Costa RC, Lima CG. Cervical spondylomyelopathy in Great Danes: a magnetic resonance imaging morphometric study. Vet J. 2014;201:64–71.
19. Shrout PE. Measurement reliability and agreement in psychiatry. Stat Methods Med Res. 1998;7:301–17.

3

Validation of an automated assay for the measurement of cupric reducing antioxidant capacity in serum of dogs

Camila Peres Rubio[1], Asta Tvarijonaviciute[1,2], Silvia Martinez-Subiela[1], Josefa Hernández-Ruiz[3] and José Joaquin Cerón[1*]

Abstract

Background: The objective of the present study was to optimize and validate an automated method to assess the total antioxidant capacity (TAC) in serum of dogs using the cupric reducing antioxidant capacity (CUPRAC) methodology (TAC_C) with bathocuproinedisulfonic acid disodium salt as chelating agent, evaluating also possible variations due to the use of two different automated analyzers. The method is based on the reduction of Cu^{2+} into Cu^{1+} by the action of the non-enzymatic antioxidants that are present in the sample.

Results: Imprecision was low in both apparatus utilized, and the results were linear across serial Trolox and canine serum samples dilutions. Lipids did not interfere with the assay; however, hemolysis increased the TAC_C concentrations. When TAC_C concentrations were determined in ten healthy (control) dogs and in twelve dogs with inflammatory bowel disease (IBD), dogs with IBD had lower TAC_C concentrations when compared with the healthy dogs.

Conclusions: The method validated in this paper is precise, simple, and fast and can be easily adapted to automated analyzers.

Keywords: Bathocuproinedisulfonic acid, CUPRAC, Dogs, Oxidative stress, Validation

Background

Oxidative stress is characterized by the inability of endogenous antioxidants to counteract the oxidative damage on biological targets [1, 2]. Antioxidant response can be monitored by analysis of individual biomarkers such as α-tocopherol (vitamin E), carotenoids, glutathione peroxidase, selenium, among others, and/or by assays that measure the total antioxidant capacity (TAC). TAC can be measured by direct methods (e.g., Trolox equivalent antioxidant capacity) [3] that are based on the ability of inhibiting the oxidation of a chemical substance, or by indirect methods based on the determination of the reductive properties of the sample such as the cupric reducing antioxidant capacity (CUPRAC) and the ferric reducing ability of plasma (FRAP) [4, 6, 16]. TAC assays provide a global measurement of the antioxidant capacity of the body, including in some cases possible in vivo interaction between different antioxidants [5, 6].

In humans, a decrease of TAC values has been reported in several conditions, including metabolic syndrome, prediabetes or surgery [7–10]. In dogs, decreased TAC values have been reported after surgery and when anaesthetized with isoflurane [11, 12]. Furthermore, increases in this analyte have been described in demodicosis, parvoviral enteritis, and lymphoma [13–15].

CUPRAC assay evaluates the capacity of the sample in reducing the Cu^{2+} to Cu^{1+} in the presence of a chelating agent. Neocuproine, bathocuproine and bathocuproinedisulfonic acid disodium salt are different chelating agents used for this purpose. This method has been applied to human serum, food, and plant extracts [16–19].

To the authors' knowledge, no CUPRAC assay has been validated for TAC measurements in canine serum samples. The objective of the present study was to optimize

* Correspondence: jjceron@um.es
[1]Interdisciplinary Laboratory of Clinical Analysis Interlab-UMU, Faculty of Veterinary Medicine, Regional Campus of International Excellence 'Campus Mare Nostrum', University of Murcia, Espinardo, Murcia 30100, Spain
Full list of author information is available at the end of the article

and validate an automated method to assess the TAC in serum of dogs using the CUPRAC methodology (TAC_c) and the bathocuproinedisulfonic acid disodium salt as the chelating agent. The evaluation was performed using two different automated analyzers; therefore possible variations of the assay due to the use of different equipment were also evaluated.

Methods

Chemicals

Trolox (6-hydroxy-2,5,7,8-tetramethylchromane-2-carboxylic acid), potassium chloride (KCl), sodium chloride (NaCl), potassium phosphate (KH_2PO_4), bathocuproinedisulfonic acid disodium salt, and copper(II) sulphate ($CuSO_4$) were obtained from Sigma-Aldrich. Di-sodium hydrogen phosphate anhydrous (Na_2HPO_4) was obtained from Panreac.

Apparatus

The analyses were performed in the Cobas Mira Plus Biochemical Auto Analyzer (ABX Diagnostic) and in the Olympus AU400 Automatic Chemistry Analyzer (Olympus Europe GmbH).

Principle of the assay

The CUPRAC assay is based on the reduction of Cu^{2+} into Cu^{1+} by the action of the non-enzymatic antioxidants presented in the sample. The oxidant complex, consisted of Cu^{2+}-bathocuproinedisulfonic acid (Cu^{2+}-BCS) reacts with the antioxidants of the sample and is reduced to a Cu^{1+}-bathocuproinedisulfonic acid (Cu^{1+}-BCS), a stable complex which has a maximum absorbance at 490 nm [19]. The antioxidant capacity of the sample is assumed to be equal to the extent of the complex Cu^{1+}-BCS formation [19]. The assay used for CUPRAC in the present study was based on the method described by Campos et al. [19] with some modifications.

Measurement procedure for the Cobas Mira Plus biochemical auto analyzer

In brief, a 5 µL volume of sample was pipetted. Then, 195 µL of the reagent 1 were added and a first read at 500 nm was taken. Subsequently, 50 µL of the reagent 2 were added to the reaction and incubated at 37 °C during 200 seconds. After incubation, a second read at 500 nm was taken and the difference between the first and the second read was used to calculate the antioxidant capacity of the sample. Distilled water was used for blanks.

Measurement procedure for the Olympus AU400 automatic chemistry analyzer

An amount of 195 µL of reagent 1 and 5 µL of sample were pipetted. A first read at 480 nm was taken before the addition of the second reagent. Then, 50 µL of reagent 2 were added to the mixture and incubated at 37 °C during 280 seconds. A second read at 480 nm was taken and the difference between the first and the second read was used for calculation of the antioxidant capacity of the sample. Distilled water was used instead of sample or standard for blanks.

Preparation of standards

Trolox solution at a concentration of 2.0, 1.0, 0.5, 0.25, 0.125, 0.0625 and 0.0 mmol/L were used. The results obtained for test samples were compared with a standard curve obtained with Trolox and were expressed as millimoles of Trolox equivalents per liter.

Optimization of reagents concentrations

To adjust the assay for measurements in canine serum, different concentrations of reagent 1 and reagent 2 were tested with the standards at different concentrations and also with different samples in the Cobas Mira Plus biochemical analyzer.

Reagent 1 was prepared at 0.1, 0.25, 1.0 and 1.6 mmol/L of bathocuproinedisulfonic acid disodium salt in 10 mmol/L phosphate buffer (pH 7.4) while reagent 2 was prepared at 0.1, 0.5, and 0.8 mmol/L of $CuSO_4$ in ultrapure water.

The optimal concentrations were selected based on the production of a higher signal with lower background and a lower intra-assay imprecision calculated after analysis of one sample five times in one assay run.

Analytical validation of the assay

For the analytical validation of the CUPRAC assay, imprecision, accuracy, and sensitivity were evaluated following previously reported protocols [19–22].

Imprecision

Imprecision was expressed as coefficient of variation (CV) and was calculated as inter- and intra-assay variations. The CV was calculated as the standard deviation (SD) divided by the mean value (X_{mean}) of analyzed replicates x 100 % in the formula CV = (SD x 100 %)/ X_{mean}. To determine inter-assay variation, four serum samples were used. Inter-assay CV was determined by analyzing the same samples in separate runs performed on five different days. Five aliquots of each serum sample were stored in plastic vials at −20 °C until analysis. On the day of analysis, the samples were brought to room temperature prior to TAC_c measurement. The intra-assay CV was calculated after analysis of four samples five times in one assay run. Intra-assay CV tests were performed for all the different combination of reagents tested, although in the results only appear the values for the final concentration selected for the assay.

Accuracy

The accuracy was evaluated through assessment of linearity and spiking recovery. The linearity was evaluated by linearity under dilution, then duplicate determinations of TAC_c were made of a canine serum diluted at 1/2, 1/4, 1/8, 1/16 and 1/32 using ultrapure water. Dilution of a Trolox solution (2.0, 1.0, 0.5, 0.25, 0.125, and 0.0625 mmol/L) was also analyzed. For the spiking recovery, two canine serum samples with a known TAC_c concentration were mixed in different percentages (12.5, 25, 50, 75 and 87.5 %). The percentages of the measured TAC_c concentrations to the expected TAC_c concentrations were then calculated.

Sensitivity

The detection limit was calculated on the basis of data from 20 replicate TAC_c determinations of ultrapure water as mean value plus 3 SDs. The lower limit of quantification (LLOQ) was calculated based on the lowest TAC_c concentration that could be measured within a CV less than 15 % [20].

Effects of hemolysis and lipemia

In order to examine the effect of hemolysis and lipemia, serum samples from three dogs were mixed with various concentrations of hemoglobin and lipids solution, respectively, and TAC_c was measured [23]. To study the effects of hemolysis, fresh hemolysate was prepared by the addition of distilled water to packed, washed canine red blood cells from one dog, followed by centrifugation to remove cell debris. The hemoglobin concentration was adjusted to 80, 40, 20, 10, 5, and 0.0 g/L. Ten μL of each concentration were added to three 90 μL samples of canine serum to produce test samples with final hemoglobin concentration of 8, 4, 2, 1, 0.5, and 0.0 g/L, respectively. The 0.0 g/L concentration was reached by adding 10 μL of distilled water to 90 μL of the serum sample. Prepared samples were used to determine the TAC_c concentrations.

To investigate the effects of lipemia, a commercial fat emulsion (Lipofundina 20 %; Braun Medical S.S.) with triglycerides concentration of 200 g/L was serially diluted to 50, 25, 12.5, 6.25,3.125 and 0.0 g/L. Ten μL of each dilution were added to 90 μL of the serum samples and were used to determine the TAC_c concentration. The final concentrations of triglycerides in the samples were 5, 2.5, 1.25, 0.625, 0.3125, and 0.0 g/L (10 μL of distilled water were added to 90 μL of the serum samples).

The TAC_c measurements to evaluate the effect of hemolysis and lipemia in the assay were made in the Olympus AU400.

Clinical validation

TAC_c levels were determined in healthy (control) dogs and dogs with inflammatory bowel disease (IBD). The control samples were from ten (seven males and three females) clinically healthy dogs of several different breeds aged between 3 and 8 years old, that were presented for routine checkups and had normal physical examination. Twelve dogs with IBD were included in this study. They were four female and eight male dogs aged between 3 and 8 years old also of different several breeds. A diagnosis of IBD was made on the basis of clinical signs (vomiting, diarrhea, and weight loss) of at least 3 weeks' duration, and detection of lymphoplasmacytic inflammation during histologic examination of duodenal biopsy samples following the criteria of Ohta et al. [24]. Exclusion of other causes of chronic gastrointestinal tract signs including urinalysis, abdominal ultrasound, fecal exam, complete blood count and serum biochemistry were made [25, 26].

Blood samples of the healthy and diseased dogs were collected from each via jugular or lateral saphenous venipuncture into tubes without anticoagulant. Samples were centrifuged at 3,500 x g for 5 min at 20 °C. The

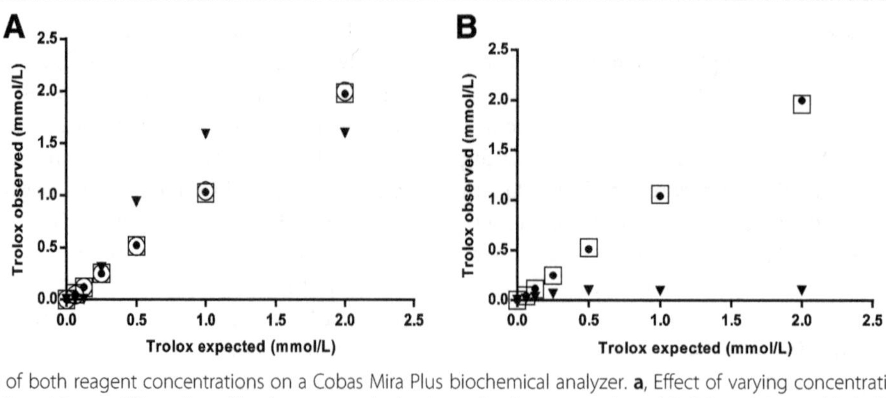

Fig. 1 Optimization of both reagent concentrations on a Cobas Mira Plus biochemical analyzer. **a**, Effect of varying concentrations of reagent 1 (▼, 0.1; ○, 0.25; ●, 1.0; □, 1.6 mmol/L) on the calibration curves obtained at a fixed concentration of $CuSO_4$ at 0.5 mmol/L. **b**, Effect of varying concentrations of reagent 2 (▼, 0.1; ●, 0.5; □, 0.8 mmol/L) on the calibration curves obtained at a fixed concentration of bathocuproinedisulfonic acid disodium salt at 0.25 mmol/L

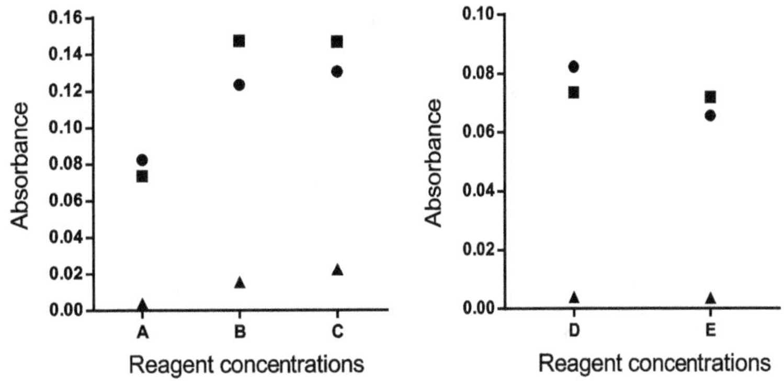

Fig. 2 Absorbance obtained of a reagent blank (H_2O instead of sample) (▲) and of two different canine serum samples (•, ■) studied with different reagent 1 (A, 0.25; B, 1.0; C, 1.6 mmol/L) and reagent 2 concentrations (D, 0.5; E, 0.8 mmol/L). When the reagent 1 was tested, the reagent 2 was fixed at 0.5 mmol/L and when the reagent 2 was tested, the reagent 1 was fixed at 0.25 mmol/L

serum samples were stored in plastic vials at - 20 °C until analysis.

Statistical analysis

Arithmetic means, medians, intra- and inter-assay CVs were calculated by use of routine descriptive statistical procedures and computer software (Excel 2013, Microsoft; GraphPad Statistics Guide). Linearity under dilution was investigated by linear regression. To compare the TAC_c results from both analyzers a Spearman correlation coefficient was used. The influence of hemolysis or lipemia on TAC_c concentration was investigated by use of 1-way ANOVA and Dunnett posttests. Interferograms were prepared to show the differences in TAC_c concentrations when hemoglobin or lipids were added. Kolmogorov-Smirnov's test was performed to assess normality of data. Comparison of the TAC_c concentrations between healthy dogs and dogs with IBD were made by use of Student's *t* test once a parametric distribution was given. For all tests, $P < 0.05$ was considered as statistically significant.

Results

Analytical validation

Results of the optimization of the reagents appear in Figs. 1 and 2. When concentrations of 0.1 mmol/L of reagent number 1 was tested with Trolox, the method lost its linearity at high Trolox concentrations. The other concentrations (0.25, 1.0 and 1.6 mmol/L) showed a similar reaction kinetic, but the background of the reaction increased with increased concentrations. When different concentrations of reagent number 2 were tested with Trolox, the concentration of 0.1 mmol/L did not produce a reaction. Concentrations of 0.5 and 0.8 mmol/L showed a similar reaction kinetic, but when 0.8 mmol/L was used, the background was higher.

When canine serum samples were tested, higher values were obtained when the concentrations of reagents 1 and 2 were increased (Fig. 2). However, the background was also higher. Also, when the reagent 2 was set at 0.8 mmol/L, the imprecision of the assay increased (data not shown). Therefore final concentrations of 0.25 mmol/L bathocuproinedisulfonic acid disodium

Table 1 Mean, standard deviation (SD), intra- and inter-assay CVs variation in TAC_c concentrations of canine serum samples (two with lower concentration and two with high concentrations) measured in the two apparatus

Apparatus	Validation parameter	Number of samples	Mean (mmol Trolox equiv./L)	SD	CV (%)
Cobas Mira Plus	Intra-assay	2	0.2325	0.004	1.9
		2	0.3823	0.007	1.8
	Inter-assay	2	0.2254	0.015	6.8
		2	0.3766	0.019	5.1
Olympus AU400	Intra-assay	2	0.2623	0.003	1.2
		2	0.3999	0.003	0.7
	Inter-assay	2	0.2533	0.022	8.6
		2	0.3842	0.030	7.8

TAC_c total antioxidant capacity using the cupric reducing antioxidant capacity methodology and the bathocuproinedisulfonic acid disodium salt, *SD* standard deviation, *CV* coefficient of variation

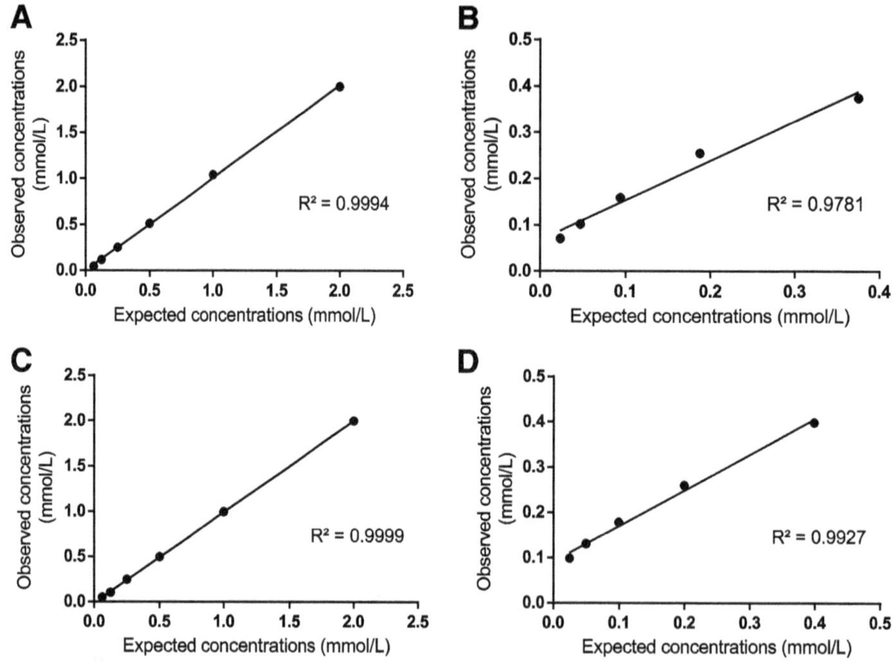

Fig. 3 **a** and **b**, Regression lines showing the TAC_c concentrations in the Cobas Mira Plus with the Trolox solution and canine serum sample, respectively. **c** and **d**, Regression lines showing the linearity of TAC_c concentrations in the Olympus AU400 with the Trolox solution and canine serum sample, respectively. Coefficients of determination (R^2) are shown

salt (reagent 1) and 0.5 mmol/L $CuSO_4$ (reagent 2) were established as optimal for the assay.

The mean, SD, and the intra- and inter-assay CVs obtained with the CUPRAC assay in the two apparatus are shown in Table 1. Intra-assay CVs were lower than 2 % in all cases. The inter-assay CVs were lower than 7 % and 9 % for the Cobas Mira Plus and Olympus AU400, respectively.

The method showed a high linearity with the Trolox and with canine serum sample in both apparatus (Fig. 3). The results of spiking recovery obtained in the Cobas Mira Plus were between 100 % and 103 % (Table 2), and in the Olympus AU400 were between 97 % and 101 % (Table 3).

The assay detection limit in the Cobas Mira Plus and Olympus AU400 were 0.017 mmol/L (mean ± SD, 0.001 ± 0.005) and 0.003 mmol/L (mean ± SD, 0.0001 ± 0.001), respectively. The lower limit of quantification could not be determined because the CVs were less than 15 % in all cases.

Data of the TAC_c obtained with the Cobas Mira Plus were significantly correlated with the data obtained in the Olympus AU400 (r = 0.973, $P < 0.001$).

Table 2 Recovery of CUPRAC assay in canine serum samples evaluated in the Cobas Mira Plus

% sample		Expected (mmol/L Trolox equiv./L)	Detected (mmol/L Trolox equiv./L)	Recovery (%)
High TAC_c	Low TAC_c			
100	0	0.3961	0.3961	100
87.5	12.5	0.3753	0.3771	101
75	25	0.3552	0.3581	101
50	50	0.3156	0.3202	102
25	75	0.2760	0.2822	103
0	100	0.2442	0.2442	100

CUPRAC cupric reducing antioxidant capacity using bathocuproinedisulfonic acid disodium salt. *TAC_c* total antioxidant capacity using the cupric reducing antioxidant capacity methodology and the bathocuproinedisulfonic acid disodium salt

Effects of hemolysis and lipemia

Lipids did not interfere with TAC_c concentrations (Fig. 4a). The addition of hemoglobin significantly increased the TAC_c concentrations, the increase being proportional with the hemoglobin concentration of the sample (Fig. 4b).

Clinical validation

The TAC_c results for serum samples in both apparatus are shown in Table 4. The TAC_c concentrations in dogs with IBD were significantly lower than those in healthy dogs when measured with both apparatus.

Discussion

In this study, an assay for evaluation of TAC by the CUPRAC method was described and validated for the first time in serum of dogs. This method is automated

Table 3 Recovery of CUPRAC assay in canine serum samples evaluated in the Olympus AU400

% sample		Expected (mmol/L Trolox equiv./L)	Detected (mmol/L Trolox equiv./L)	Recovery (%)
High TAC_c	Low TAC_c			
100	0	0.2346	0.2346	100
87.5	12.5	0.2571	0.2584	101
75	25	0.2796	0.2785	100
50	50	0.3245	0.3136	97
25	75	0.3695	0.3687	100
0	100	0.4144	0.4144	100

CUPRAC cupric reducing antioxidant capacity using bathocuproinedisulfonic acid disodium salt. *TAC_c* total antioxidant capacity using the cupric reducing antioxidant capacity methodology and the bathocuproinedisulfonic acid disodium salt

and uses bathocuproinedisulfonic acid disodium salt. The preparation of the reagents and measurement steps are simpler and faster compared to what has reported in other CUPRAC assays [16], making easier its application on routine analysis. Although in this paper the description of the assay is for automated analyzers, the method can be easily adapted to other formats such as 96 microplate well.

The optimal reagent concentrations determined in this work were different from those described in humans. Campos et al. [19] reported that the final established concentrations were 0.2 and 0.1 mmol/L for reagent number 1 and 2, respectively. Another study reported that the optimal concentrations for the reagent number 1 and 2 were 0.7 and 0.128 mmol/L, respectively [27]. In our study, it was found that higher concentrations of both reagents, especially reagent 2, were needed for the development of an optimal reaction (lower background and higher difference in absorbance between healthy and diseased individuals, and lower imprecision) in dog serum.

The validation results showed that the method has a good precision since all the intra- and inter-assay CVs in both apparatus were lower than 9 %. The method showed a good linearity with dog samples and with serial dilutions of Trolox. Campos et al. [19] also reported a linearity of this assay with Trolox dilutions. The assay showed recovery rates of around 100 % when canine serum samples were mixed at different proportions, indicating that the assay was accurate when measuring the TAC_c in canine serum samples.

The validation was performed in two different automated analyzers, the Cobas Mira Plus and Olympus AU400 in order to evaluate their agreement [28] and the repeatability of method in different equipment [29]. In this study, a high correlation between the TAC_c results obtained using the Cobas Mira Plus and Olympus AU400 was achieved revealing that this assay can be performed in both apparatus. Regarding the analytical validation results, the two automated equipment also gave similar results with the exception of the detection limit that was higher in the Cobas Mira Plus compared with the Olympus AU400. However, both detection limits were lower than the values usually observed in routine analyses and do not compromise the analytical sensitivity of the assay.

The presence of lipemia and hemolysis can interfere with the results of various analytes leading to an erroneous interpretation if the effect is unknown [23]. In the case of the CUPRAC assay, the lipemia did not interfere with the assay, which is an advantage to use it in clinical setting. However, hemolysis resulted in higher TAC_c concentrations. Therefore, results of this assay should be interpreted with caution when hemolytic samples are used.

Dogs with IBD had lower TAC_c concentrations than healthy dogs. The IBD is a progressive gastrointestinal tract disorder of unknown cause [25, 30]. During active episodes of IBD, the uncontrolled overproduction of reactive oxygen species could easily overwhelm the antioxidants, which are protective mechanisms, resulting in oxidative damage to cells and tissue. It was suggested that, this event may play a role in the pathogenesis of the disease [31–33]. In humans, the serum TAC, evaluated by the crocin bleaching method, was significantly reduced in IBD patients compared to healthy controls [32]. This is in line with the results of the present study, where our assay was able to demonstrate

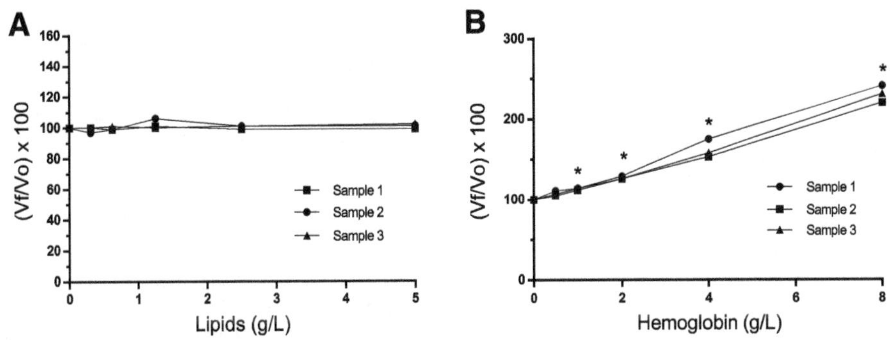

Fig. 4 Interferogram for the effect of lipids (**a**) and hemoglobin (**b**) on TAC_c concentration. Values for each given concentration (*Vf*) are reported as a percentage of the original value (V_O).* Significantly increased ($P < 0.05$)

Table 4 Mean ± SD TAC_c (mmol/L Trolox equiv./L) concentrations determined in 10 healthy dogs and 12 dogs with IBD

	Healthy dogs	Dogs with IBD	*P* value
Olympus AU400	0.3626 ± 0.02	0.3015 ± 0.07	0.0181
Cobas Mira Plus	0.3904 ± 0.03	0.2936 ± 0.08	0.0049

TAC_c total antioxidant capacity using the cupric reducing antioxidant capacity methodology and the bathocuproinedisulfonic acid disodium salt. $P < 0.05$ was considered significant

diminished concentrations of total antioxidants likely in response to oxidative stress in dogs with IBD.

Conclusions

In conclusion, the automated CUPRAC assay validated in this study can measure the TAC in serum of dogs in a simple, fast and reliable manner and could be adapted to two common automated analyzers. It is expected that this assay could contribute to a wider use of TAC_c measurements and therefore the evaluation of the antioxidant status in canine medicine.

Acknowledgements
Not applicable.

Funding
The National Council for Scientific and Technological Development (CNPq) of Brazil funded the PhD scholarship of CPR. The Ministerio de Economia y Competitividad of Spain funded AT through a postdoctoral grant (Juan de la Cierva). This study was also funded by the Seneca Foundation of Murcia Region (19894/GERM/15).

Authors' contributions
CPR and JJC designed and led the project, and wrote the manuscript; SMS, JHR and AT contributed to the interpretation of the data and revised the manuscript. All authors read and approved the final manuscript.

Competing interests
The authors declare that they have no financial or personal relationship(s) which may have inappropriately influenced them in writing this article.

Consent for publication
Not applicable.

Author details
[1]Interdisciplinary Laboratory of Clinical Analysis Interlab-UMU, Faculty of Veterinary Medicine, Regional Campus of International Excellence 'Campus Mare Nostrum', University of Murcia, Espinardo, Murcia 30100, Spain. [2]Department of Animal Medicine and Surgery, Veterinary School, University Autonoma of Barcelona, Barcelona, Spain. [3]Department of Plant Biology (Plant Physiology), Faculty of Biology, University of Murcia, Murcia, Spain.

References

1. López-Alarcón C, Denicola A. Evaluating the antioxidant capacity of natural products: A review on chemical and cellular-based assays. Anal Chim Acta. 2013;763:1–10.
2. Sies H. Oxidative stress: a concept in redox biology and medicine. Redox Biol. 2015;4:180–3.
3. Miller NJ, Rice-Evans C, Davies MJ, Gopinathan V, Milner A. A novel method for measuring antioxidant capacity and its application to monitoring the antioxidant status in premature neonates. Clin Sci. 1993;84:407–12.
4. Benzie IF, Strain JJ. The ferric reducing ability of plasma (FRAP) as a measure of "antioxidant power": the FRAP assay. Anal Biochem. 1996;239:70–6.
5. Rice-Evans CA, Diplock AT, Symons MC. Techniques in free radical research. Laboratory techniques in biochemistry and molecular biology. London: Elsevier; 1991.
6. Bartosz G. Non-enzymatic antioxidant capacity assays: limitations of use in biomedicine. Free Radic Res. 2010;44:711–20.
7. Glantzounis GK, Tselepis AD, Tambaki AP, Trikalinos TA, Manataki AD, Galaris DA, Tsimoyiannis EC, Kappas AM. Laparoscopic surgery-induced changes in oxidative stress markers in human plasma. Surg Endosc. 2001;15:1315–9.
8. Zulfikaroglu B, Koc M, Soran A, Isman FK, Cinel I. Evaluation of oxidative stress in laparoscopic cholecystectomy. Surg Today. 2002;32:869–74.
9. Hopps E, Canino B, Montana M, Lo Presti R, Averna MR, Caimi G. Behavior of the total antioxidant status in a group of subjects with metabolic syndrome. Diabetes Metab Syndr. 2014;8:166–9.
10. Mohieldein AH, Hasan M, Al-Harbi KK, Alodailah SS, Azahrani RM, Al-Mushawwah SA. Dyslipidemia and reduced total antioxidant status in young adult Saudis with prediabetes. Diabetes Metab Syndr. 2015;9:287–91.
11. Lee JY. Evaluation of the total oxidant and antioxidant status of the plasma of dogs anaesthetised with isoflurane. Vet Rec. 2013;173:96.
12. Lee JY, Kim MC. Comparison of oxidative stress status in dogs undergoing laparoscopic and open ovariectomy. J Vet Med Sci. 2014;76:273–6.
13. Martínez-Subiela S, Bernal LJ, Tvarijonaviciute A, Garcia-Martinez JD, Tecles F, Cerón JJ. Canine demodicosis: the relationship between response to treatment of generalised disease and markers for inflammation and oxidative status. Vet Dermatol. 2014;25:72–e24.
14. Kocaturk M, Tvarijonaviciute A, Martinez-Subiela S, Tecles F, Eralp O, Yilmaz Z, Ceron JJ. Inflammatory and oxidative biomarkers of disease severity in dogs with parvoviral enteritis. J Small Anim Pract. 2015;56:119–24.
15. Winter JL, Barber LG, Freeman L, Griessmayr PC, Milbury PE, Blumberg JB. Antioxidant status and biomarkers of oxidative stress in dogs with lymphoma. J Vet Intern Med. 2009;23:311–6.
16. Apak R, Güçlü K, Özyürek M, Karademir SE, Altun M. Total antioxidant capacity assay of human serum using copper (II)-neocuproine as chromogenic oxidant: the CUPRAC method. Free Radic Res. 2005;39:949–61.
17. Güçlü K, Sözgen K, Tütem E, Özyürek M, Apak R. Spectrophotometric determination of ascorbic acid using copper (II)–neocuproine reagent in beverages and pharmaceuticals. Talanta. 2005;65:1226–32.
18. Özyürek M, Güçlü K, Bektaşoğlu B, Apak R. Spectrophotometric determination of ascorbic acid by the modified CUPRAC method with extractive separation of flavonoids–La (III) complexes. Anal Chim Acta. 2007;588:88–95.
19. Campos C, Guzmán R, López-Fernández E, Casado Á. Evaluation of the copper (II) reduction assay using bathocuproinedisulfonic acid disodium salt for the total antioxidant capacity assessment: The CUPRAC–BCS assay. Anal Biochem. 2009;392:37–44.
20. Tiwari G, Tiwari R. Bioanalytical method validation: An updated review. Pharm Methods. 2010;1:25–38.
21. Tvarijonaviciute A, Tecles F, Caldin M, Tasca S, Cerón J.-Validation of spectrophotometric assays for serum paraoxonase type-1 measurement in dogs. Am J Vet Res. 2012;73:34–41.
22. Kjelgaard-Hansen M, Jacobsen S. Assay validation and diagnostic applications of major acute-phase protein testing in companion animals. Clin Lab Med. 2011;31:51–70.
23. Martínez-Subiela S, Cerón JJ. Effects of hemolysis, lipemia, hyperbilirrubinemia, and anticoagulants in canine C-reactive protein, serum amyloid A, and ceruloplasmin assays. Can Vet J. 2005;46:625–9.
24. Ohta H, Sunden Y, Yokoyama N, Osuga T, Lim SL, Tamura Y, Morishita K, Nakamura K, Yamasaki M, Takiguchi M. Expression of apical junction complex proteins in duodenal mucosa of dogs with inflammatory bowel disease. Am J Vet Res. 2014;75:746–51.
25. Washabau RJ, Day MJ, Willard MD, Hall EJ, Jergens AE, Mansell J, Minami T, Bilzer TW. Endoscopic, biopsy, and histopathologic guidelines for the evaluation of gastrointestinal inflammation in companion animals. J Vet Intern Med. 2010;24:10–26.

26. Rossi G, Cerquetella M, Antonelli E, Pengo G, Magi GE, Villanacci V, Rostami-Nejad M, Spaterna A, Bassotti G. The importance of histologic parameters of lacteal involvement in cases of canine lymphoplasmacytic enteritis. Gastroenterol Hepatol Bed Bench. 2015;8:33–41.
27. Gosmaro F, Bagnati M, Berto S, Bellomo G, Prenesti E. Measurement of total antioxidant capacity of human plasma: setting and validation of the CUPRAC–BCS method on routine apparatus ADVIA 2400. Talanta. 2013;115: 526–32.
28. Sutton A, Dawson H, Hoff B, Grift E, Shoukri M. Analyte comparisons between 2 clinical chemistry analyzers. Can Vet J. 1999;40:255.
29. Baral R, Morton J, Dhand NK, Krockenberger MB, Govendir M. Repeatability of results from three in-house biochemistry analyzers and a commercial laboratory analyzer used in small animal practice. Comp Clin Path. 2015;24:755–765.
30. Jackson M, Jewell D. Metabolomic and clinical disturbances in canine inflammatory bowel disease. FASEB J. 2015;29:265–7.
31. Pavlick KP, Laroux FS, Fuseler J, Wolf RE, Gray L, Hoffman J, Grisham MB. Role of reactive metabolites of oxygen and nitrogen in inflammatory bowel disease 1,2. Free Radic Biol Med. 2002;33:311–22.
32. Koutroubakis I, Malliaraki N, Dimoulios PD, Karmiris K, Castanas E, Kouroumalis EA. Decreased total and corrected antioxidant capacity in patients with inflammatory bowel disease. Dig Dis Sci. 2004;49:1433–7.
33. Minamoto Y, Otoni CC, Steelman SM, Büyükleblebici O, Steiner JM, Jergens AE, Suchodolski JS. Alteration of the fecal microbiota and serum metabolite profiles in dogs with idiopathic inflammatory bowel disease. Gut Microbes. 2015;6:33–47.

4

Morphological, densitometric and mechanical properties of mandible in 5-month-old Polish Merino sheep

Anna Szabelska[1], Marcin R. Tatara[2*] and Witold Krupski[3]

Abstract

Background: Among bones building the axial and appendicular skeleton, the mandible is characterized by unique morphological and functional traits. The aim of the study was to evaluate morphological, densitometric and mechanical properties of mandible in 5-month-old Polish Merino sheep. Using quantitative computed tomography, volumetric bone mineral density (vBMD) and calcium hydroxyapatite density of the cortical bone (Cb_{Ca-HA}), mean vBMD (MvBMD) and total bone volume were determined. Using computed tomography cross-sectional scans of the mandible, cross-sectional area, second moment of inertia, mean relative wall thickness and cortical index were determined. Three-point bending test was applied to determine mechanical properties. Serum concentration of insulin-like growth factor I (IGF-I) and bone-specific alkaline phosphatase (BAP) was also measured.

Results: All the investigated morphometric, densitometric and mechanical parameters of the right and left mandibular halves were not significantly different ($P > 0.05$). There was no correlation of final body weight, MvBMD, Cb_{Ca-HA}, BAP and IGF-I with all the analyzed parameters of mandible ($P > 0.05$). However, positive correlations between the other investigated morphometric, densitometric and mechanical parameter of mandible were found ($P < 0.05$).

Conclusions: Relationships between morphological, densitometric and mechanical parameters of the mandible indicate that the elaborated experimental model may serve for further studies on metabolic responses of skeletal system to physiological, nutritional, pharmacological, toxicological and environmental factors.

Keywords: Sheep, Mandible, Volumetric bone mineral density, Quantitative computed tomography (QCT), Animal model

Background

Osteoporosis in animals and humans is a metabolic disorder of skeletal system characterized by low bone mass and microarchitectural deterioration of bony tissue with consequent increased risk of bone fracture [1–3]. Considering that peak bone mass (PBM) in mature mammals is genetically determined in 70–80%, approximately 20–30% of the variation in PBM is determined by environmental factors such as nutrition, physical activity, exposure to sunlight, external temperature and other [4]. Thus, manipulations of the environmental factors during growth and development period in vertebrates may result in the attainment of higher bone mass of skeletal system expressed by superior bone mineral density, morphological and the mechanical properties of bones [5]. Among bones building the axial and appendicular skeleton, mandible is characterized by unique morphological and functional traits. Whereas vertebral bodies consist mainly trabecular bone, long bones are composed of trabecular and cortical bone types [6]. Mandible in mammals is built of cortical bone mainly and it is equipped with teeth physiologically [7]. It is susceptible to bone loss occurring with age and in response to endocrine and metabolic impairments, medications or locally acting factors [8–11]. In humans, after 50 years of age, there is an observed bone loss of the cortical bone compartment with subsequent thinning of the lower jaw and an increase in its porosity. The rate of mandibular bone loss is sex-dependent, with females having a lower mandibular size, volume and bone mass compared to males [12, 13]. Considering the importance of mandibular functions in animals and humans, the aim of the study was to elaborate original experimental model for

* Correspondence: matatar99@gazeta.pl
[2]Department of Animal Physiology, Faculty of Veterinary Medicine, University of Life Sciences in Lublin, ul. Akademicka 12, 20-950 Lublin, Poland
Full list of author information is available at the end of the article

experimental studies focused on bone metabolism regulation. There is a dearth of information on the basic anatomical and physiological characteristics of the mandible of lambs. Thus, in this study, morphological, densitometric, and mechanical properties of mandible in 5-month-old Polish Merino male sheep was investigated.

Methods

Experimental design and sampling procedure

The study was carried out on growing Polish Merino male lambs ($N = 7$) which were reared intensively from birth to 5 months of age under standard rearing conditions. Lambs and ewes were provided with drinking water *ad libitum* and fed a standard diet. During neonatal and postnatal period (up to 10 weeks of life) ram lambs were fed maternal milk. Between the fourth week and the fifth month of life, lambs were fed commercial concentrate and hay *ad libitum*. At the age of 5 months of life, the animals were euthanized to obtain whole mandible for morphometric, densitometric and mechanical analyses. Bone samples were isolated postmortally and cleaned of remaining soft tissues, including periosteum. Morphological properties of the whole mandible (including teeth) such as bone weight and bone length were measured. To avoid sample dehydration, mandibles were wrapped in plastic bags and stored frozen at –25 °C until further analyses. Bone samples were thawed at room temperature for 2 h before further morphometric, densitometric and mechanical analyses.

Densitometric evaluation of mandible

Quantitative computed tomography (QCT) technique and Somatom Emotion Siemens apparatus (Siemens, Erlangen, Germany), equipped with Somaris/5 VB10B software (version B10/2004A) were used to determine volumetric bone mineral density (vBMD) of the cortical bone (Cd), mean volumetric bone mineral density (MvBMD) and total bone volume (Bvol) of the whole mandible with teeth (Volume Evaluation application package, Siemens, Erlangen, Germany). The measurement of Cd was performed on cross-sectional scan of mandibular body positioned in the half distance of the diastema (half distance between canine (the fourth incisor) and premolar, approximately 50 mm measuring from the extremity of the mandible determined by the external alveolar margin of the first lower incisor) (Fig. 1a and b). Using the same measuring scan and Osteo CT application package (Software Version B10/2004A), calcium hydroxyapatite (Ca-HA) density of the cortical bone ($Cb_{Ca\text{-}HA}$) compartment was determined (Fig. 1c). Volumetric bone mineral density of the cortical bone of mandible and $Cb_{Ca\text{-}HA}$ were measured on the same cross-sectional scans for both the right and left mandibular halves. Mean volumetric bone mineral density of mandible and Bvol were determined using volume-of-interest (VOI) limited by minimum and maximum density of the investigated samples at 0 and 3071 Hounsfield units, respectively. The measurements of MvBMD and Bvol were performed for the whole mandible (combined right and left halves) and the results obtained reflect MvBMD measured for all the anatomical structures including teeth.

Determination of geometrical properties of mandible

Geometrical properties of the right and left mandibular body were determined on the basis of measurements of horizontal and vertical diameters (both external and internal) of the mid-diastemal cross-sections of the bone (the same measuring scans which were used for densitometric evaluation) obtained from computed tomography multiplanar reconstructions (Fig. 1d). The values of cross-sectional area (A), second moment of inertia (Ix), mean relative wall thickness (MRWT) and cortical index (CI) were determined in accordance to the following mathematical formulas:

$$A = 3.14(HV\text{–}hv)/4$$

$$Ix = 3.14\left(V^3H\text{–}v^3h\right)/64$$

$$MRWT = [(V\text{–}v)/v + (H - h)/h]/2$$

$$CI = \{[H\text{-}h/H + (V - v)/V]/2\}100$$

where: H – horizontal external diameter, h – horizontal internal diameter, V – vertical external diameter, v – vertical internal diameter [14–16].

Mechanical analysis of mandible

Using an INSTRON 3367 apparatus and Bluehill 2 software (Instron Corp., Canton, USA) the relationship between the loading force and bone displacement in the three-point bending test was recorded. Right and left halves of mandible (separated at the mandibular symphysis) were placed separately on flat bone supports on the lateral mandibular surface and the measuring head loaded bone samples on the medial surface at 50% of its length with the constant speed of 50 mm/min. Mechanical parameters such as maximum elastic strength (Wy) and ultimate strength (Wf) of both mandibular halves were determined. The distance between bone supports was set at 40% of mandible length.

Biochemical analysis of serum

Blood samples were collected from the lambs at 5 months of age for serum analysis. Insulin-like growth factor I (IGF-I) was determined in serum using IGF-I ELISA kit and two-site IEMA (Immunodiagnostic Systems Ltd., Boldon, Tyne & Wear, UK). Serum concentration of bone-specific alkaline phosphatase (BAP) was measured using Ostase® BAP immunoenzymometric assay (IEMA; Immunodiagnostic Systems

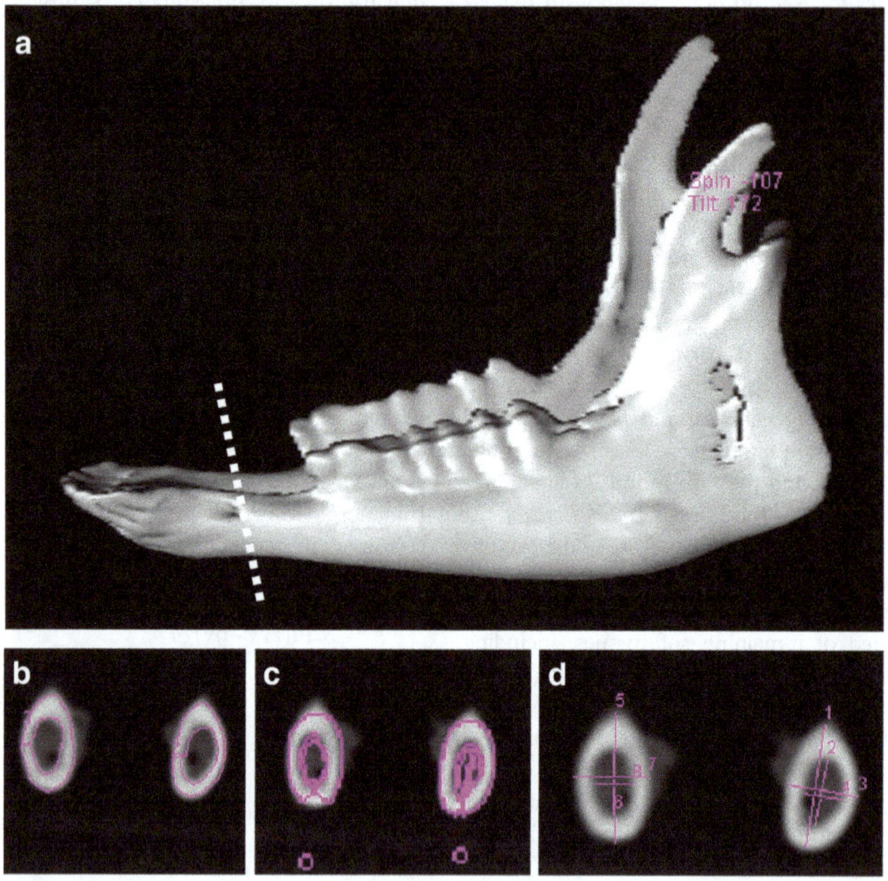

Fig. 1 Three dimensional (3D) computed tomography reconstruction of mandible in 5-month-old Polish Merino sheep showing the placement of the measuring scans (**a**). Measurement of volumetric bone mineral density (vBMD) of the cortical bone (Cd) of the right and left mandibular body on cross-sectional measuring scans (**b**) using quantitative computed tomography (QCT). Volumetric bone mineral density of the cortical bone of mandible was measured on 2 mm thick scans positioned in the half distance of the diastema (half distance between canine (the fourth incisor) and premolar). Calcium hydroxyapatite density of the cortical bone ($Cb_{Ca\text{-}HA}$) was measured at the same position on 10 mm thick cross-sectional measuring scan of mandible (**c**). Results of $Cb_{Ca\text{-}HA}$ measurements were expressed in mg of Ca-HA/ml. Geometrical parameters of the right and left mandibular body were determined on the basis of measurements of horizontal and vertical diameters (both external and internal) of the mid-diastemal cross-sections of the bone obtained from computed tomography multiplanar reconstructions (**d**). All these measurements were performed using Somatom Emotion Siemens scanner supplied with Somaris/5 VB10B software and Osteo CT application package (Siemens, Erlangen, Germany)

Ltd., Boldon, Tyne & Wear, UK). Results of biochemical evaluation of serum were obtained with the use of Benchmark Plus microplate spectrophotometer supplied with Microplate Manager Software Version 5.2.1 (Bio-Rad Laboratories, Inc., Hercules, CA, USA).

Statistical analysis

Statistical analysis of data collected was performed using Statistica software (version 6.0). Data are presented as means ± SEM. The comparison of mean values of the investigated variables between right and left halves of the mandible was performed using paired Student's *t*-test for dependent variables. *P*-value < 0.05 was considered as statistically significant for all comparisons. Pearson's correlation coefficient (r) was determined between all the investigated mandibular variables, final body weight, IGF-1 and BAP serum concentrations and $P < 0.05$ was considered as statistically significant.

Results

Results of morphological, densitometric and mechanical properties of the mandible in 5-month-old ram lambs are presented in Table 1. All the investigated morphometric, densitometric and mechanical parameters of right and left mandibular halves were not significantly different ($P > 0.05$). The values of Pearson's correlation coefficient between all the investigated parameters of mandible, final body weight, and serum concentration of BAP and IGF-1 in 5-month old sheep are shown in Table 2. Mandibular weight was observed to be positively correlated with mandibular length, Bvol, Cd, A, Ix and Wy ($P < 0.05$). Mandibular length was positively correlated with Bvol and Cd ($P < 0.05$). Total bone volume was positively correlated

Table 1 Morphometric, densitometric and mechanical properties of mandible in 5-month-old Polish Merino sheep

Investigated parameter	Right mandible	Left mandible	Whole mandible
Bone weight (g)	-	-	116.3 ± 5.6
Bone length (mm)	218.9 ± 2.8	218.6 ± 2.9	218.7 ± 2.9[a]
Total bone volume (cm^3)	-	-	71.7 ± 3.3
Volumetric bone mineral density of the cortical bone (g/cm^3)	2.457 ± 0.027	2.446 ± 0.025	2.451 ± 0.024[a]
Calcium hydroxyapatite density of the cortical bone (g/ml)	1043 ± 26	1065 ± 35	1054 ± 26[a]
Mean volumetric bone mineral density (g/cm^3)	-	-	1.864 ± 0.017
Cross-sectional area (mm^2)	51.7 ± 1.9	56.0 ± 2.8	53.9 ± 2.3[a]
Second moment of inertia (mm^4)	254 ± 21	276 ± 22	265 ± 21[a]
Mean relative wall thickness	0.756 ± 0.020	0.843 ± 0.025	0.797 ± 0.017[a]
Cortical index	42.9 ± 0.6	45.6 ± 0.7	44.3 ± 0.5[a]
Maximum elastic strength (N)	801 ± 31	844 ± 69	823 ± 42[a]
Ultimate strength (N)	1121 ± 105	1312 ± 135	1216 ± 106[a]

Values are means ± standard error of the mean
[a]Values obtained as means of right and left halves of mandible

with Cd, A, Ix, and Wf ($P < 0.05$). Cross-sectional area and Ix were found to be positively correlated ($r = 0.97$; $P < 0.001$) and both parameters were positively correlated with Cd ($P < 0.05$). Volumetric bone mineral density of the cortical bone was found to be also positively correlated with Wy and Wf ($P < 0.05$). Positive correlations between MRWT and CI as well as between Wy and Wf were found (all $P < 0.05$).

Discussion

In this study, a new experimental model to investigate bone metabolism regulation and skeletal system properties in mammals was introduced. Using quantitative computed tomography technique, for the first time Bvol and MvBMD of mandible in sheep was determined. While Bvol represents morphometric parameter, MvBMD is a densitometric parameter characterizing all anatomical structures of the

Table 2 The values of Pearson's correlation coefficient between the investigated parameters of mandible, final body weight and serum concentration of bone-specific alkaline phosphatase (BAP) and insulin-like growth factor 1 (IGF-1) in ram lambs at the age of 5 months

Investigated parameter	Body weight	Mandibular weight	Mandibular length	MvBMD	Bvol	Cd	Ca-HA	A	Ix	MRWT	CI	Wy	Wf	BAP	IGF-1
Body weight	x	0.58	0.45	- 0.06	0.51	0.72	0.32	0.75	0.68	0.39	0.38	0.65	0.55	- 0.61	- 0.64
Mandibular weight	0.58	x	0.77[a]	0.29	0.98[a]	0.91[a]	0.02	0.89[a]	0.94[a]	0.10	0.12	0.66	0.86[a]	- 0.42	- 0.50
Mandibular length	0.45	0.77[a]	x	0.69	0.81[a]	0.77[a]	0.35	0.61	0.62	0.08	0.10	0.59	0.68	- 0.47	- 0.07
MvBMD	- 0.06	0.29	0.69	x	0.33	0.40	0.69	- 0.01	- 0.02	0.22	0.24	0.51	0.50	0.15	0.46
Bvol	0.51	0.98[a]	0.81[a]	0.33	x	0.89[a]	- 0.01	0.88[a]	0.93[a]	0.03	0.04	0.61	0.80[a]	- 0.41	- 0.48
Cd	0.72	0.91[a]	0.77[a]	0.40	0.89[a]	x	0.37	0.88[a]	0.83[a]	0.43	0.44	0.80[a]	0.86[a]	- 0.27	- 0.44
Ca-HA	0.32	0.02	0.35	0.69	- 0.01	0.37	x	- 0.03	- 0.18	0.68	0.68	0.61	0.34	0.21	0.29
A	0.75	0.89[a]	0.61	- 0.01	0.88[a]	0.88[a]	- 0.03	x	0.97[a]	0.20	0.20	0.54	0.64	- 0.48	- 0.69
Ix	0.68	0.94[a]	0.62	- 0.02	0.93[a]	0.83[a]	- 0.18	0.97[a]	x	0.02	0.03	0.52	0.70	- 0.54	- 0.71
MRWT	0.39	0.10	0.08	0.22	0.03	0.43	0.68	0.20	0.02	x	0.99[a]	0.33	0.21	0.27	0.19
CI	0.38	0.12	0.10	0.24	0.04	0.44	0.68	0.20	0.03	0.99[a]	x	0.34	0.22	0.28	0.20
Wy	0.65	0.66	0.59	0.51	0.61	0.80[a]	0.61	0.54	0.52	0.33	0.34	x	0.90[a]	- 0.12	- 0.43
Wf	0.55	0.86[a]	0.68	0.50	0.80[a]	0.86[a]	0.34	0.64	0.70	0.21	0.22	0.90[a]	x	- 0.21	- 0.40
BAP	- 0.61	- 0.42	- 0.47	0.15	- 0.41	- 0.27	0.21	- 0.48	- 0.54	0.27	0.28	- 0.12	- 0.21	x	0.40
IGF-1	- 0.64	- 0.50	- 0.07	0.46	- 0.48	- 0.44	0.29	- 0.69	- 0.71	0.19	0.20	- 0.43	- 0.40	0.40	x

MvBMD mean volumetric bone mineral density, *Bvol* total bone volume, *Cd* volumetric bone mineral density of the cortical bone, *Ca-HA* calcium hydroxyapatite density of the cortical bone, *A* cross-sectional area, *Ix* second moment of inertia, *MRWT* mean relative wall thickness, *CI* cortical index, *Wy* maximum elastic strength, *Wf* ultimate strength
[a]Statistically significant values for $P < 0.05$

mandible, including the teeth. Similarly to bone weight determination, both Bvol and MvBMD measurements were performed for whole mandible without its separation into two halves. The methodological advantage resulting from the determination of Bvol and MvBMD for whole mandible is that both these parameters may be evaluated both ex vivo and in vivo, while mandibular weight may be determined precisely on ex vivo isolated samples only. As opposed to the parameters characterizing whole mandible, densitometric, geometric and mechanical properties in this bone were determined for the right and left halves separately. As the results of densitometric evaluation of the right and left mandibular body, it was shown that Cd and Ca-HA values were not significantly different in both these halves of the bone. Noteworthy is the fact that anatomical shape and structure of mandible in sheep and physiological occurrence of the diastema enable volumetric bone mineral density determination (in terms of Cd and Ca-HA) exclusively for cortical bone compartment. The reference measuring point of the densitometric parameters in mandible is recommended at the half length of the diastema, since at this point also geometrical parameters for the right and left halves may be evaluated [17]. In this study, computed tomography evaluations of serial cross-sections of the whole mandible along its longitudinal axis have not provided the reference point for the separate determination of vBMD of the trabecular bone compartment. Moreover, it was not possible to exclude non-invasively teeth from bone tissue of the mandible for measurements of bone weight, Bvol and MvBMD. As opposed to sheep model, studies in pigs have revealed that vBMD of the cortical bone in mandible may be measured on cross-sectional scan of the mandibular body positioned just after the 4th premolar tooth [18]. It is interesting that at this reference point in mandible of pigs, cortical bone area and mechanical properties may be also evaluated. The loading head acts on the mandible in pigs exactly at this reference point in three-point bending test [10]. Mechanical testing of mandible in sheep using three-point bending test can not be performed in the reference point used for Cd and Ca-HA determinations, which makes this model different from the mandibular models in pigs. Both densitometric parameters are measured approximately 5 cm from proximal extremity of mandible in sheep (determined by the external alveolar margin of the first lower incisor), while the loading head should act on bone sample at 50% of its length [14, 16]. In this study, the length of mandible varied between 205 and 228 mm. The separation of the right and left halves of the mandible enabled their separate evaluation. Bone length measured for the right and left halve of mandible did not revealed significant differences. Analogical results were obtained evaluating geometrical parameters of mandible. Cross sectional area, Ix, MRWT and CI had no significant differences in the values obtained in both mandibular halves. As opposed to anatomical traits of mandible in other animal species like pig, dog, fox and rodents, oval shape of the cross section of the middle part of the diastema in sheep enables determination of geometrical parameters in accordance to the principles applied in case of long bones such as tibia, femur, humerus and ribs [16, 19–23]. While A and Ix are considered as geometrical indices of mechanical endurance of bone shaft to acting forces, MRWT and CI reflect the amount of bone tissue accumulated in the midshaft ring in relation to the medullary cavity size [14–16]. Besides morphological, densitometric and geometrical parameters, mechanical testing of both halves of mandible was performed in this study. Based on three-point bending test, neither Wy nor Wf were found to be differentiated between the right and left halves of mandible. Considering the observed lack of the differences of mechanical endurance of the right and left halves of mandible and the fact that mandible in sheep may be classified as flat bone, precise mechanical testing of the bone may include the three-point and four-point bending tests; however, in such case both halves undergo structural disintegration [24]. Separate evaluation of the right and left halves of mandible gives possibility to take average from both measurements, improving methodological precision. Moreover, separate evaluation of bone weight, Bvol and MvBMD for the right and left halves of mandible is possible; however, all these measurements must be repeated after the separation of bone halves at the symphysis.

In this study, the correlations between all the investigated parameters of mandible, final body weight and serum BAP and IGF-1 concentration were evaluated. Final body weight and serum indices of bone metabolism were not significantly correlated with the other investigated parameters of mandible in lambs and these observations are similar to the results obtained in pigs were such correlations also were not found. However, in the previous study on pigs, serum IGF-1 concentration was associated with the final body weight [18]. Lack of correlations of MvBMD and Ca-HA with all the other investigated parameters were stated in this study that is partially in agreement with studies on pigs, where MvBMD of mandible were not correlated with final body weight, bone weight, bone length and Bvol. However, except for the insignificant correlation between Bvol and Cd in pigs, all the other evaluated parameters of mandible were significantly positively correlated [10]. The current study revealed also that mandibular weight and volume are positively correlated with morphometric, densitometric and mechanical properties of mandible, while mandibular length, A and Ix were correlated only with morphometric (bone weight and volume) and densitometric (Cd) indices. Volumetric bone mineral density of the cortical bone was positively correlated with morphometric parameters (bone weight, length, Bvol, A and Ix) and has shown the most prognostic value for bone mechanical strength prediction, since its value was positively correlated with both Wy and Wf. Besides listed above relationships, significant positive correlations between geometrical (A and Ix as well as MRWT and CI) and mechanical (Wy and Wf) parameters of mandible were stated.

The results obtained in this study indicate that mandible in sheep provide possibility to investigate effects of experimental manipulations on bone tissue metabolism and skeletal system properties with a use of physiological, nutritional, pharmacological, toxicological and environmental factors. Even though mandibular samples were harvested from ram lambs in this study, the same analytical procedures may be applied for mandible from ewes. Except for ovariectomy-induced osteopenia and osteoporosis, experimental evaluation of mandible from ram lambs may provide valuable data on prevention and treatment of metabolic bone disorders resulting from malnutrition, glucocorticoid treatment, androgen deficiency, mineral and vitamin deficiency and impaired environmental conditions. Metabolic effects of positive or negative factors influencing bone tissue properties in mammals may be more apparent when acting during systemic growth and development period than later in skeletally matured or older animals [25]. The elaborated experimental model in this study is characterized by numerous advantages in comparison to other animal models. In rodents, serial blood collection, small size of mandible and existing differences in bone growth and mineralization pattern in comparison to humans make these experimental models and data interpretation less attractive than in case of sheep or other small ruminants [26–29]. Bone size, histological characteristic and bone remodeling activity, as well as bone metabolism responses to hormonal manipulations in sheep skeleton is similar to humans [30, 31]. Moreover, in sheep serial blood sampling, housing, handling and experimental procedures are relatively easy to perform and similarity of the hormonal profile with humans favors sheep model for studies on bone metabolism [32, 33]. The other rationale for the use of mandible in experimental studies on bone metabolism regulation results from impact of bone loss in maxillofacial bones on health and quality of the stomatognathic system and whole body both in animals and humans. Maxillar and mandibular bone loss most commonly results from periodontal disease, resorption of alveolar ridges following tooth extraction, or a combination of both [34]. Apart from these similarities, the differences such as gastrointestinal structure and digestion process in ruminants and quadruped posture must be also considered as potential limitations in some experimental approaches using the sheep model. However, during the neonatal and postnatal period of systemic growth and development, gastrointestinal tract anatomy and digestion and absorption processes in sheep are similar to monogastric mammals like pigs, dogs and humans. The quadruped posture in sheep appears not to be a limitation in studies on bone metabolism regulation and bone quality with the use of mandibular model, since the body posture has no impact on craniofacial bones characteristics [13, 23, 33].

Conclusions

In conclusion, this study presents basic morphological, densitometric and mechanical characteristics of mandible in 5-month-old Polish Merino sheep. Significant differences of the evaluated parameters between the right and left halves of the mandible were not shown. Common relationships between morphological, densitometric and mechanical parameters of the mandible indicate that the originally elaborated experimental model may serve for further studies on metabolic responses of bone tissue and skeletal system to physiological, nutritional, pharmacological, toxicological and environmental factors influencing bone tissue metabolism. Moreover, quantitative computed tomography may be also used for in vivo and ex vivo evaluation of morphometric and densitometric properties of bones of the stomatognathic system in sheep.

Abbreviations

A: Cross-sectional area; BAP: Bone-specific alkaline phosphatase; Bvol: Total bone volume; Ca-HA: Calcium hydroxyapatite; $Cb_{Ca\text{-}HA}$: Calcium hydroxyapatite density of the cortical bone; Cd: Volumetric bone mineral density of the cortical bone; CI: Cortical index; IGF-I: Insulin-like growth factor I; Ix: Second moment of inertia; MRWT: Mean relative wall thickness; MvBMD: Mean volumetric bone mineral density; PBM: Peak bone mass; QCT: Quantitative computed tomography; vBMD: Volumetric bone mineral density; VOI: Volume of interest; Wf: Ultimate strength; Wy: Maximum elastic strength

Acknowledgments

Not applicable.

Funding

Study financed by Medical University of Lublin.

Authors' contributions

AS was responsible for the concept of the study, collection and interpretation of data, statistical analysis, references collection, and writing the manuscript. MT was responsible for the concept of the study, supervised all stages of the study, participated in animal management, collection and interpretation of data, as well as writing the manuscript. WK performed QCT analysis of bones and was responsible for interpretation of data and supervised all stages of the study. All authors participated in the preparation of, and have approved the final version of the manuscript.

Competing interests

The authors declare that they have no competing interests.

Consent for publication

Not applicable.

Author details

[1]Department of Prosthetic Dentistry, Medical University in Lublin, ul. Karmelicka 7, 20-081 Lublin, Poland. [2]Department of Animal Physiology, Faculty of Veterinary Medicine, University of Life Sciences in Lublin, ul. Akademicka 12, 20-950 Lublin, Poland. [3]II Department of Radiology, Medical University in Lublin, ul. Staszica 16, 20-081 Lublin, Poland.

References

1. Anonymous. Prevention and management of osteoporosis. World Health Organ Tech Rep Ser. 2003;921:1–164.
2. Webster AB. Welfare implications of avian osteoporosis. Poult Sci. 2004;83:184–92.
3. Thompson KG. Skeletal diseases of sheep. Small Rumin Res. 2008;76:112–9.
4. Eastell R, Lambert H. Diet and healthy bones. Calcif Tissue Int. 2002;70:400–4.
5. Tatara MR. Neonatal programming of skeletal development in sheep is mediated by somatotrophic axis function. Exp Physiol. 2008;93:763–72.
6. Seeman E, Wahner HW, Offord KP, Kumar R, Johnson WJ, Riggs BL. Differential effects of endocrine dysfunction on the axial and the appendicular skeleton. J Clin Invest. 1982;69:1302–9.
7. Tatara MR, Szabelska A, Krupski W, Tymczyna B, Luszczewska-Sierakowska I, Bieniaś J, Ostapiuk M. Morphometric, densitometric and mechanical properties of mandibular deciduous teeth in 5-month-old Polish Merino sheep. BMC Vet Res. 2014;10:45.
8. Groen JJ, Duyvensz F, Halsted JA. Diffuse alveolar atrophy of the jaw (non-inflammatory form of paradental disease) and pre-senile osteoporosis. Gerontol Clin. 1960;2:68–86.
9. Bellido M, Lugo L, Castañeda S, Roman-Blas JA, Rufián-Henares JA, Navarro-Alarcón M, Largo R, Herrero-Beaumont G. PTH increases jaw mineral density in a rabbit model of osteoporosis. J Dent Res. 2010;89:360–5.
10. Tymczyna B, Bachanek T, Tatara MR, Krupski W, Tyczyna-Sobotka M, Łuszczewska-Sierakowska I. Interrelationships between morphometric, densitometric, and mechanical properties of mandible in 6-month-old male pigs. Bull Vet Inst Pulawy. 2012;56:177–81.
11. Raubenheimer EJ, Noffke CE, Hendrik HD. Recent developments in metabolic bone diseases: a gnathic perspective. Head Neck Pathol. 2014;8:475–81.
12. Ulm CW, Solar P, Ulm MR, Matejka M. Sex-related changes in the bone mineral content of atrophic mandibles. Calcif Tissue Int. 1994;54:203–7.
13. Drozdowska B, Michno M, Michno A. The relationships between mandibular bone mass and skeletal osteopenia/osteoporosis – a review. Nowa Stomatol. 2002;3:127–30.
14. Ferretti JL, Capozza RF, Mondelo N, Zanchetta JR. Interrelationships between densitometric, geometric and mechanical properties of rat femora: inferences concerning mechanical regulation of bone modelling. J Bone Miner Res. 1993;8:1389–96.
15. Brodzki A, Silmanowicz P, Tatara MR, Brodzki P, Orzelski M. Cortical index (CI) of dogs' femur assessment in determining mechanical and geometrical properties of the skeletal system. Med Weter. 2004;60:1056–60.
16. Tatara MR, Sierant-Rożmiej N, Krupski W, Majcher P, Śliwa E, Kowalik S, Studziński T. Quantitative computed tomography for the assessment of mineralization of the femur and tibia in turkeys. Med Weter. 2005;61:225–8.
17. Krupski W, Tatara MR, Szabelska A, Łuszczewska-Sierakowska I, Tymczyna B. Interrelationships between morphometric, densitometric and mechanical properties of mandible in 5-month old Polish Merino sheep. Bone Abstracts. 2013;1:PP79.
18. Tymczyna B, Tatara MR, Krupski W, Tymczyna-Sobotka M, Łuszczewska-Sierakowska I, Bachanek T. Relationships between biochemical bone metabolism indices and morphometric, densitometric and mechanical properties of mandible in 6-month-old pigs. Ann Agric Environ Med. 2012;19:535–9.
19. Tatara MR, Krupski W, Majcher P, Studziński T. Long-term denervation of the humerus in turkeys as an experimental model for osteopenia. Poult Sci. 2005;84:718–22.
20. Krupski W, Tatara MR. Interrelationships between densitometric, morphometric, and mechanical properties of the tibia in turkeys. Bull Vet Inst Pulawy. 2007;51:621–6.
21. Tatara MR, Krupski W, Śliwa E, Maciejewski R, Dąbrowski A. Fundectomy-evoked osteopenia in pigs is mediated by the gastric-hypothalamic-pituitary axis. Exp Biol Med. 2007;232:1449–57.
22. Tatara MR, Tygesen MP, Sawa-Wojtanowicz B, Krupski W, Majcher P, Harrison AP. Bone development: the effect of short term alpha-ketoglutarate administration on long term mechanical properties of ribs in ram lambs. Small Rumin Res. 2007;67:179–83.
23. Tatara MR, Krupski W, Tymczyna B, Majcher P, Rosenbeiger P, Niedziela D. Interrelationships between densitometric, morphometric, and mechanical properties of the femur in male Polish Merino sheep. Bull Vet Inst Pulawy. 2011;55:795–9.
24. Abu-Serriah M, Kontaxis A, Ayoub A, Harrison J, Odell E, Barbenel J. Mechanical evaluation of mandibular defects reconstructed using osteogenic protein-1 (rhOP-1) in a sheep model: a critical analysis. Int J Oral Maxillofac Surg. 2005;34:287–93.
25. Tatara MR, Krupski W, Majer-Dziedzic B, Szabelska A. Novel and current approaches to dietary and non-dietary bone metabolism regulation. In: Watson RR, Mahadevan D, editors. Handbook of nutrition and diet in therapy of bone diseases. Wageningen: Wageningen Academic Publishers; 2016. p. 129–90.
26. Long J, Tang W, Fan YB, Tian WD, Feng F, Liu L, Zheng XH, Jing W, Wu L. Effects of rapid distraction rate on new bone formation during mandibular distraction osteogenesis in goats. Injury. 2009;40:831–4.
27. Jing XL, Farberg AS, Monson LA, Donneys A, Tchanque-Fossuo CN, Buchman SR. Radiomorphometric quantitative analysis of vasculature utilizing micro-computed tomography and vessel perfusion in the murine mandible. Craniomaxillofac Trauma Reconstr. 2012;5:223–30.
28. Bozzini CE, Champin GM, Alippi RM, Bozzini C. Biomechanical properties of the mandible, as assessed by bending test, in rats fed a low-quality protein. Arch Oral Biol. 2013;58:427–34.
29. Shimizu Y, Ishida T, Hosomichi J, Kaneko S, Hatano K, Ono T. Soft diet causes greater alveolar osteopenia in the mandible than in the maxilla. Arch Oral Biol. 2013;58:907–11.
30. Fortune CL, Farrugia W, Tresham J, Scoggins BA, Wark JD. Hormonal regulation of osteocalcin plasma production and clearance in sheep. Endocrinology. 1989;124:2785–90.
31. Pastoureau P, Arlot ME, Caulin F, Barier JP, Meunier PJ, Delmas PD. Effects of oophorectomy on biochemical and histological indices of bone turnover in ewes. J Bone Miner Res. 1989;4 Suppl 1:477.
32. Lill CA, Fluegel AK, Schneider E. Effect of ovariectomy, malnutrition and glucocorticoid application on bone properties in sheep: a pilot study. Osteoporos Int. 2002;13:480–6.
33. Turner AS. The sheep as a model for osteoporosis in humans. Vet J. 2002;163:232–9.
34. Turner AS. Animal models of osteoporosis - necessity and limitations. eCM. 2001;1:66–81.

5

A prospective follow up of age related changes in the subchondral bone density of the talus of healthy Labrador Retrievers

W. Dingemanse[1*], M. Müller-Gerbl[2], I. Jonkers[3], J. Vander Sloten[4], H. van Bree[1] and I. Gielen[1]

Abstract

Background: During growth, the skeletal structures adapt to the increased loading conditions and mature to a fully-grown skeleton. Subchondral bone density reflects the effect of long-term joint loading and it is expected to change over time. The aim of this study was to describe the long-term changes in the density distribution of the subchondral bone of the talus of healthy Labrador Retrievers in a prospective study.

Results: The subchondral bone density distribution was evaluated using computed tomographic osteoabsorptiometry (CTOAM). Visually, all joints showed very similar density distribution patterns. No significant differences in the topography of the density maxima were found between t_1 and t_2. The mean density, maximum density, and maximum area ratio (MAR) were significantly increased with increasing age.

Conclusions: The subchondral bone density of the talus of healthy Labrador Retrievers increases with increasing age. It is likely an adaptive response of the subchondral bone due to increased joint loading during growth.

Keywords: CTOAM, Dog, Growth, Subchondral bone, Talus

Background

Skeletal structures play an important role in vertebrate limb mechanics: apart from allowing locomotion, they have an import role in weight bearing and the associated transfer of forces through joints. In general, bones continually adapt in response to loads and these adaptive modeling and remodelling responses are guided by specific strain-related objectives [1–3]. The bone strains, induced by loads acting on the bones as a result of weight bearing and muscle action [1, 4] are dedicated mechanical stimuli for bone adaptations. This adaptive process is referred to as mechano-transduction and induces geometrical adaptation of the bone as well as tissue-level adaptations [5–7].

The same principles apply to the subchondral bone, which supports the overlying joint cartilage, and transmits forces from the joint surface to the trabecular structures [8]. Although the initial skeletal anatomy is formed in utero, almost all mechanical adaptations take place after birth [4]. These adaptations are necessary for the bones to fulfil their load bearing function and to withstand the mechanical stress during locomotion [4].

At the level of the joints, it is the subchondral bone plate (SBP) that continually adapts to loading magnitude, direction and penetration depth. Indeed, the subchondral bone density in joints is highly correlated with joint loading and reflects the loading history of the joint [9–12]. Bone density can be evaluated using dual-energy x-ray absorptiometry (DEXA) or peripheral quantitative computed tomography (pQCT) [13], but they lack the regional detail required to evaluate subchondral bone density at the joint surface. Using computer tomographic osteoabsorptiometry (CTOAM), the density distribution of the subchondral bone can be visualised and evaluated in detail [9–12].

The goal of this study was to evaluate subchondral bone density, using CTOAM, in the talus of healthy Labrador Retrievers at different ages, using a longitudinal study design, in order to document the adaptation of the subchondral bone plate with increasing age. An

* Correspondence: walter.dingemanse@ugent.be
[1]Department of Medical Imaging of Domestic Animals and Orthopaedics of Small Animals Faculty of Veterinary Medicine, Ghent University, Merelbeke, Belgium
Full list of author information is available at the end of the article

increase in subchondral bone density with increasing age is hypothesised.

Methods

Study population

In this study 10 healthy Labrador Retrievers were used that were included in a study on hip dysplasia and elbow dysplasia at the Faculty of Veterinary Medicine, Ghent University. The study was approved by the ethical committee of the Faculty of Veterinary Medicine, Ghent University (approval nr. EC2011/193) and verbal owner consent was obtained in each case. Inclusion criteria for this study were no abnormalities on orthopaedic examination and lameness evaluation and no abnormalities on radiographs of hips, elbows and tarsal joints. For screening of elbow dysplasia a group of Labrador Retrievers had a CT examination between 8 and 10 months of age (t_1), and between 20 and 22 months of age (t_2). After the CT examination of the elbow joint, the tarsal joints were scanned as well.

Image acquisition

Under general anaesthesia, computer tomographic (CT) images were acquired from the tarsal joints using a 4 slice helical CT scanner (Lightspeed Qx/i, General Electric Medical Systems, Milwaukee, WI). The CT parameters were 120 kVp and 300 mAs. Contiguous, 1,25 mm collimated, transverse images were obtained in a soft tissue reconstruction algorithm. Dogs were positioned in ventral recumbency and left and right tarsal joints were scanned simultaneously, with the tarsal joints in extension, according to patient protocol [14]. A calibration phantom (Bone Density Calibration Phantom, QRM GmbH, Germany) was placed between the scanning table and the tarsal joints as a density reference standard. Based on the calibration phantom, the Hounsfield Units (HU) in the final measurements were converted to mg hydroxyapatite (HA)/cm^3. The use of a calibration phantom reduces the inter-scan variability [15] and can be used to convert the apparent density measures to absolute values.

Correct positioning was confirmed on the laterolateral and dorsoplantar scout view. Acquisition time was approximately five minutes, including repositioning after CT examination of the elbow joints.

Image analysis

The CT images were exported in DICOM format to commercially available software (Analyze 11.0, Biomedical Imaging Resource, Mayo Foundation, Rochester, MN, USA), used to complete the CTOAM workflow (Fig. 1). The workflow results in an articular surface representation of the underlying subchondral bone density.

In the first step, the talus was segmented using the segmentation algorithm in Analyze. On the transverse images, the bone structure of the talus is manually outlined, to select only the talus. Based on the segmented transverse images, two different three-dimensional (3D) views of the joint surface of the talus were reconstructed, more specific a proximal and a dorsal view of the joint surface of the talus (Fig. 2). A proximal view was reconstructed first, and the dorsal view was obtained by tilting the proximal view backwards approximately 90°. This allowed the evaluation of the entire joint contact area of the lateral and medial trochlear ridge. These two images were created for each individual joint, and were used in further analysis. Subsequently, the SBP of the articulating surface was isolated and reconstructed in exactly the same orientations. The maximum bone density was projected onto the articular surface using a maximum intensity projection (MIP) with a depth of 1,5 mm. With a MIP, the three-dimensional

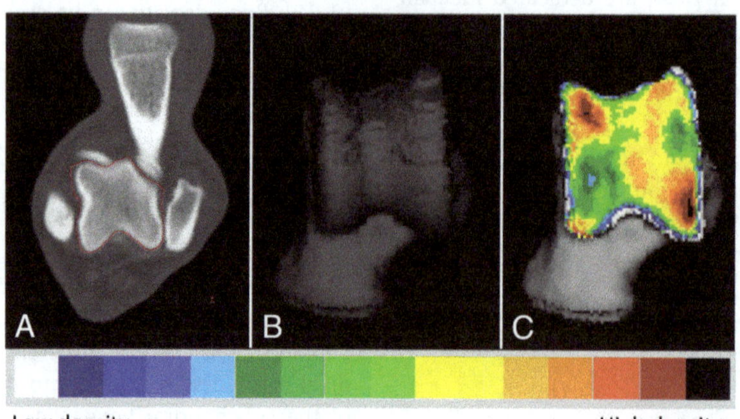

Fig. 1 The CTOAM workflow. Segmentation (isolation) of the talus bone on transverse images (**a**), 3D reconstruction of the dorsal view (**b**), and the MIP with false-colour scale visualizing the distribution of the subchondral bone density on a dorsal view of the talus (**c**)

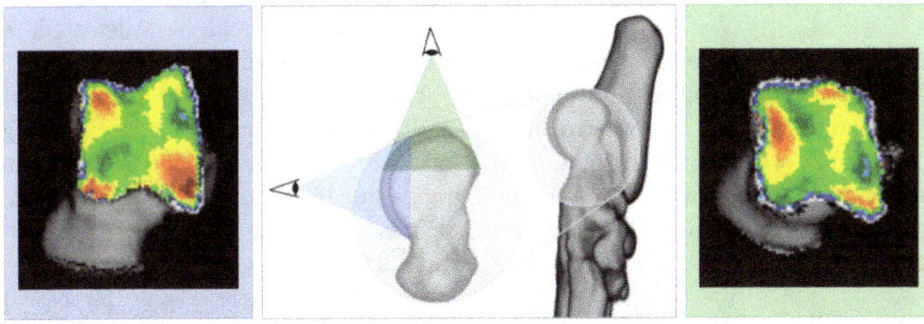

Fig. 2 Three dimensional reconstruction of the tarsal and metatarsal bones of the right foot, medial view. Line of sight for the two 3D reconstructions that are reconstructed from the segmented images, proximal view (*green*) and dorsal view (*blue*). The use of these two views provides full visualisation of the trochlear ridges with the typical distribution shown for the proximal (*right*) and dorsal (*left*) view

(3D) data volume (in voxels) is converted to a 2D image (in pixels) in which each pixel represents the maximum value (based on the HU). This maximum value is obtained from the voxels along the line perpendicular to the pixel in the 2D image plane, the length of this line is equal to the depth of the MIP. This MIP view was then converted to a false colour scale, where the range of 200 – 1200 HU was divided in value ranges of 100 HU. This resulted in a visual representation of the density distribution (densitogram), which was further evaluated. For both views, the overall mean density and the maximum density were recorded at t_1 and t_2.

For quantification purposes, the density values (in HU) were converted to 8-bit values, i.e. 256 density values, which were split equally over 8 bins, according to literature [16]. Thus, each bin contains a range of 32 density values. A density maximum was defined as an area with density values in the two highest density bins of the densitogram. To quantify the density maxima, a 30×30 unit grid was projected onto the densitogram of the proximal and dorsal view. The grid edges were positioned to ensure that the entire joint surface could fit within. The number of units in each grid was kept the same, to standardize the coordinates of the density maxima. The density maxima were characterized by their x- and y-coordinates (Fig. 3).

In addition, the maximum was described as a ratio of the area of the density maximum and the joint surface area of the proximal or dorsal view respectively, and defined as the maximum area ratio (MAR).

$$\text{MAR} = \text{number of pixels of the density maximum} \,/\, \text{number of pixels of the total joint surface}$$

The use of MAR allows a relative comparison between individuals, and accounts for size-differences.

Statistics

Using commercially available software (SPSS Statistics 22), the location of the density maxima, the mean density, the maximum density, and the MAR was compared between t_1 and t_2. In addition mean density and maximum density were compared. Data was checked for normality with Shapiro-Wilk test and was further evaluated using a paired Student's T-test. Significance was set at $P < .05$.

Results

Study population

Ten Labrador Retrievers had a CT scan at two different time points. Six were male, 4 were female, age at t_1 was 8.7 (0.8) months, age at t_2 was 20.8 months (0.75) and time between scans was 12.1 (1.0) months, mean weight increase was 21% (range 17–28%).

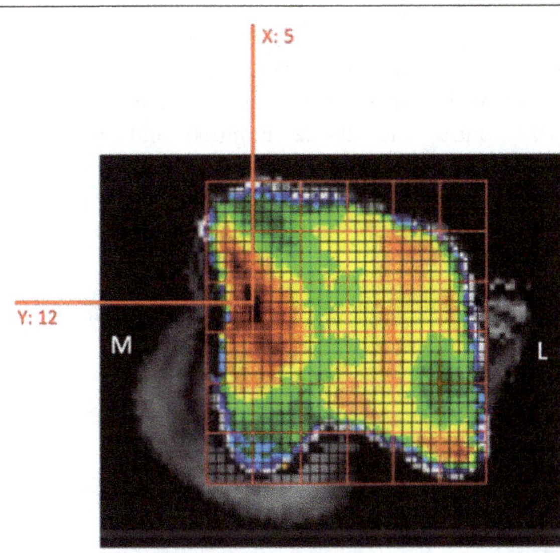

Fig. 3 Positioning of the grid and description of the subchondral bone density maximum by x- and y-coordinates

Qualitative interpretation of the subchondral bone density distribution

Based on the false colour scale, the overall density increased between t_1 and t_2 over the entire joint contact area. The density maximum on the medial trochlear ridge was located proximally, whereas the maximum on the lateral trochlear ridge was located more distally (Fig. 3). The distribution pattern remained unchanged with increasing age.

Quantitative comparison of the subchondral bone density distribution

The overall mean density was significantly higher at t_2 compared to t_1 on both the proximal and the dorsal view. The maximum density was also significantly higher at t_2 compared to t_1 on both the proximal and the dorsal view (Table 1). There was no significant difference in the location (x- and y-coordinates) between t_1 and t_2 on the proximal (*p*-value .752) and dorsal view (*p*-value .111) (Fig. 4). The MAR increased significantly with age, for both the proximal and dorsal view (Table 1).

Discussion

For the first time in bone density research in dogs, CTOAM data from a longitudinal study, using follow-up of the same individuals is presented. The authors hypothesise an increase in subchondral bone density with increasing age.

Other studies have used cross-sectional study designs with the classification of the study population into age groups [17], with a comparison between three different groups and an age range from 2 months to 17 years. Although in this study only 2 groups are compared and the age ranges from 8 to 22 months, the authors feel this data provides a valuable addition to the field of veterinary orthopaedic research, because of the longitudinal study design. In this study, 10 Labrador Retrievers had a CT scan of the tarsal joint at two different time points (8–10 months and 20–22 months) and subsequent evaluation of the subchondral bone density of the talus, using CTOAM. The use of a calibration phantom with known densities allowed a comparison of different scans with minimal inter-scan variability. In addition, absolute density values could be calculated, facilitating future comparisons in subchondral bone density research.

The subchondral bone adapts to loading conditions and undergoes important remodelling during skeletal maturation [4, 13, 18]. The age range in this study is the range in which the dogs still grow, mean weight increase in this study was 21%, and significant changes in subchondral bone density can be expected.

For all dogs, there was an increase in overall density and maximum density of the subchondral bone. An increase in loading will cause an increase in subchondral bone density, which is commonly seen during growth or increased exercise [1, 4]. The mechano-biological adaptations are a life-long process. In dogs, the bone mineral content of femurs increased, with increasing age [13]. A similar process is likely to take place in all load-bearing bones, including the subchondral bone underlying the joint surface. The increased density is most likely due to increased loading of the limbs due to an increase in body weight and an increase in physical activity. The dogs used in this study were guide dogs in training, and the level and amount of training increases towards the end of their training period.

In humans, an increased adaptive response in bones is seen in the peripubertal years and is linked to the number and functional competence of estrogen receptor α in bones [19, 20]. This age-dependent response to bone strain may also be present in dogs. In growing horses, the mineral density of the bone matrix increased with age. These changes can be purely age-related, i.e. maturation of the bone matrix, or linked to weight gain (21% in this study). It was noted that these effects could not be evaluated separately due to the non-linear character of the growth curve in a growing individual [18]. The same applies to our results and the increase in subchondral bone density is most likely due to a combined effect of increased loading and bone maturation. The pathways for adaptive response to bone strains by osteoblasts is the pathways of which have been described in detail elsewhere [21].

Interestingly, the location of the density maxima did not differ significantly between t_1 and t_2. This implies that the loading pattern, i.e. the distribution of the load over the articular surface and the cartilage-subchondral bone interface, remains similar during growth. The major adaptations in density distribution itself take place in the early post-natal months [4, 18]. So, the joint loading distribution at 8 months of age is very similar to the final joint loading distribution at 20 months.

The alterations described in this study will likely be a response to an increase in loads. This increase in load also explains the increased MAR, as the area of maximum density increases to accommodate the increasing

Table 1 Results summary

		t_1	t_2	*p*-value
Overall density (mg HA/cm^3)	Proximal view	664.5 (51.1)	736.0 (46.3)	.001
	Dorsal view	696.1 (47.3)	761.5 (36.9)	.001
Maximum density (mg HA/cm^3)	Proximal view	1049.5 (68.7)	1122.2 (77.9)	.01
	Dorsal view	1094.2 (78.0)	1186.6 (78.0)	.01
MAR	Proximal view	12.0 (5.2)	19.0 (6.6)	.002
	Dorsal view	18.9 (5.7)	26.8 (3.9)	.000

Overall density (in mg hydroxyapatite/cm^3), maximum density and maximum area ratio (MAR) for both time points (t_1 and t_2). Values displayed as mean (SD)

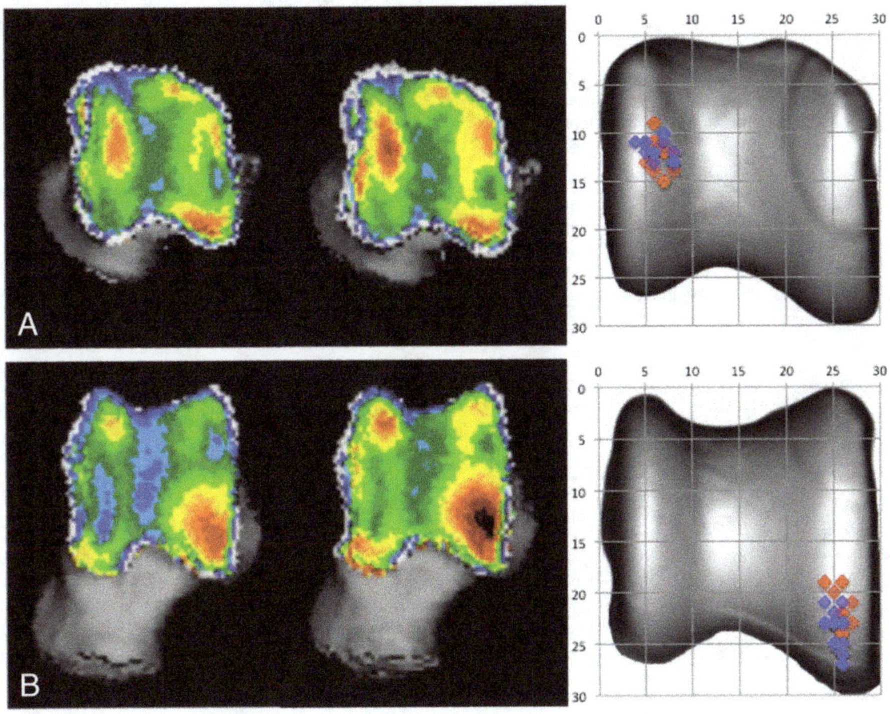

Fig. 4 Summation picture of the location of the subchondral bone density maximum on a proximal (**a**) and dorsal (**b**) view of the talus. Values at t_1 are displayed in *blue*, values at t_2 are displayed in *red*

biomechanical needs of the subchondral bone plate. The use of a ratio (MAR) allowed controlling for differences in size. These differences can be caused by absolute size differences (i.e. larger or smaller talus), although in this study this effect will be very minimal since all dogs were Labrador Retrievers of approximately the same size, weight and age. The second reason is differences the size of the field of view (FOV). The FOV was always 512x512, so pixel size depends on the size of the scanned object and FOV for the scan. Again, the effect will be minimal due to a standardised position of the joint, and minimal size differences between the dogs used in this study.

Of course, the statements above are only true in healthy individuals without orthopaedic disease, as orthopaedic pathology can alter joint loading distribution and thus alter the subchondral bone density distribution [8, 10]. Indeed, altered joint biomechanics can also lead to orthopaedic disease, e.g. the development of osteochondrosis (OC). It is important to remember that changes in loading and biomechanical properties of bones, play a key-role in the development and progression of orthopaedic disease [22].

A possible drawback of using CTOAM for the evaluation of subchondral bone density is the representation of a 3D volume (voxels of the subchondral bone plate) in a 2D densitogram. Data from dogs younger than 8 months old, might provide additional information on the development of the subchondral bone density distribution pattern. However, this was not possible in the current study.

Conclusions

This study reports on the evolution of the subchondral bone density distribution of the talus in healthy Labrador Retrievers during an important phase of skeletal maturation. Based on current findings, the physiological joint loading distribution does not change significantly during this period, but the subchondral bone density increased, at least for most part, in response to increased joint loading, consistent with increased weight. The morphological and pathological consequences of a non-physiological joint loading distribution remain subject to further research. The strength of CTOAM is that is allows the evaluation of temporal changes and the morphological consequences of (altered) joint loading and changes over time. This makes CTOAM a valuable addition to veterinary orthopaedic research.

Abbreviations

3D: Three-dimensional; CT: Computed tomographic; CTOAM: Computed tomographic osteoabsorptiometry; FOV: Field of view; HU: Hounsfield units; MAR: Maximum area ratio; MIP: Maximum intensity projection; OC: Osteochondrosis; SBP: Subchondral bone plate

Funding

Research funded by a Ph.D. grant of the Agency for Innovation by Science and Technology (IWT).

Authors' contributions

WD carried out the data collection and data processing and drafted the manuscript. MMG participated in the data processing and study design. HvB and IG participated in the conceiving and design of the study, the statistical analysis, as well as drafting the manuscript. IJ and JVS participated in the study design and helped to draft the manuscript. All authors read and approved the final manuscript. Preliminary results were presented in part at the EVDI congress, Utrecht, The Netherlands, August 27–30th, 2014, by WD.

Competing interests

The authors declare that they have no competing interests.

Consent for publication

Not applicable.

Author details

[1]Department of Medical Imaging of Domestic Animals and Orthopaedics of Small Animals Faculty of Veterinary Medicine, Ghent University, Merelbeke, Belgium. [2]Institute of Anatomy, Basel University, Basel, Switzerland. [3]Human Movement Biomechanics Research Group, Faculty of Kinesiology and Rehabilitation Sciences, KU Leuven, Leuven, Belgium. [4]Biomechanics Section, Faculty of Engineering Science, KU Leuven, Leuven, Belgium.

References

1. Lanyon LE. Control of bone architecture by functional load bearing. J Bone Miner Res. 1992;7:S369–75.
2. Boskey AL, Coleman R. Aging and bone. J Dent Res. 2010;89(12):1333–48. doi:10.1177/0022034510377791.
3. Lanyon LE, Goodship AE, Pye CJ, Macfie JH. Mechanically adaptive bone remodeling. J Biomech. 1982;15(3):141–54. doi:10.1016/0021-9290(82)90246-9.
4. Frost HM. A 2003 update of bone physiology and Wolff's Law for clinicians. Angle Orthod. 2004;74(1):3–15.
5. Gefen A, Seliktar R. Comparison of the trabecular architecture and the isostatic stress flow in the human calcaneus. Med Eng Phys. 2004;26(2):119–29. doi:10.1016/J.Medenghy.2003.10.003.
6. Main RP, Biewener AA. In vivo bone strain and ontogenetic growth patterns in relation to life-history strategies and performance in two vertebrate taxa: goats and emu. Physiol Biochem Zool. 2006;79(1):57–72. doi:10.1086/498184.
7. Polk JD, Blumenfeld J, Ahluwalia D. Knee posture predicted from subchondral apparent density in the distal femur: an experimental validation. Anat Rec. 2008;291(3):293–302. doi:10.1002/Ar.20653.
8. Madry H, van Dijk CN, Mueller-Gerbl M. The basic science of the subchondral bone. Knee Surg Sports Traumatol Arthrosc. 2010;18(4):419–33. doi:10.1007/S00167-010-1054-Z.
9. Frost HM. The Utah paradigm of skeletal physiology: an overview of its insights for bone, cartilage and collagenous tissue organs. J Bone Miner Metab. 2000;18(6):305–16. doi:10.1007/s007740070001.
10. Müller-Gerbl M, Putz R, Hodapp N, Schulte E, Wimmer B. Computed-tomography-osteoabsorptiometry - a method of assessing the mechanical condition of major joint in a living subject. Clin Biomech. 1990;5(4):193–8. doi:10.1016/0268-0033(90)90002-n.
11. Müller-Gerbl M, Putz R, Kenn R. Demonstation of subchondral bone density patterns by three-dimensional CT osteoabsorptiometry as a noninvasive method for in vivo assessment of individual long-term stresses in joints. J Bone Miner Res. 1992;7(S2):411–8.
12. Eckstein F, Jacobs CR, Merz BR. Mechanobiological adaptation of subchondral bone as a function of joint incongruity and loading. Med Eng Phys. 1997;19(8):720–8. doi:10.1016/s1350-4533(97)00031-3.
13. Schneider S, Breit SM, Grampp S, Kunzel WWF, Liesegang A, Mayrhofer E, et al. Comparative assessment of bone mineral measurements obtained by use of dual-energy x-ray absorptiometry, peripheral quantitative computed tomography, and chemical-physical analyses in femurs of juvenile and adult dogs. Am J Vet Res. 2004;65(7):891–900. doi:10.2460/Ajvr.2004.65.891.
14. Gielen I, van Bree H, Van Ryssen B, De Clercq T, De Rooster H. Radiographic, computed tomographic and arthroscopic findings in 23 dogs with osteochondrosis of the tarsocrural joint. Vet Rec. 2002;150(14):442–7.
15. Cann CE. Quantitative Ct for determination of bone-mineral density - a review. Radiology. 1988;166(2):509–22.
16. Patel BA, Carlson KJ. Habitual use of the primate forelimb is reflected in the material properties of subchondral bone in the distal radius. J Anat. 2006; 208:659–70.
17. Dickomeit MJ, Bottcher P, Hecht S, Liebich HG, Maierl J. Topographic and age-dependent distribution of subchondral bone density in the elbow joints of clinically normal dogs. Am J Vet Res. 2011;72(4):491–9.
18. Holopainen JT, Brama PAJ, Halmesmaki E, Harjula T, Tuukkanen J, van Weeren PR, et al. Changes in subchondral bone mineral density and collagen matrix organization in growing horses. Bone. 2008;43(6):1108–14. doi:10.1016/J.Bone.2008.07.254.
19. Bass SL, Saxon L, Daly RM, Turner CH, Robling AG, Seeman E, et al. The effect of mechanical loading on the size and shape of bone in pre-, peri-, and postpubertal girls: a study in tennis players. J Bone Miner Res. 2002; 17(12):2274–80. doi:10.1359/Jbmr.2002.17.12.2274.
20. Lee KCL, Lanyon LE. Mechanical loading influences bone mass through estrogen receptor alpha. Exerc Sport Sci Rev. 2004;32(2):64–8. doi:10.1097/00003677-200404000-00005.
21. Ehrlich PJ, Lanyon LE. Mechanical strain and bone cell function: a review. Osteoporos Int. 2002;13(9):688–700. doi:10.1007/S001980200095.
22. Colborne GR. Bringing canine biomechanics research out of the dark ages. Vet J. 2007;173(3):469–70. doi:10.1016/j.tvjl.2006.01.002.

6

Subchondral bone density distribution of the talus in clinically normal Labrador Retrievers

W. Dingemanse[1*], M. Müller-Gerbl[2], I. Jonkers[3], J. Vander Sloten[4], H. van Bree[1] and I. Gielen[1]

Abstract

Background: Bones continually adapt their morphology to their load bearing function. At the level of the subchondral bone, the density distribution is highly correlated with the loading distribution of the joint. Therefore, subchondral bone density distribution can be used to study joint biomechanics non-invasively. In addition physiological and pathological joint loading is an important aspect of orthopaedic disease, and research focusing on joint biomechanics will benefit veterinary orthopaedics. This study was conducted to evaluate density distribution in the subchondral bone of the canine talus, as a parameter reflecting the long-term joint loading in the tarsocrural joint.

Results: Two main density maxima were found, one proximally on the medial trochlear ridge and one distally on the lateral trochlear ridge. All joints showed very similar density distribution patterns and no significant differences were found in the localisation of the density maxima between left and right limbs and between dogs.

Conclusions: Based on the density distribution the lateral trochlear ridge is most likely subjected to highest loads within the tarsocrural joint. The joint loading distribution is very similar between dogs of the same breed. In addition, the joint loading distribution supports previous suggestions of the important role of biomechanics in the development of OC lesions in the tarsus. Important benefits of computed tomographic osteoabsorptiometry (CTOAM), i.e. the possibility of in vivo imaging and temporal evaluation, make this technique a valuable addition to the field of veterinary orthopaedic research.

Keywords: CTOAM, Dog, Joint loading, Osteochondrosis, Subchondral bone, Talus

Background

Joint loading, including tensile and compressive stresses, is an important factor in cartilage and subchondral bone physiology and pathology [1–3]. Changes in loading and biomechanical properties of these important load-bearing structures, play a key-role in the development and progression of orthopaedic disease [4].

In recent years, different methods have been applied to study joint biomechanics both in vitro and in vivo. The initial studies presented detailed anatomical descriptions of joint structures [5, 6], followed by studies describing pressure distributions and contact areas [7, 8]. These studies were often done on cadaveric specimens and required a certain degree of dissection, thus altering joint kinematics. In vivo biomechanics are often limited to kinetic and kinematic research using marker data and pressure plates [4]. Actual joint loading cannot easily be assessed non-invasively in vivo, since it requires intra-articular insertion of pressure films [9] making it difficult to apply in studies using larger populations and patient populations. Subchondral bone density is directly influenced by joint biomechanics and limb function and can be used to evaluate joint biomechanics.

The stresses acting on the joint surface induce modelling and remodelling of the bony tissue, depending on whether the local strains either exceed the modelling threshold or stay below the remodelling threshold. Because of that, increased joint loading leads to increased local strains and bone modelling ensures an increase in subchondral bone density to withstand the increased loading [1, 3]. In addition, altered joint biomechanics

* Correspondence: walter.dingemanse@ugent.be
[1]Department of Medical Imaging of Domestic Animals and Orthopaedics of Small Animals Faculty of Veterinary Medicine, Ghent University, Merelbeke, Belgium
Full list of author information is available at the end of the article

lead to altered joint loading distribution, leading in turn to alterations in the subchondral bone density distribution [10, 11].

The subchondral bone density in joints is highly correlated with joint loading and reflects the loading history of the joint [3, 11–13]. Using computer tomographic osteoabsorptiometry (CTOAM), the density distribution of the subchondral bone can be visualised and evaluated [3, 11–13]. In order to evaluate subchondral bone density and changes associated with orthopaedic conditions, the normal, physiological subchondral bone density distribution has to be described first.

In addition, this type of biomechanical research can help to elucidate the role of joint biomechanics in the development of osteochondrosis (OC) [14]. Osteochondrosis is an orthopaedic condition in dogs that is considered to be multifactorial, with hereditary, dietary and environmental factors playing a role [15]. An environmental factor likely to influence the occurrence of OC is joint biomechanics, since OC lesions are often found in specific locations within the joint [16–19]. In the tarsocrural joint, lesions can be found medially (medial trochlear ridge tarsocrural osteochondrosis (MTRT-OC)) and laterally (lateral trochlear ridge tarsocrural osteochondrosis (LTRT-OC)) [14, 20, 21]. The specific joint anatomy likely affects the location of the OC lesions, and this study can aid in the understanding of the pathophysiology of this condition.

This study was conducted to describe the subchondral bone density distribution of the talus of healthy Labrador Retrievers non-invasively, as a parameter reflecting long-term joint loading in the tarsocrural joint, using CTOAM. The authors hypothesise an inhomogeneous distribution of the density of the subchondral bone.

Methods

Study population

A total of 20 tarsal joints (ten left and ten right) from ten adult (age 24–28 months) Labrador Retrievers, submitted for computer tomographic (CT) examination of the elbow joint for the screening of elbow dysplasia, were included in this study. The study was approved by the ethical committee of the Faculty of Veterinary Medicine, Ghent University (approval nr. EC2011/193) and informed, written owner consent was obtained in each case. Inclusion criteria for this study were no abnormalities on orthopaedic examination and lameness evaluation and no abnormalities on radiographs of hips, elbows and tarsal joints. After CT examination of the elbow joint, the tarsal joints were scanned as well.

Image acquisition

Under general anaesthesia and the dog positioned in ventral recumbency, CT images were acquired from the tarsal joints using a four slice helical CT scanner (Lightspeed Qx/i, General Electric Medical Systems, Milwaukee, WI, USA). The CT parameters were 120 kVp and 300 mAs. Contiguous, 1,25 mm collimated, transverse images were obtained in a soft tissue reconstruction algorithm. Left and right tarsal joints were scanned simultaneously, with the tarsal joints in extension, according to patient protocol [21]. Acquisition time was approximately five minutes, including repositioning after CT examination of the elbow joints.

Image analysis

The CT images were exported in DICOM format to commercially available software (Analyze 11.0, Biomedical Imaging Resource, Mayo Foundation, Rochester, MN, USA), used to complete the CTOAM workflow (Fig. 1). In the first step, the talus was segmented using the segmentation algorithm in 'Analyze'. Based on the segmented images, two different three-dimensional (3D) views of the trochlear ridges were reconstructed (Fig. 2). A proximal view was reconstructed first, and the distal view was obtained by tilting the proximal view backwards approximately 90 degrees. This allowed the evaluation of the entire proximal talar joint surface of the lateral and medial trochlear ridge (Fig. 3). Subsequently, the subchondral bone plate of the articulating surface was isolated and reconstructed in exactly the same orientations. The maximum bone density was projected onto the articular surface using a maximum intensity projection (MIP). With a MIP, the three dimensional (3D) data volume (in voxels) of the subchondral bone plate is converted to a 2D image (in pixels) in which each pixel represents the maximum value (based on the HU). This maximum value is obtained from the voxels along the line perpendicular to the pixel in the 2D image. The length of this line, i.e. the depth of the MIP, is based on the thickness of the subchondral bone plate and was set at 1.5 mm. This MIP view was then converted to a false colour scale, where the range of 200 – 1200 Hounsfield Units (HU) was divided in value ranges of 100 HU each representing a colour. In descending order these colours were black, dark red, light red, orange, yellow, dark green, light green, dark blue, light blue, and white. This resulted in a densitogram (Figs. 1 and 3), which displays lines of isodensities, i.e. lines connecting regions of equal density. This densitogram is a visual representation of the apparent density distribution and was further evaluated.

For quantification purposes, the density values (in HU) were converted to 8-bit values, i.e. 256 density values, which were split equally over eight bins, according to literature [22]. Thus, each bin contains a range of 32 density values. A density maximum was defined as an area with density values in the two highest density bins of the densitogram. To allow the comparison of the

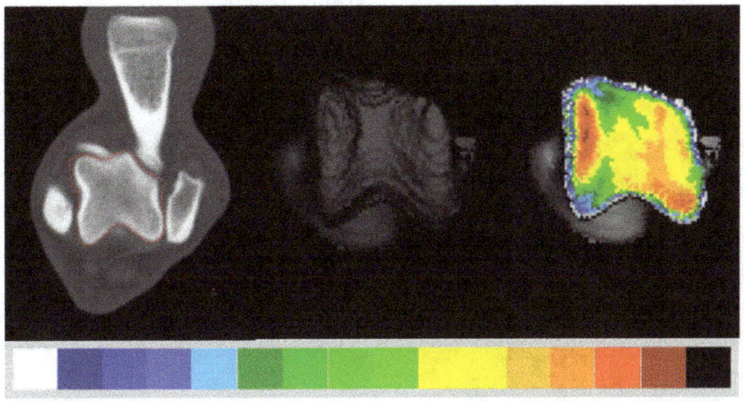

Fig. 1 CTOAM workflow in Analyze. From left to right: segmentation of the talus; 3D rendering of the proximal view; overlay of the false-colour map of the subchondral bone density distribution

individual subchondral bone density distributions, a 30 × 30 unit grid was projected over the densitogram of the proximal and dorsal view of the trochlear ridges. The grid edges were positioned thus the entire joint surface could fit within. The number of units in each grid was kept the same, to standardize the coordinates of the density maxima. The x- and y-coordinates (Fig. 4) were used to describe the location of the density maxima on the joint surface.

In addition, the size of the maximum was described as a ratio of the area of the density maximum and the joint surface area of the proximal and distal view respectively, and defined as the maximum area ratio (MAR).

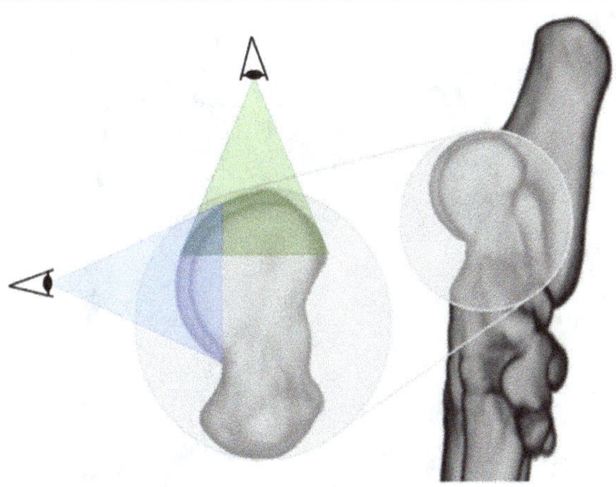

Fig. 2 Three dimensional reconstruction of the tarsal and metatarsal bones of the right foot, medial view. Line of sight for the two 3D reconstructions, proximal view (green) and distal view (blue). The use of these two views provides full visualisation of the trochlear ridges

$$\text{MAR} = \text{number of pixels of the density maximum} \div \text{number of pixels of the total joint surface}$$

The use of MAR allows a relative comparison between individuals, and accounts for size-differences.

Statistics

Using commercially available software (SPSS Statistics 22), the location of the density maxima and the MAR were compared between left and right and between dogs. Data was evaluated using a Student's *T*-test and ANOVA (with Bonferroni post-hoc) and significance was set at $P < .05$.

Results

Regional variation of subchondral bone density

The proximal and distal reconstructions provided full visualization of the subchondral bone, with a small visual overlap in the transitional area (proximodorsal area) (Fig. 2). The subchondral bone density distribution showed considerable regional differences in both the

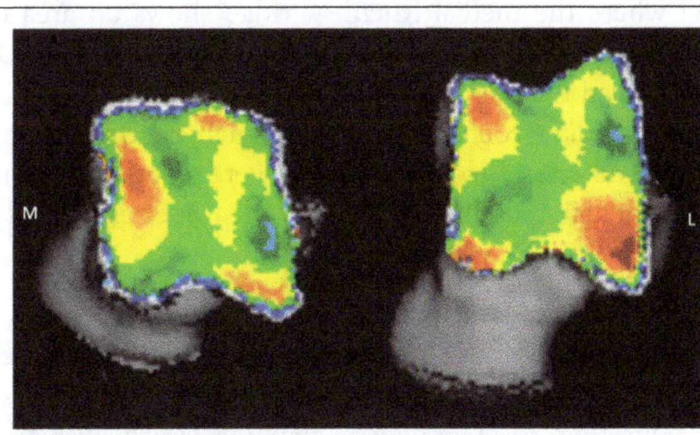

Fig. 3 Typical subchondral bone density distribution of the talus. Left talus in a proximal (left) and distal (right) view

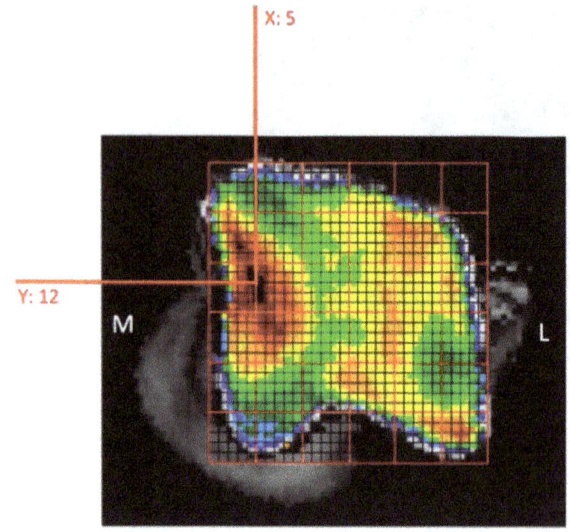

Fig. 4 Positioning of the grid on a proximal view of the talus and description of the subchondral bone density maximum by x- and y-coordinates

medial and the lateral trochlear ridge. Hounsfield Units generally ranged from 200–1200, although in some dogs ($n = 2$) the upper range was limited to around 1000 HU.

Differences in subchondral bone density distribution between medial and lateral trochlear ridge

In general, the lateral trochlear ridge had a higher apparent density in comparison to the medial trochlear ridge, as illustrated by the colour map (Fig. 3). The medial and lateral trochlear ridges showed a distinctly different density pattern.

The medial trochlear ridge had a density maximum in its proximal part. More distally, density values were lower. In 80 % of the joints ($n = 16$), a focal additional density maximum was present at the most distal part of the trochlear ridge.

On the lateral trochlear ridge, the density maximum was found at the distal part of the trochlear ridge at the level where the medial trochlear ridge shows an area of low density. This density maximum was larger (Table 1) and showed a larger variety in shape than the maximum on the medial trochlear ridge. The density maxima on medial and lateral trochlear ridges were located adjacent to the medial and lateral border of the ridge respectively.

Quantification of density maxima

The location of the density maxima on the standardized grid is displayed in a summary view for both views of the talus (Fig. 5). The density maxima clearly display a very similar distribution in all dogs. No significant differences in the coordinates were found between left and

Table 1 Results summary

		Left	Right	*P*-value
Proximal view	Total # pixels	2254.8 (482.1)	2226.4 (494.9)	.909
	Area max # pixels	737.9 (212.4)	716.5 (218.0)	.845
	MAR	32.4 (4.3)	31.6 (3.9)	.720
Distal view	Total # pixels	2348.1 (404.2)	2288.8 (366.4)	.763
	Area max # pixels	919.9 (184.4)	944.4 (208.5)	.807
	MAR	39.5 (5.0)	41.5 (6.6)	.495

Total number of pixels, number of pixels of the density maximum and MAR. Values displayed as mean (SD)

right joints (p-values .607 and .540) and between different dogs (p values .755 and .367).

Comparison of MAR

There was no significant difference in the MAR between left and right (Table 1). Between dogs, there was no significant difference for the MAR in the proximal view

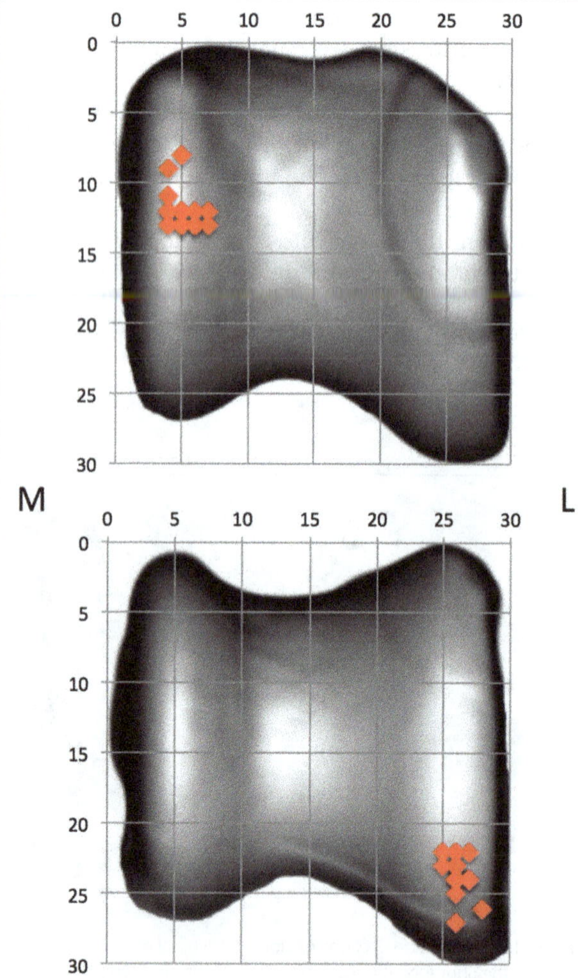

Fig. 5 Summation view of the density maxima coordinates. Proximal (top) and distal (bottom) view, right coordinates were mirrored to left

(p-value .505), but a significant difference was found in the distal view (p-value .003).

Discussion

This study describes the subchondral bone density distribution of the talus in a group of healthy Labrador Retrievers, using conventional CT data and CTOAM. In addition to a description and visual representation of the subchondral bone density distribution. Density maxima were described using a standardised grid overlay and the maximum area ratio (MAR) was calculated.

Previous studies in humans have shown regional subchondral bone density variations in many different joints [11, 12, 23], but studies in dogs have been limited to the elbow and stifle joint [24–26]. In this study, considerable regional differences of subchondral bone density were found in the convex surface of the talus, articulating with the distal tibia.

The density distribution of the trochlear ridges of the proximal talus is characterized by two density maxima. One is located at the proximal part of the medial trochlear ridge and the other one is located more distally on the lateral trochlear ridge. In addition, the apparent density of the lateral trochlear ridge is higher than the apparent density of the medial trochlear ridge. A possible explanation for this is the fact that the lateral trochlear ridge in the dog is more pronounced and is more likely to endure increased loads during gait. Geometry plays a major role in the development of subchondral bone density patterns, as it determines the magnitude and direction of the dynamic loads, which in turn will guide the modelling process, leading to morphological adaptations [3, 27], which is in this case an increase in apparent density.

Both the location of the density maxima and the MAR showed no significant differences between left and right limbs. A recent study described asymmetry in limb and joint mechanics in orthopedically sound Labrador Retrievers [28]. Mechanical dominance has been described in various species, and in dogs right hind limb dominance appears to be most common [29]. These conclusions are based on the calculation of the total support moment of the limbs, and showed that the tarsal joint moment was significantly larger on the dominant side. Mechanical dominance was not evaluated using gait analysis in the dogs used in this study. Based on our findings, we assume that the dogs used in this study have symmetrical gait, or that the differences in case of asymmetry due to hind limb dominance, did not significantly effect subchondral bone density distribution. Whether or not hind limb dominance in dogs has an influence on subchondral bone density is a very interesting topic, and is subject of further research.

On the proximal view there was no significant difference found for the MAR between dogs, whereas on the distal view there was a significant difference for the MAR. As mentioned above, the maximum on the lateral trochlear ridge was located distally, so it was visualised best on the distal view, and showed more variety in shape compared to the maximum on the medial trochlear ridge. This explains the difference in MAR between dogs in the distal view. A possible explanation is that the proximal part of the medial trochlear ridge is subjected to more homogeneous loading. Another possibility, that is likely to play a simultaneous role, is that the force-transmitting area of the medial trochlear ridge is much more constant between dogs, whereas for the lateral trochlear ridge this can vary more between dogs.

Possible drawback of CTOAM for the evaluation of subchondral bone density is that the density distribution of a 3D volume (the voxels) is displayed in 2D (pixels). Because the density is evaluated over the thickness of the subchondral bone plate, perpendicular to the line of sight on the joint surface, this will cause no problems on flat articular surfaces. On more curved articular surfaces, the use of multiple views is necessary to evaluate the subchondral bone density distribution.

Differences in the size of the area of maximum density can be caused by absolute size differences (i.e. larger or smaller talus) but in this study this effect will be very minimal since all dogs were Labrador Retrievers of approximately the same size, weight, and age. Another reason is differences in scanning parameters, specifically the size of the field of view (FOV). Pixel size depends on the size of the scanned object and FOV used for the scan. Since we used consistently a FOV of 512×512, this effect will be minimal due to a standardised position of the joint, and minimal size differences between the dogs used in this study. The use of the MAR, allows a relative comparison of the area of maximum density, accounting for the above confounders when using absolute size values.

When considering joint loading and joint congruency, another important factor is the joint cartilage. Joint cartilage has the important biomechanical role to provide an even distribution of the joint loading on the articular surface [30]. Thicker cartilage is found in places with higher biomechanical loads. A study by Brunnberg et al. supports our conclusion that the lateral trochlear ridge is most likely subjected to higher loads. The cartilage of the lateral trochlear ridge is significantly thicker than the cartilage at the medial trochlear ridge [31].

The location of the density maximum on the medial trochlear ridge is the same location where the majority of MTRT-OC lesions are found [14]. Repetitive loading above the bone modelling threshold, can cause accumulation of microdamage to the bone [32]. Areas with increased subchondral bone density, and thus increased loading conditions, are more likely to be subjected to loading causing microdamage as well. On the talus, these areas subjected to high loading coincide with the location of MTRT-OC lesions. Thus, this study supports previous suggestions that repetitive microdamage [33] is an important factor in the development of OC, although more research is necessary to elucidate the exact pathophysiology.

Lesions on the lateral trochlear ridge (LTRT-OC lesions), are larger than MTRT-OC lesions and have a larger variation in size [14]. Interestingly, the subchondral bone density maximum on the lateral trochlear ridge is larger and shows more variation compared to the medial trochlear ridge, and similar distribution as the OC lesions.

However, changes in subchondral bone density can be cause or effect of OC lesions. A local increase in subchondral bone density, as is the case at the level of a subchondral bone density maximum, may increase the discrepancy between the biomechanical properties of two articulating surfaces. In humans, this mismatch has been suggested to contribute to the development of OC lesions [33, 34].

Conclusion

This study shows a distinct pattern of subchondral bone density in the talus of healthy, adult Labrador Retrievers. This pattern, or density distribution, provides more information on the biomechanical aspects of the tarsocrural joint and the morphological adaptations under normal joint loading conditions. The influence of altered joint kinematics, bone geometry and leg conformation on the subchondral bone density distribution remains subject of further research.

Although the evaluation of the subchondral bone density distribution pattern supports previous suggestions on the role of joint biomechanics in the development of tarsocrural OC, more research is needed to determine cause and effect. Therefore, research should focus on early stages of OC lesions and systematically review all factors contributing to the biomechanical joint loading.

In the field of veterinary biomechanics, CTOAM could provide new insights in physiological joint loading distribution, and alterations in pathological conditions. The technique can be used in vivo, in patient populations, and to evaluate temporal changes, for instance following orthopaedic surgery. This implies significant advantages compared to more traditional and invasive techniques used to evaluate joint loading.

Abbreviations

3D: three-dimensional; CT: computed tomographic; CTOAM: computed tomographic osteoabsorptiometry; HU: hounsfield units; LTRT-OC: lateral trochlear ridge tarsocrural osteochondrosis; MAR: maximum area ratio; MIP: maximum intensity projection; MTRT-OC: medial trochlear ridge tarsocrural osteochondrosis; OC: osteochondrosis.

Competing interests

The authors declare they have no financial or personal relationships with other people or organisations that could inappropriately influence their work.

Authors' contributions

WD carried out the data collection and data processing and drafted the manuscript. MMG participated in the data processing and study design. IJ and JVS participated in the study design and helped to draft the manuscript. HvB and IG participated in the conceiving and design of the study, the statistical analysis, as well as drafting the manuscript. All authors read and approved the final manuscript.

Acknowledgements

Research funded by a Ph.D. grant of the Agency for Innovation by Science and Technology (IWT).

Author details

[1]Department of Medical Imaging of Domestic Animals and Orthopaedics of Small Animals Faculty of Veterinary Medicine, Ghent University, Merelbeke, Belgium. [2]Institute of Anatomy, Basel University, Basel, Switzerland. [3]Human Movement Biomechanics Research Group, Kinesiology Department, KU Leuven, Leuven, Belgium. [4]Biomechanics Section, Faculty of Engineering Science, KU Leuven, Leuven, Belgium.

References

1. Burton NJ, Ellis JR, Burton KJ, Wallace AR, Colborne GR. An ex vivo investigation of the effect of the TATE canine elbow arthroplasty system on kinematics of the elbow. J Small Anim Pract. 2013;54(5):240–7. doi:10.1111/Jsap.12060.
2. Turner CH. Three rules for bone adaptation to mechanical stimuli. Bone. 1998;23(5):399–407. doi:10.1016/s8756-3282(98)00118-5.
3. Frost HM. The Utah paradigm of skeletal physiology: an overview of its insights for bone, cartilage and collagenous tissue organs. J Bone Miner Metab. 2000;18(6):305–16. doi:10.1007/s007740070001.
4. Colborne GR. Bringing canine biomechanics research out of the dark ages. Vet J. 2007;173(3):469–70. doi:10.1016/j.tvjl.2006.01.002.
5. Barone R. Anatomie Comparèe des mammifères domestiques. Tome 2: Arthrologie et myologie. Paris: Vigot; 2000.
6. Aron DN, Purinton PT. Collateral ligaments of the tarsocrural joint - an anatomic and functional study. Vet Surg. 1985;14(3):173–7. doi:10.1111/j.1532-950X.1985.tb00857.x.
7. Mason DR, Schulz KS, Fujita Y, Kass PH, Stover SM. Measurement of humeroradial and humeroulnar transarticular joint forces in the canine elbow joint after humeral wedge and humeral slide osteotomies. Vet Surg. 2008;37(1):63–70. doi:10.1111/j.1532-950X.2007.00349.x.
8. Preston CA, Schulz KS, Kass PH. In vitro determination of contact areas in the normal elbow joint of dogs. Am J Vet Res. 2000;61(10):1315–21. doi:10.2460/ajvr.2000.61.1315.
9. Coughlin KM, Peura GD, Fleming BC, Hallock S, Beynnon BD. In vivo loads in the medial compartment of the rabbit knee. Clin Biomech. 2005;20(9):1007–9. doi:10.1016/j.clinbiomech.2005.06.015.
10. Giunta RE, Krimmer H, Krapohl B, Treutlein G, Lanz U, Müller-Gerbl M. Patterns of subchondral bone mineralization in the wrist after midcarpal fusion. J Hand Surg-Am Vol. 1999;24A:138–47.
11. Müller-Gerbl M, Putz R, Hodapp N, Schulte E, Wimmer B. Computed-tomography-osteoabsorptiometry - A method of assessing the mechanical condition of major joint in a living subject. Clin Biomech. 1990;5(4):193–8. doi:10.1016/0268-0033(90)90002-n.
12. Müller-Gerbl M, Putz R, Kenn R. Demonstation of subchondral bone density patterns by three-dimensional CT osteoabsorptiometry as a noninvasive method for in vivo assessment of individual long-term stresses in joints. J Bone Miner Res. 1992;7(S2):411–8.
13. Eckstein F, Jacobs CR, Merz BR. Mechanobiological adaptation of subchondral bone as a function of joint incongruity and loading. Med Eng Phys. 1997;19(8):720–8. doi:10.1016/s1350-4533(97)00031-3.
14. Dingemanse W, Gielen I, Duchateau L, van Bree H. Comparison of morphological and clinical features between medial and lateral trochlear ridge talar osteochondrosis dissecans in dogs. Vet Surg. 2013;42:340–5.
15. Ytrehus B, Carlson CS, Ekman S. Etiology and pathogenesis of osteochondrosis. Vet Pathol. 2007;44(4):429–48. doi:10.1354/vp.44-4-429.
16. Dammrich K. Relationship between nutrition and bone-growth in large and giant dogs. J Nutr. 1991;121(11):S114–21.

17. van Ee RT, Gibson K, Roberts ED. Osteochondritis dissecans of the lateral ridge of the talus in a dog. J Am Vet Med Assoc. 1988;193(10):1284–6.
18. Dingemanse W, Gielen I, van Bree H. Diagnosis and treatment of tarsocrural osteochondrosis in the dog. Vlaams Diergenskund Tijds. 2011;80(3):223–32.
19. Kuroki K, Cook JL, Stoker AM, Turnquist SE, Kreeger JM, Tomlinson JL. Characterizing osteochondrosis in the dog: potential roles for matrix metalloproteinases and mechanical load in pathogenesis and disease progression. Osteoarthr Cartil. 2005;13(3):225–34. doi:10.1016/j.joca.2004.11.005.
20. Montgomery RD, Hathcock JT, Milton JL, Fitch RB. Osteochondritis dissecans of the canine tarsal joint. Compend Contin Educ Pract Vet. 1994;16(7):835–45.
21. Gielen I, van Bree H, Van Ryssen B, De Clercq T, De Rooster H. Radiographic, computed tomographic and arthroscopic findings in 23 dogs with osteochondrosis of the tarsocrural joint. Vet Rec. 2002;150(14):442–7.
22. Patel BA, Carlson KJ. Habitual use of the primate forelimb is reflected in the material properties of subchondral bone in the distal radius. J Anat. 2006; 208:659–70.
23. Kraljevic M, Zumstein V, Hugli R, Müller-Gerbl M. A comparison of subchondral bone mineralization between the glenoid cavity and the humeral head on 57 cadaverous shoulder joints. Surg Radiol Anat. 2013;35: 295–300.
24. Bottcher P, Zeissler M, Grevel V, Oechtering G, Maierl J. Mapping Subchondral Bone Density of Selected Donor and Recipient Sites for Autologous Osteochondral Transplantation in the Canine Stifle Joint Using Computed Tomographic Osteoabsorptiometry. Vet Surg. 2010;39(4):496–503. doi:10.1111/j.1532-950X.2010.00674.x.
25. Samii VF, Les CM, Schulz KS, Keyak JH, Stover SM. Computed tomographic osteoabsorptiometry of the elbow joint in clinically normal dogs. Am J Vet Res. 2002;63(8):1159–66. doi:10.2460/ajvr.2002.63.1159.
26. Dickomeit MJ, Bottcher P, Hecht S, Liebich HG, Maierl J. Topographic and age-dependent distribution of subchondral bone density in the elbow joints of clinically normal dogs. Am J Vet Res. 2011;72(4):491–9.
27. Madry H, van Dijk CN, Mueller-Gerbl M. The basic science of the subchondral bone. Knee Surg Sports Traumatol Arthrosc. 2010;18(4):419–33. doi:10.1007/s00167-010-1054-z.
28. Colborne GR, Good L, Cozens LE, Kirk LS. Symmetry of hind limb mechanics in orthopedically normal trotting Labrador Retrievers. Am J Vet Res. 2011; 72(3):336–44. doi:10.2460/Ajvr.72.3.336.
29. Colborne GR. Are sound dogs mechanically symmetric at trot? No, actually. Vet Comp Orthop Traumatol. 2008;21(3):294–301.
30. Ebel CMI, Prodinger PM, Muhlhofer H, Muller-Gerbl M, Linsenmaier U, Putz R. Morphological adaptation of the tarso-metatarsal joints onto load transmission in the foot. Surg Radiol Anat. 2010;32(2):107–13. doi:10.1007/s00276-009-0554-3.
31. Brunnberg MM, Engelke E, Gielen IM, van Bree HJ, Hoffmann JE, Brunnberg L, et al. Cartilage thickness of the trochlea of the talus, with emphasis on sites predisposed to osteochondrosis dissecans, in clinically normal juvenile and adult dogs. Am J Vet Res. 2011;72(10):1318–24.
32. Frost HM. A 2003 update of bone physiology and Wolff's Law for clinicians. Angle Orthod. 2004;74(1):3–15.
33. Schenck RC, Goodnight JM. Current Concept Review - Osteochondritis Dissecans. J Bone Joint Surg. 1998;78:439–56.
34. Athanasiou KA, Niederauer GG, Schenck RC. Biomechanical Topography of Human Ankle Cartilage. Ann Biomed Eng. 1995;23(5):697–704. doi:10.1007/Bf02584467.

7

Scrotal granulomatous aspergillosis in a dromedary camel (*Camelus dromedarius*)

Frine Eleonora Scaglione[1*], Andrea Peano[1], Sara Piga[2], Stefano Meda[2], Enrico Bollo[1], Francesca Tiziana Cannizzo[1], Mario Pasquetti[1] and Henrik Elvang Jensen[3]

Abstract

Background: This report describes a case of primary subcutaneous aspergillosis in a 7-year-old neutered male dromedary camel (*Camelus dromedarius*).

Case presentation: The animal developed a large nodular lesion in the right scrotum two years after surgical intervention for neutering. The mass had a firm consistency and was painful at palpation. Histopathology revealed dermal granulomatous inflammation with a necrotic centre, surrounded by plasma cells, macrophages, neutrophils, and sparse fungal hyphae characterised by parallel cell walls, distinct septa, and dichotomous branching. Fungal culture was not performed, but a panel of mono- and polyclonal antibodies specific for different fungal genera identified the hyphae as *Aspergillus* sp.

Conclusions: The occurrence of subcutaneous lesions is a rare manifestation of aspergillosis in animals, and this appears to be the first case reported in the dromedary camel.

Keywords: Dromedary, Camelids, Immunohistochemistry, *Aspergillus*, Scrotum

Background

Aspergillus species are ubiquitous environmental fungal organisms [1]. They have been found worldwide in humans, in almost all domestic animals, birds as well as in many wildlife species, causing a wide range of diseases from localized infections to fatal disseminated forms [2]. Invasive aspergillosis in humans is typically associated with pulmonary infection in immunosuppressed patients [3]. However, a number of extrapulmonary localizations has been reported, sometimes in immunocompetent individuals [1]. Cutaneous aspergillosis occurs relatively less frequently, as either primary or secondary infection [3, 4]. Primary cutaneous aspergillosis usually involves sites of skin injury of various nature, while secondary lesions result either from contiguous extension to the skin from infected underlying structures or from widespread blood-borne infections [3].

In the same way aspergillosis in animals is mainly a disease of the respiratory tract (nasal cavities and lungs in mammals; trachea, lungs and air sacs in birds), although other localizations typical of particular hosts have been recognized (e.g. the guttural pouches and the cornea in horses; the retro-orbital space in cats; the intervertebral disk in dogs) [2]. Cases with cutaneous involvement are hardly found in the literature [2]. The present report describes a case of primary subcutaneous aspergillosis in a dromedary camel (*Camelus dromedarius*).

Case presentation

A captive 7-year-old neutered male dromedary camel, living in a zoological garden in northern Italy (Zoom Torino) and sharing the habitat with two conspecifics (a male and a female), developed a subcutaneous nodular mass in the right scrotum. The animal had been neutered two years before. A blood sample was taken from the left jugular vein and a full blood screening was performed. Differential diagnoses taken in account included an abscess and a neoplastic process. The animal was treated with antibiotics (Enrofloxacin2,5 mg/kg) given orally for 2 weeks and with anti-inflammatory drugs (Meloxicam 0,4 mg/kggiven orally for 7 days. After two months, the mass had increased (about 10 cm in diameter) (Fig. 1). At that time, it was decided to proceed with surgery. The animal was anaesthetized

* Correspondence: frineeleonora.scaglione@unito.it
[1]Dipartimento di Scienze Veterinarie, Università degli Studi di Torino, Largo Paolo Braccini 2, 10095 Grugliasco (To), Italy
Full list of author information is available at the end of the article

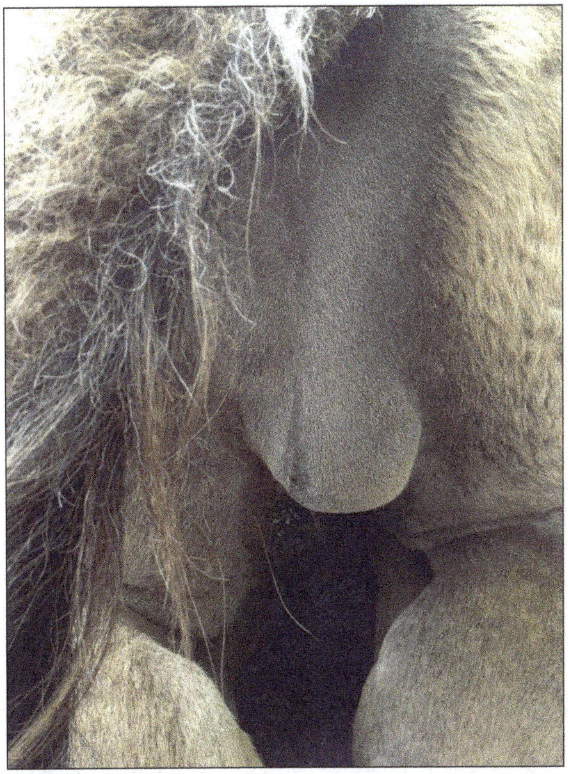

Fig. 1 Clinico-pathological evidence of the mass in the scrotum of a dromedary camel (*Camelus dromedarius*). Subcutaneous nodular mass in the scrotum of a dromedary camel (*Camelus dromedarius*)

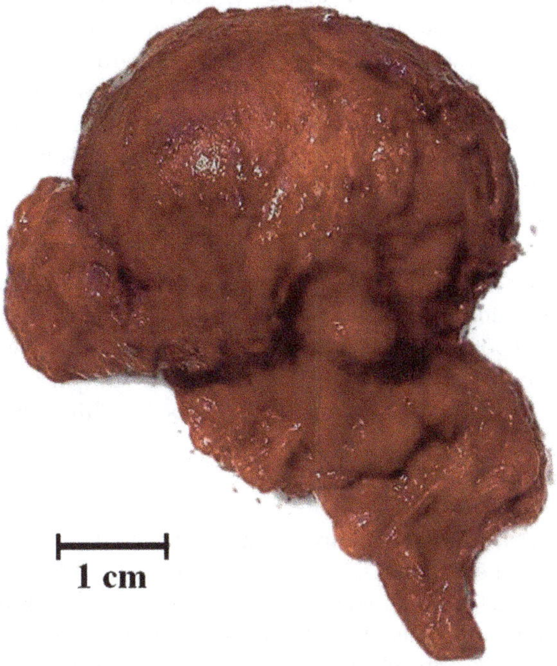

Fig. 2 Macroscopical appearance of the mass. Encapsulated mass removed out of the scrotum of a dromedary camel

with a xylazine-ketamine combination and the surgical area was scrubbed with chlorhexidine solution. Both the mass and the capsule were removed. The scrotum was flushed with sterile saline solution and a drainage was placed to prevent fluid accumulation. The drainage was removed after four days, and after seven days the antibiotic therapy was discontinued. The mass (Fig. 2) was fixed in 10% neutral buffered formalin and referred to the Department of Veterinary Sciences of the University of Turin (Italy) for histological and histochemical examination. The mass was paraffin-embedded and sections of 4 μm were stained with hematoxylin and eosin.

Because fungal cultures were not performed at the time of surgery, an immunohistochemical study was carried out in order to identify of the organism. Sections of the mass were mounted on adhesive slides and kept at +4 °C until processed. Sections were examined with a panel of mono- and polyspecific anti-fungal reagents applied in various immunohistochemical techniques. In the techniques, primary reagents for immunostaining included genus-specific monoclonal and polyclonal antibodies reacting with species of *Aspergillus*, Mucorales, *Candida*, *Geotrichum*, *Fusarium* and *Scedosporium*, respectively [5–7]. The detecting system PowerVision + (Part No. DPVB +110AEC; Immuno Vision Technologies Co. USA) was used for signal-amplification and applied according to the manufacturer's instructions. Sections were counterstained in Meyer's hematoxylin for 10 s, and washed for 1 min in tap water and 4 min in distilled water. Finally, sections were mounted with glycerol-gelatin. To ensure specific reactivity of antibodies, sections were run in parallel with sections from laboratory animals experimentally infected with homologous and heterologous fungi. Moreover, in all series of staining, negative controls were run without primary reagents and with substitution of the primary antiserum or monoclonal antibody of identical isotypes, respectively, raised towards nonsense antigens.

Results

At palpation the mass had a firm consistency and was painful. It measured 4 cm in diameter and was firmly adherent to the inner surface of the scrotum. Haematology indicated leukocytosis suggestive of a chronic inflammation, while no biochemical abnormality was detected. At the opening of the scrotum through a vertical incision, the mass appeared to be surrounded by a capsule and showed a solid appearance at the cut surface. Histopathology revealed dermal granulomatous inflammation with a necrotic centre, surrounded by plasma cells, macrophages, neutrophils, and sparse fungal hyphae. The mass was surrounded by a thick fibrous layer with multifocal lymphocytic infiltrate and haemorrhages. In order to improve the visualization of the fungal elements, periodic acid-Schiff and Grocott stains were applied to selected sections of the mass. Hyphae were characterised by parallel cell walls, distinct septa, and a dichotomous branching pattern (Figs. 3 and 4). Fungal hyphae were present only in the encapsulated granulomatous mass and no invasion of the epidermis and adjacent structures has been observed. Within the nodule removed from the dromedary the fungal hyphae only stained positive (Fig. 5) with the monoclonal antibody (clone WF-AF-1, LSBio) reacting specifically with *Aspergillus* [7, 8]. At follow up, one year after the excision of the mass, the animal was in good health with no sign of recurrence of infection.

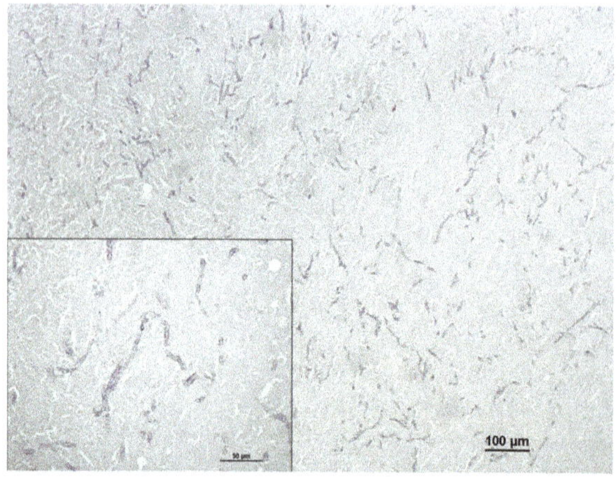

Fig. 4 Histopathology of the mass (HE). Histopathology of a scrotal mass removed from a dromedary camel. Fungal hyphae characterized by parallel cell walls, distinct septa, and dichotomous branching (HE staining)

Discussion

This case of aspergillosis appears to be the first with a subcutaneous localization ever reported in the dromedary camel, and represents a rarity with regards to aspergillosis in animals [2]. In the dromedary, *Aspergillus* has been found associated to post-traumatic buccal infections and osteomyelitis in consequence of mandibular fractures [9] and to a clinical syndrome with multi-organic involvement, skin excluded [10]. Cases of pulmonary aspergillosis have also been reported in other camelids, such as alpaca [11], and lama [12].

Given the localization of the mass, the present case had likely a traumatic origin, represented by the surgical procedure employed to neuter the animal. The subcutaneous tissues exposed during surgery were probably colonized by spores of *Aspergillus* that induced a slow granulomatous reaction. The granulomatous inflammation with abundant fibrosis is a typical finding of chronic aspergillosis [13]. Reports in human medicine frequently describe a more rapid development of different lesions, represented by erythematous to violaceous papules or plaques that may progress to form necrotic ulcers with a central eschar, pustules and subcutaneous abscesses [14, 15]. However, also infections characterized by subcutaneous chronically slow-growing nodules have been reported [3]. In the present case it is somewhat surprising that two years after surgery the nodular mass grew to only 4 cm diameter and then a further 6 cm diameter in just two months. However, cases with a similar trend have been already described in human medicine. For example Cheetham [16] reported a patient with a subcutaneous infection by *Aspergillus* attributed to the inoculation of fungal spores occurred

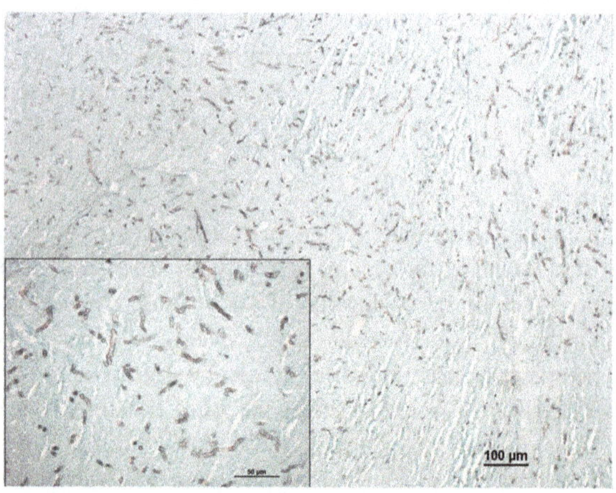

Fig. 3 Histopathology of the mass (Grocott). Histopathology of a scrotal mass removed from a dromedary camel. Fungal hyphae characterized by parallel cell walls, distinct septa, and dichotomous branching (Grocott staining)

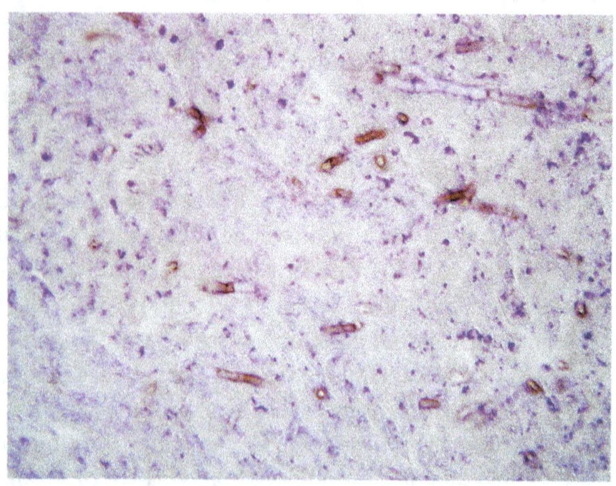

Fig. 5 Immunohistochemical features of the mass. Specific immunolabelling of *Aspergillus* sp. in the lesion from a dromedary camel

about one and a half year before during a course of penicillin injections. The authors speculated that the fungus lay dormant, or only developed slowly, during the year before lesion was first noted, and that the more rapid development of the mass in the later stages may have been due to the appearance of a mutant more adapted to growth in the body than the original strain [16]. Even more extreme is the case described by Lakhanpal et al. [14], regarding a 30-year-old male who developed a subcutaneous nodule due to *Aspergillus* infection over a period of 15 years.

As noted above, cases of aspergillosis with cutaneous involvement are rarely found in veterinary literature. In cats, the occurrence of skin nodules has been reported as the result of contiguous extension to the skin from infected underlying structures (nasal cavity and retro-orbital space) [2, 17]. In other cases, mostly regarding birds, the suspected pathogenesis was more similar to that of our case, i.e. on traumatic base. For example, Abrams et al. [18] described a case of *Aspergillus* blepharitis and dermatitis in a Peregrine Falcon-Gyrfalcon Hybrid (*Falco peregrinus* x *Falco rusticolus*) likely due to a trauma occurred during hunting. Copetti et al. [13] reported an outbreak of aspergillosis in some Pekin mallards (*Anas platyrhynchos*), with the involvement of different organs including the skin. The skin presented multiple elevated, yellowish brown, crusted, multifocal lesions located at the base of the feather follicles in the breast. The infection was attributed to skin trauma in cited by the poultry litter [13]. Chute et al. [19] described a systemic fatal infection by *Aspergillus fumigatus* in White Rock cockerels, that was attributed to the contamination of the cutaneous incision performed to caponize the animals. Finally, in a case of some chickens, cutaneous aspergillosis was seen with generalized, tumor-like swellings, the infection being limited to the skin [20].

Primary "traumatic" aspergillosis is a well characterized condition, although rare if compared with pulmonary and systemic infections, in human medicine [3, 4]. Lesions usually develop in cutaneous sites traumatized in course of accidents or burns, but also due to surgery or minor medical procedures (positioning of intravenous catheter, drug injections, use of occlusive dressings and tapes, etc.) [3]. Most of the cases occur in patients with deficiencies in their immunological status of various reasons (AIDS, corticosteroids use, chemotherapy and immunosuppressive therapy used in organ transplants, diabetes, neonatal period and hematological disorders) [21], although primary cutaneous aspergillosis has been reported also in immunocompetent individuals [15].

Conclusions

Although culture isolation remains the gold standard for the identification of fungi involved in human and animal infections [11], many cases are not cultured because a fungal etiology is not suspected when biological samples are sent to the laboratory [5, 6]. Even when submitted, cultures often fail to isolate the fungus responsible of the infection [8]. Despite the lack of culture in the present case, a definitive diagnosis of aspergillosis was upheld by the application of specific immunohistochemical staining techniques.

Acknowledgements
The authors gratefully acknowledge the Centro di Referenza di Patologia Comparata "Bruno Maria Zaini". The case was presented as poster at the congress of the European Association of Zoo and Wildlife Veterinarians, Vienna (Austria), 8-11 May 2013.

Funding
No funding source has been employed to perform this research.

Authors' contributions
FES was the mentor and principal advisor and proposed the concept of the study, EB and FTC performed histological examination and diagnosis, HEJ performed immunohistochemical investigation, SP and SM were responsible for the surgical procedure. AP and MP were involved in the drafting and writing of the manuscript. All authors have read, commented and approved the final article.

Authors' information
Not applicable.

Competing interests
None of the authors of this paper has a financial or personal relationship with other people or organisations that could inappropriately influence or bias the content of the paper.

Consent for publication
Not applicable.

Author details
[1]Dipartimento di Scienze Veterinarie, Università degli Studi di Torino, Largo Paolo Braccini 2, 10095 Grugliasco (To), Italy. [2]Zoom Torino, Strada Piscina 36, 10040 Cumiana, Italy. [3]Department of Veterinary Disease Biology, University of Copenhagen, Ridebanevej 3, DK-1870 Frederiksberg C, Copenhagen, Denmark.

References

1. Paterson DL. New clinical presentations of invasive aspergillosis in non-conventional hosts. Clin Microbiol Infect. 2004;10:24–30.
2. Seyedmousavi S, Guillot J, Arné P, de Hoog GS, Mouton JW, Melchers WJG, Verweij PE. *Aspergillus* and aspergilloses in wild and domestic animals: a global health concern with parallels to human disease. Medical Mycol. 2015;53:765–97.
3. Van Burik JA, Colven R, Spach DH. Cutaneous Aspergillosis. J Clin Microbiol. 1998;36:3115–21.
4. Perusquía-Ortiz AM, Vázquez-González D, Bonifaz A. Opportunistic filamentous mycoses: aspergillosis, mucormycosis, phaeohyphomycosis and hyalohyphomycosis. J Dtsch Dermatol Ges. 2012;10:611–21.
5. Jensen H, Schonheyder HC, Hotchi M, Kaufman L. Diagnosis of systemic mycosis by specific immunohistochemical tests. APMIS. 1996;104:241–58.

6. Jensen HE, Salonen J, Ekfors TO. The use of immunohistochemistry to improve sensitivity and specificity in the diagnosis of systemic mycosis in patients with haematological malignancies. J Pathol. 1997;181:100–5.
7. Jung J, Park YS, Sung H, Song JS, Lee S-O, Choi S-H, Kim YS, Woo JH, Kim S-H. Using immunohistochemistry to assess the accuracy of histomorphologic diagnosis of aspergillosis and mucormycosis. Clin Infect Dis. 2015;11:1664–70.
8. Choi JK, Mauger J, McGowan L. Immunohistochemical detection of Aspergillus species in pediatric tissue samples. Am J Clin Pathol. 2004;121:18–25.
9. Al-Dughaym AM, Ramadan RO, Mohamed GE, Fadlelmula A, Abdin-Bey MR. Post-traumatic buccal infection and osteomyelitis associated with mandibular fractures in the dromedary camel. J camel pract res. 2003;10:57–60.
10. El-Khouly AB, Gadir FA, Cluer DD, Manefield GW. Aspergillosis in camels affected with a specific respiratory and enteric syndrome. Aust Vet J. 1992;69:182–6.
11. Hughes K, Mueller K. Pathologic lesions of mycotic pneumonia in an alpaca following third compartment ulceration. J Vet Diagn Investig. 2008;20:672–5.
12. Quist CF, Dutton DM, Schneider DA, Prestwood AK. Gastrointestinal ulceration and pulmonary aspergillosis in a llama treated for parelaphostrongylosis. J Am Vet Med Assoc. 1998;212:1438–41.
13. Copetti MV, Barcelos Ada S, Kommers GD, Santurio JM, Oliveira FN, Lovato M. Cutaneous, respiratory and hepatic aspergillosis in Brazilian white Pekin mallards (*Anas platyrhynchos*). Mycopathologia. 2015;179:321–5.
14. Lakhanpal S, Pandhi RK, Khaitan BK, Iyer VK, Bannerjee U. Primary cutaneous aspergillosis in an immunocompetent host. Acta Derm Venereol. 2000;80:74–5.
15. Venugopal TV, Venugopal PV. Primary cutaneous aspergillosis from Tamilnadu diagnosed by fine needle aspiration cytology. Med Mycol Case Rep. 2012;1:103–6.
16. Cheetham HD. Subcutaneous infection due to *Aspergillus terreus*. J Clin Pathol. 1964;17:251–3.
17. Giordano C, Gianella P, Bo S, Vercelli A, Giudice C, Della Santa D, Tortorano AM, Peruccio C, Peano A. Invasive mould infections of the naso-orbital region of cats: a case involving *Aspergillus fumigatus* and an aetiological review. J Feline Med Surg. 2010;12:714–23.
18. Abrams GA, Paul-Murphy J, Ramer JC, Murphy CJ. *Aspergillus* Blepharitis and Dermatitis in a Peregrine Falcon-Gyrfalcon Hybrid (*Falco peregrines x Falco rusticolus*). J Avian Med Surg. 2001;15(2):114–20.
19. Chute HL, Witter JF, Rountree JL. O' meara DC. The pathology of a fungous infection associated with a caponizing injury J Am Vet Med Assoc. 1955;127:207–9.
20. Mohammed MA, Sokkar SM, Batrawi A, Refaie MK, Ahmed AA. Natural and experimental nodular dermatomycosis in chickens. Avian Pathol. 1980;9:185–92.
21. Galimberti R, Kowalczuk A, Hidalgo Parra I, Gonzalez Ramos M, Flores V. Cutaneous aspergillosis: a report of six cases. Br J Dermatol. 1998;139:522–6.

8

Serum proteomic profiles in CKCS with Mitral valve disease

Chiara Locatelli[1†], Cristian Piras[1†], Giulia Riscazzi[1], Isabella Alloggio[1], Ilaria Spalla[1], Alessio Soggiu[1], Viviana Greco[2], Luigi Bonizzi[1], Paola Roncada[1,3] and Paola G. Brambilla[1*]

Abstract

Background: Myxomatous mitral valve disease (MVD) is the most common acquired heart disease in dogs, and the Cavalier King Charles Spaniel (CKCS) is the most studied breed because of the high prevalence, early onset and hereditary component evidenced in the breed. MVD has different severity levels, and there are many practical limitations in identifying its asymptomatic stages. Proteomic techniques are valuable for studying the proteins and peptides involved in cardiovascular diseases, including the period prior to the clinical onset of the disease. The aim of this study was to identify the serum proteins that were differentially expressed in healthy CKCS and those affected by MVD in mild to severe stages. Proteomics analysis was performed using two-dimensional gel electrophoresis separation and a bioinformatics analysis for the detection of differentially expressed spots. In a comparative analysis, protein spots with a $p < 0.05$ (ANOVA) were considered statistically significant and were excised from the gels for analysis by MALDI–TOF–MS for protein identification.

Results: Eight proteins resulted differentially expressed among the groups and significantly related to the progression of the disease.
In mild affected group versus healthy dogs complement factor H isoform 2, inhibitor of carbonic anhydrase, hemopexin, dystrobrevin beta isoform X7 and CD5 molecule-like resulted to be down-regulated, whereas fibronectin type-III domain-containing protein 3A isoform X4 was up-regulated.
In severe affected dogs versus healthy group complement factor H isoform 2, calpain-3 isoform *X*2, dystrobrevin beta isoform X7, CD5 molecule-like and l-2-hydroxyglutarate dehydrogenase resulted to be down-regulated. Complement factor H isoform 2, calpain-3 isoform *X*2, dystrobrevin beta isoform X7, CD5 molecule-like and hydroxyglutarate dehydrogenase were found to be down-regulated in mild affected group versus healthy dogs. All of these proteins except complement factor H followed a decreasing trend according to the progression of the pathology.

Conclusion: The differential expression of serum proteins demonstrates the possibility these might be valuable for the detection and monitoring of the disease. Further longitudinal studies are required to determine whether differential protein expression occurs sufficiently early in the progression of the disease and with sufficient predictive value to allow proteomics analysis to be used as an early detection and on-line diagnostic tool.

Keywords: Proteomic analysis, Mitral valve disease, Dog, Cavalier King Charles Spaniel

* Correspondence: paola.brambilla@unimi.it
[†]Equal contributors
[1]DIMEVET, Department of Veterinary Medicine, University of Milan, Milan, Italy
Full list of author information is available at the end of the article

Background

Myxomatous mitral valve disease (MVD) is the most prevalent acquired heart disease in dogs, and is the most common cause of left heart failure, particularly in older and small breed dogs [1].

The Cavalier King Charles Spaniel (CKCS) is an exception, and the interesting in study MVD in this breed comes from the evidence that CKCS shows the youngest onset and the highest incidence, compared with other breeds [1–5].

The cause of canine MVD is currently unknown, although a genetic predisposition has been proven [2, 4, 6].

MVD has also been increasingly considered as the result of certain effector proteins released in response to mechanical or chemical stimuli through signalling pathways rather than only an age-related disease [6]. The signalling mechanisms at the core of MVD have been investigated by the use of new technologies, and advances in proteomic techniques have improved the tools available for studying cardiovascular diseases [7]. The proteome reflects all proteins and peptides that may be related to certain genes and allows a more detailed evaluation of disease status [8, 9]. In 2009, Lacerda et al. conducted the first proteomic study on canine mitral valve leaflet tissue obtained postmortem from healthy dogs and from dogs with early and end-stage MVD. More than 300 proteins were identified, and 117 of these that were over- or under-expressed, which could provide mechanistic clues into the pathogenesis of MVD [3, 10].

In 2013, Gao et al. investigated plasma protein expression in human patients affected by degenerative or rheumatic valvular disease and compared it with healthy subjects [8]. They reported that few proteomic studies on MVD have been done, and most of them studied tissue, whereas the serum or plasma are ideal sources for proteome analysis, as they are easily sampled and are able to analyse processes in specific anatomical compartments because blood flows in all tissues and is therefore able to take up proteins secreted or shed by tissues [8]. Authors used a similar experimental approach with the difference that they used the depletion of high abundant proteins and described that Carbonic anhydrase protein was over-represented.

In 2013, Tan et al. applied proteomic methods to plasma samples collected from humans with mitral regurgitation (MR) and with or without mitral valve prolapse (MVP) [11]. This study revealed four proteins differentially expressed with a presumptive role in the pathogenesis of MVP: haptoglobin, platelet basic protein and complement component C4b were down-regulated and fibronectin was up-regulated in MR patients with MVP versus the control cases (MR) [11]. In 2014, Xuan et al. applied his experience in plasma proteomic studies to identify plasma protein changes in congenital heart disease with regard to potential clinical significance [8, 9, 11].

At present, in veterinary medicine there is no treatment for the disease itself that can be applied on a large population of patients (i.e. valve replacement and repair surgery), and so the prevention of its occurrence is the only strategy to reduce the incidence in dogs.

To date in order to reduce the prevalence of MVD in CKCS, a breeding program has been conducted in Sweden since 2001. This program was based on heart auscultation, on pedigree analysis and on the indication that dogs under the age of four years should not be bred [12]. The effects of the breeding program were evaluated by comparing the prevalence of heart murmur in CKCS at 6 years of age in 2007 and 2009. No decrease in the prevalence of the murmur was detected, indicating that the breeding program did not achieve the desired effects [12, 13].

In 2016 the results of a mandatory breeding scheme based on cardiac auscultation and on echocardiographic detection of mitral valve prolapse, performed in Denmark from 2002 to 2011 were published. The study evidenced a significant reduction in risk of having a mitral regurgitation murmur caused by MVD after a 8 to 10 year period [13]. Nevertheless same authors reported of limitations to a wide application of the program, and that may affect the use of this method in breeding schemes including multicentre clinical examinations (differences in echocardiographic equipment, technical settings, replacing of the operators, and the changing in the overall observer performance) [13].

To our knowledge there has been extensive research into attempting to diagnose MVD, and more particularly, to diagnose the onset of heart failure in dogs, but none in which proteomic techniques on CKCD clinical patients have been used. To date, there are no reports of serum proteomic changes in dogs affected by MVD. The aim of this study was to evaluate the serum protein profile of healthy and MVD affected CKCS in order to evaluate the physiological changes and the modifications caused by MVD. These findings could provide new insights into our understanding of the underlying mechanisms and the changes from mild to severe stages. The differential expression of the serum proteins moreover could be helpful together with the current techniques in the evaluation of the stage of the pathology, of the drug administration outcome and of the disease progression.

Methods

The study was conducted on privately owned CKCS prospectively recruited at the Cardiology Unit of the Department of Veterinary Medicine, University of Milan (DiMeVet).

A convenience sample of 12 CKCS was enrolled, 4 healthy dogs (control group) and 8 dogs affected by MVD.

All of the owners signed an informed consent before enrolling their dogs in the study. Each dog underwent a complete physical examination aimed at evaluating the general physical condition. The cardiovascular system was evaluated by checking for the presence/absence of a murmur, type and intensity of the murmur (grade I-VI/VI), if present, and the point of maximum intensity. Blood pressure was indirectly measured with a Doppler method according to the ACVIM consensus statement [14]. Once reliable consecutive readings were obtained, the mean of five consecutive blood pressure measurements was calculated [12, 15]. Blood was collected from the jugular vein into 5-mL serum tubes and 2.5-mL EDTA tubes after a 12-h fasting. A complete blood count (CBC) was performed for each dog, and serum samples were centrifuged within 30 min after collection at 3000 × g for 5 min, followed by aliquoting of the plasma. The total protein content and the blood glucose of each sample were immediately evaluated. Serum protein amount was determined using the Bradford dye-binding method (Protein Assay kit 2, Bio-Rad catalogue n° 5000002) according to the manufacturer's instructions. Subsequently, serum biochemistry, including creatinine, urea and serum calcium, potassium, sodium and chloride levels, was analysed. The remaining serum was harvested and transferred into 1.5-mL plastic cryotubes, and the samples were stored at -80°C for subsequent analysis.

Thoracic radiographs in right lateral and dorsoventral recumbency were obtained for all of the dogs included. Each radiograph was evaluated for the presence/absence of cardiomegaly, left atrial/ventricle enlargement, venous congestion, and pulmonary edema.

Echocardiographic examination (2-D, M-mode, spectral, and colour-flow Doppler) was performed by two well-trained investigators using a machine equipped with a multi-frequency phased array probe (2.5–3.5 MHz)[1].

The exam was performed according to a standard procedure with concurrent continuous electrocardiographic monitoring [16]. High-quality video clips were acquired and stored using the echo machine software for off-line measurements. All measurements of interest were repeated on 3 consecutive cardiac cycles, and the mean value was used in the statistical analysis [17].

B-mode and M-mode echocardiography were used to define valve morphology and structures, including the type of lesions and the presence/absence of valvular prolapse, while the degree of mitral regurgitation (MR), if present, was assessed by the use of colour Doppler, calculating the maximal ratio of the regurgitant jet area signal to LA area (ARJ/LAA ratio) [17]. The left atrial to aortic root ratio (LA/Ao) was measured as previously described [4, 18]. Diagnosis of MVD was based on 2-D and colour Doppler echocardiographic findings: characteristic valvular lesions of the mitral valve apparatus and a demonstrated MR on the colour Doppler echocardiogram were considered as the definitive diagnostic criteria, as previously described [17].

The M-mode-derived end-diastolic volume index (EDVI) and the end-systolic volume index (ESVI) were calculated for each patient using the Teichholtz method [19]. The area length method was used for the calculation of 2-D derived parameters: EF%, EDVI and ESVI for each patient.

Based on body weight, the values for LVIDad (left ventricle internal diameter allometric diastole) and LVIDas (left ventricle internal diameter allometric systole) were also calculated according the formulas proposed by Cornell et al. (2004) [20].

The 12 enrolled subjects were stratified into three groups according to the guidelines for the diagnosis and treatment of chronic valvular heart disease established by the American College of Veterinary Internal Medicine Consensus Statement (ACVIM) [21].

Group H included 4 healthy subjects (stage A of ACVIM) with a normal clinical history, examination, thoracic radiography, echocardiography, serum biochemistry, and complete blood count (CBC) [21].

Group M included 4 asymptomatic affected dogs (stages B1 and B2 of ACVIM) with a systolic heart murmur, echocardiographic evidence of MVD and no radiographic signs of venous congestion or pulmonary edema [21].

Group S included 4 symptomatic CKCS (stage C and D of ACVIM) with clinical and radiographic signs of heart failure and echocardiographic evidence of MVD [21]. All of the dogs of the S group were treated with chronic pharmacologic therapy for heart failure including furosemide, angiotensin-converting enzyme inhibitors and pimobendan at the recommended dosage (Atkins et al. 2009). None of them received spironolactone or other potassium-sparing diuretics.

Serological proteome analysis (SERPA)

Before analysis, the frozen serum was thawed slowly at room temperature [22, 23]. The serum samples were analysed through 2D electrophoresis. The first-dimensional analysis was performed using Immobiline Dry strips (pH 3-7 NL, length 7 cm, GE-Healthcare). Immobiline Dry strips were rehydrated overnight in a buffer containing 7 M urea, 2 M thiourea, 4% 3-[(3-Cholamidopropyl) dimethylammonio]-1-propanesulfonate hydrate (CHAPS), 1% threo-1,4-Dimercapto-2,3-butanediol, DL-Dithiothreitol, Cleland's reagent (DTT), 2% ampholine pH 3.5–10 and 0.002% bromophenol blue. One hundred µg of protein was loaded on each IPG strip by cup loading at the cathodic side. Isoelectric focusing was performed using the Protean IEF (Isoelectric Focusing) Cell System (Bio-Rad). For IEF, the following protocol was used: 100 V (4h), 250 V (2h), 5000 V (5h), 5000 V (50000 Volt-hrs).

After the first dimension run was completed, the strips were equilibrated with a solution containing 6 M urea, 20% glycerol, 2% SDS and 50 mM Tris–HCl (pH 8.8), with the addition of 1% w/v DTT in the first step and 2.5% w/v iodoacetamide in the second step. For the second dimension, the proteins were separated by SDS-PAGE on 10% polyacrylamide gels using the Mini Protean System (Biorad, USA). Molecular weight protein markers (Precision Plus - BioRad) were applied on one end of the IPG strips. In the second dimension, the gels were run at 7.5 mA/gel for 20 min and then at 15 mA/gel until the bromophenol blue ran off of the gel. The gels were stained with Coomassie G250.

All images were acquired using an Image Scanner III (GE Healthcare, Uppsala). The gel images were imported into Progenesis SameSpot v4.5 software (Nonlinear Dynamics, UK) for analysis. All of the imported images were processed with Progenesis SameSpots to check image quality (saturation and dimension). The aligned images were then automatically analysed using the 2D analysis module for spot detection, background subtraction, normalization, and spot matching, and all spots were manually reviewed and validated to ensure proper detection and matching.

Statistical analysis

The statistical analysis of the echocardiographic variables, the electrolyte concentrations and the haematological parameters was performed using SAS statistical software (SAS version 11 SW; SAS Institute, Cary, North Carolina, USA). Medians and ranges were calculated, and p-values less than 0.05 were considered statistically significant. The differences among the categories were assessed using the Kruskal-Wallis test, followed by a paired Wilcoxon test.

Statistical analysis of the proteomic data was performed using the Progenesis Stats module on the log-normalized volumes for all spots. The Stats module automatically performed a one-way ANOVA on each spot to evaluate the p-value between different groups, with p-values under 0.05 considered statistically significant.

MALDI TOF MS protein identification

Single spots were excised from the Coomassie-stained 2DE gels, and the spots, previously reduced and alkylated, were digested with a solution of 0.01 μg/μl of porcine trypsin at 37 °C for 16 h. The reaction was stopped with 1% TFA in H_2O (v/v). The peptides were desalted and concentrated by a C18 ZipTip (Millipore) and then co-crystallized with a solution of 0.5 mg/ml α-ciano-4-hydroxycinnamic acid (HCCA) on a Ground Steel plate (Bruker-Daltonics, Bremen, Germany) previously spotted with a thin layer of a 10 mg/ml HCCA solution. Mass spectra were acquired with an Ultraflex III MALDI-TOF/TOF spectrometer (Bruker-Daltonics) in a positive reflectron mode and processed with FlexAnalysis 3.1 software (Bruker-Daltonics) for the selection of the monoisotopic peptide masses. External and internal calibrations were performed. After exclusion of contaminant ions (known matrix and human keratin peaks), the created peak lists were analysed by the MASCOT v.2.4.1 algorithm (www.matrixscience.com) against the NCBI_201410 database restricted to Canis Lupus Familiaris (class: Other Mammalia). The query for database searching was performed with the carbamidomethylation of cysteines as a fixed modification, the oxidation of methionines as a variable modification, and one missed cleavage site allowed for trypsin at 70 ppm as a maximal tolerance. Mascot protein scores greater than 74 were considered significant ($p < 0.05$) for protein identification assignment. To confirm PMF identifications, the instrument was switched to LIFT mode; MS/MS spectra were acquired and processed by Flex-Analysis 3.0 software (Bruker-Daltonics).

Results

The 4 dogs in the H group were significantly younger than those in the M group (2.3 vs 6.1 years, $p = 0.0380$) and those in the S group (9 versus 2.3 years, $p = 0.0284$). There were no significant differences by sex and weight between the three groups (Table 1). The normal reference values, the medians and ranges of the echocardiographic

Table 1 Population characteristics

ID	Age (years)	Sex	Weight (kg)	MVD severity
1	3	F	11,5	H
2	2	F	6,8	H
3	1,5	F	9	H
4	3	F	7	H
5	2	M	7,5	M
6	5,5	F	5	M
7	10	FS	9	M
8	7	F	9	M
9	9	M	8	S
10	7	M	12	S
11	11	FS	9,5	S
12	9	M	8	S

MVD mitral valve disease, *F* female, *M* male, *FS* neutered female, *H* healthy dogs, *M* mild affected, *S* severe affected

variables for all of the dogs included and for the different groups are reported in Table 2 [20, 24, 25].

The electrolyte normal values and their levels in the H, M and S groups are reported in Table 3 [26]. Serum sodium levels showed a statistically significant decrease in subjects in the S group compared with the M and the H groups ($p = 0.0228$ and $p = 0.0256$, respectively), and serum calcium levels also decreased significantly in subjects belonging to the S group compared to the H group ($p = 0.0304$).

Serum potassium and chloride and the levels of other biochemical analytes (creatinine and urea) were not significantly different among the three groups.

Red blood cells and haematocrit values decreased in group S versus the M and H groups, but the differences were not statistically significant (Table 3) [27].

Proteomics analysis (SERPA 2DE and MALDI-TOF-MS)

Proteomics analysis highlighted a total of eight proteins differentially expressed among the groups (data shown in Table 4). Figure 1 shows the relative 2D map with differentially expressed proteins excised from the gel for MALDI- TOF MS analysis.

Five proteins were found to be down-regulated and one protein was up-regulated ($p \leq 0.05$) in group M versus H. The down-regulated proteins included complement factor H isoform 2 (gi|74005944), inhibitor of carbonic anhydrase (gi|545538999), haemopexin (gi|73988725), dystrobrevin beta isoform X7 (gi|545527237) and CD5 molecule-like (gi|545505255). Fibronectin type-III domain-containing protein 3A isoform X4 (gi|545537390) was found to be up-regulated in the M group versus the H group.

Five proteins were found to be down-regulated in group S versus group H: complement factor H isoform 2 (gi|74005944), calpain-3 isoform *X*2 (gi|545549554), dystrobrevin beta isoform X7 (gi|545527237), CD5 molecule-like (gi|545505255) and l-2-hydroxyglutarate dehydrogenase (mitochondrial isoform 2, gi|345804340). As shown in Table 4, complement factor H isoform 2, calpain-3 isoform *X*2, dystrobrevin beta isoform X7, CD5 molecule-like and hydroxyglutarate dehydrogenase were found to be down-regulated in group M versus group H. All of these proteins except complement factor H followed a decreasing trend according to the progression of the pathology.

Discussion

To our knowledge, this is the first proteomic study on serum proteins in CKCS affected by MVD. In this study, the differential proteomic profiles of CKCS dogs affected by MVD with different degrees of severity, as well as healthy controls, has been analysed.

This study was focused mostly on proteins differentially expressed in mildly affected dogs (group M) in comparison to healthy controls in order to provide complementary tools for the early detection of this pathology and/or in the evaluation of its stage/severity.

The group M (or the mildly affected dogs) represented a valuable pool of samples for the study of this pathology in its subclinical status. Nevertheless, all groups have been analysed and, the proteomics profiling of advanced stages provided a more complete overview of the trends of the expression of each protein. The average expression of each protein in all groups of CKCS has been represented in Table 4.

Table 2 Echocardiographic variables in all dogs and in each groups of severity

Variables M mode	Normal value	Over all population (12 dogs)	Group H (4 dogs)	Group M (4 dogs)	Group S (4 dogs)
LVIDs (mm)	* 15.2 ± 4.8	19.8 (15.9-31.4)	19.1 (16.2-20.7)	19.2 (17.7-22.6)	19.45 (15.9-31.4)
LVIDd (mm)	* 26 ± 4.7	30.95 (25.1-49.8)	29.75 (25.1-31.1)	30.1 (25.3-33.9)	39.65 (34.6-49.8)
LVIDas	0.71-1.26	0.94 (0.82-1.63)	0.92 (0.87-1.12)	1.11 (0.93-1.15)	0.92 (0.82-1.63)
LVIDasd	1.27-1.85	1.77 (1.22-2.7)	1.61 (1.22-1.77)	1.65 (1.30-1.91)	1.97 (1.86-2.7)
ESVI (ml/m^2)	<30	31.9 (17-96)	23.9 (19.9-37.1)	37.9 (39.3-23.8)	36.5 (17.4-96.1)
EDVI (ml/m^2)	<100	105.8 (43-287)	84.9 (43.4-104.7)	91.3 (59-125.7)	157.5 (120-287.9)
EF%	* 70 ± 9.20	67.5 (38-86)	69 (38-78)	61.5 (51-69)	83 (66-86)
Variables 2D					
LA/Ao	* 1.22 ± 0.31	1.3 (0.9-3.1)	1.2 (0.9-1.3)	1.2 (0.9-1.6)	2.14 (1.6-3.1)
ESVI (ml/m^2)	<30	24 (18-42)	24.5 (18-30)	20 (17-26)	41 (40-42)
EDVI (ml/m^2)	<70	53.5 (31-167)	45 (37-54)	54.5 (31-68)	123.5 (80-167)

LVIDd was significantly increased in dogs in group S compared with dogs in group H ($p = 0.0304$) and with dogs in group M ($p = 0.0304$). LVIDad was increased in group S compared with group H ($p = 0.0304$). M-mode-derived EDVI was significantly increased in dogs in group S compared with dogs in group H ($p = 0.0304$). The ratio of left atrial to aorta root was significantly increased in dogs in group S than in group M ($p = 0.0304$) and group H ($p = 0.0304$). No statistically significant difference was found in the LVIDs, LVIDas, ESVI (M-mode), ESVI and EDVI (2-D) FS% and EF% (M-mode and 2-D) among the groups
Data are reported as median and ranges (minimum-maximum). *Data are expressed as means values ± standard deviation

Table 3 Electrolytes levels, red blood cells count (RBCC) and hematocrit reported as median and ranges (minimum–maximum) in all dogs and in each groups of severity

	Normal Value	Over all population	Group H (4 dogs)	Group M (4 dogs)	Group S (4 dogs)
Serum Calcium (mg/dl)	8.98-11.82	10.6 (9-12.2)	11.65 (11.3-11.9)	10.6 (9.3-12.2)	9.75 (9-10.1)
Serum Potassium (mmol/l)	3.7 – 5.8	4.6 (4.3-5.2)	4.75 (4.5-4.9)	4.65 (4.3-5.2)	4.45 (4.3-4.6)
RBCC (x10^6/ µl)	5.5-8.5	6.23 (5.64-7.08)	6.45 (6.16-6.87)	6.1 (5.64-7.08)	6 (5.45-6.28)
Hematocrit (%)	35 - 55	37.4 (32.2-40.1)	36.55 (33.8-40.1)	37.6 (37.4-38.4)	35.9 (32.2-40.1)

Among all differentially expressed proteins, Hemopexin was found to be down-regulated in M group in comparison to H group. It is an acute-phase protein that can bind and transport haeme to the liver for breakdown and iron recovery, after which the free hemopexin returns to circulation [8]. Hemopexin also acts as a multifunctional agent in important processes such as iron homeostasis, antioxidant protection, and signalling pathways to promote cell survival and gene expression. This has important implications in several pathologic conditions not only associated with the release of heme but also in the control of the immune response and in the pathogenesis of renal and cardiovascular diseases [28]. The haemopexin down-regulation found in CKCS belonging to the M group is in accordance with the results reported by Ge Gao et al. [8]. In humans affected by degenerative mitral valve disease; however, these authors did not advance any hypothesis on the underlying mechanisms, and more studies were advocated [8, 29]. Moreover, Krekken et al. reported the relationship between hemopexin and angiotensin II through the regulation of the vascular angiotensin II type 1 receptor (AT1-R) [28]. These evidences could provide new hypotheses on the remodelling processes induced by this pathology especially in the light of their correlation with the disease. Finally, the decreased levels of the hemopexin we found in asymptomatic dogs could be related to the binding of the free heme produced by the haemolysis described in dogs affected by MVD due to the blood turbulences in the left atrium [30].

The carbonic anhydrase family (CAs) includes zinc metalloenzymes that catalyse the reversible hydration-

Table 4 Protein identification by MALDI-TOF-TOF analysis

Spot no.	Protein description^a	Accession no.^{b}	Regulation among experimental groups: H M S	Significance	CV %	Theoretical M_r(kDa)/pI	PMF: Mascot score^c	PMF: %Seq. coverage^d	PMF: Matched peptides^e	MS/MS: Peptide sequence^f	MS/MS: m/z^g
118	complement factor H isoform 2	gi|74005944	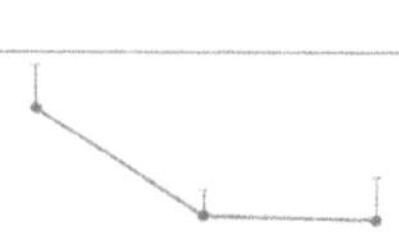	H vs M: p=0.005 H vs S: p=0.010	24.4	144.3/6.1	97	26	25/106	^{401}KNYYQGQSVR^{410} ^{110}VVYTCNEGYQLIGR^{123}	1242.61 1671.81
329	inhibitor of carbonic anhydrase-like	gi|545538999	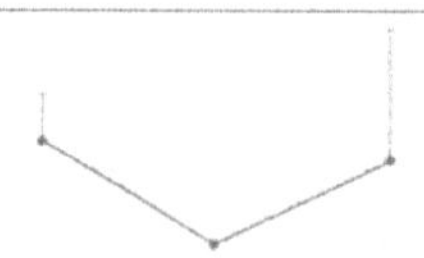	H vs M: p=0,005 H vs S: p=n.s.	18.7	79.1/ 6.2	119	32	19/72	^{271}DLLFTDATDGFLR.V^{283} ^{292}LYVGYEYFSAIQR^{304}	1483.72 1608.79
348	calpain-3 isoform X2	gi|545549554	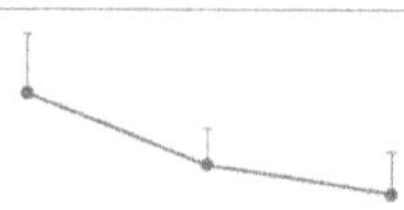	H vs M: p=n.s. H vs S: p=0.032	21.3	95.2/ 5.8	94	25	18/90	^{789}LEGMFRAFNAFDK^{801} ^{293}NMDNSQLRDSDLVPR^{307}	1561.78 1775.79
408	hemopexin	gi|73988725	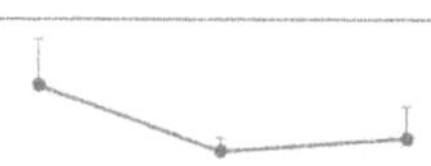	H vs M: p=0.034 H vs S: p=n.s.	15.4	52.0/ 7.0	86	33	17/118	^{399}VDGALCIEK^{407} ^{216}YPLDVRDYFIPCPGR^{230}	1004.53 1867.94
496	dystrobrevin beta isoform X7	gi|545527237	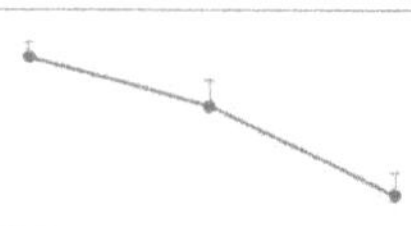	H vs M: p=0.016 H vs S: p=5.7805E-05	10.3	67.7/ 4.9	106	36	11/70	^{66}ARPAEDGMRLR^{77} ^{157}GNVGVVLFNFGKEK^{170}	1287.77 1507.8

H healthy, *M* medium, *S* severe, *CV* variation coefficient, *Mr* relative Mass, *pl* isolectric point, [a]Name of identified proteins; [b]Accession No. according to database [c]Peptide Mass Fingerprinting score calculated by MASCOT 2.4.1 algorithm (http://www.matrixscience.com) after database search; [d] sequence coverage; [e] Number of experimental peptides matched versus searched peptides; [f]Aminoacidic sequence of the peptides identified by MS/MS analysis; [g]Monoisotopic masses of the parent iones used for MS/MS analysis

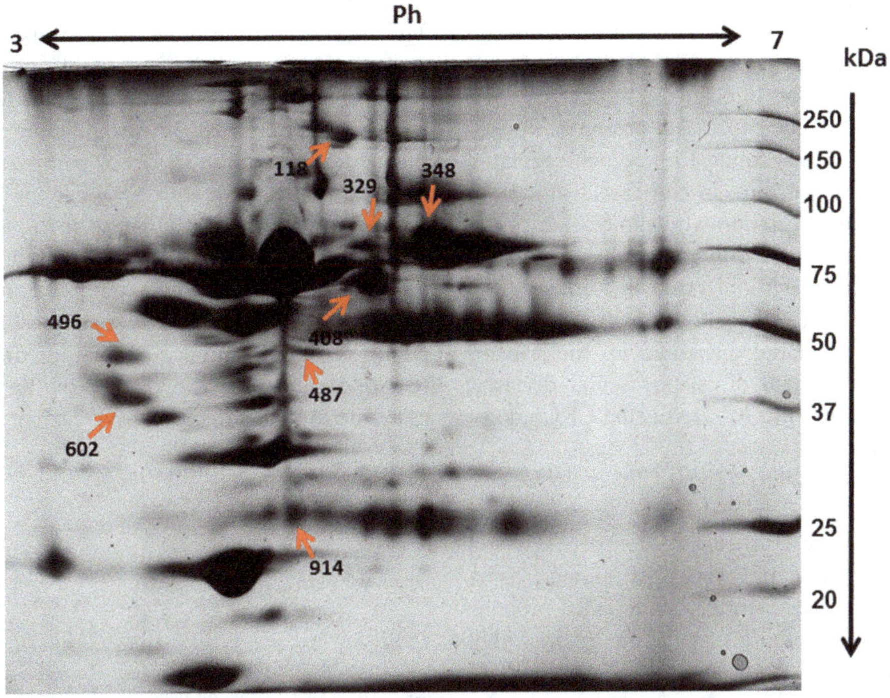

Fig. 1 2D map showing the position of the protein spots analyzed by MALDI TOF MS. The red arrows and the numbers indicated correspond to the dataset showed in Table 3 indicating the differential expression pattern among experimental groups

dehydration of carbon dioxide and bicarbonate. CAs has a role in many physiological and biological processes including calcification, acid-base balance, ion transport, and bone absorption; in vitro, it also promotes the formation of $CaCO_3$. Calcium salt precipitation is an important step in tissue calcification, and valvular calcification is one of the common and key pathological changes in MVD [8]. Using the same experimental approach, Gao and colleagues [8] identified the over-representation of Carbonic anhydrase 1 in human patients of Valvular Heart Diseases. This result seems to be consistent with the down-regulation of the inhibitor of carbonic anhydrase we found in mildly affected dogs. This result could be linked to the expression of calcium and to an improper mineralization process by the acceleration of calcium salt deposition on the mitral valve leaflets [8]. Moreover, the negative trend in the calcium levels in the serum from healthy dogs to those severely affected is in accordance with the down-regulation of the inhibitor of carbonic anhydrase evidenced in our study.

The fibronectin type-III domain-containing protein 3A isoform X4 was found to be over-represented in M vs H experimental group. This protein contains in its sequence domains of fibronectin that has been already described to be up-regulated [11] and its function is related to cell adhesion and is involved in the processes of tissue remodelling [11, 31].

In humans, the fibronectin type-III domain-containing protein 3A is as well involved in cell-cell adhesion among cells of the same organism according to GO annotations. Its putative role in this pathology is still unknown and needs further investigation but it can be considered important in the process of cardiac tissue remodelling.

In severely affected dogs, a significantly low sodium concentration was found in comparison with other groups; according to the literature, this could be due to the influence of the therapy, as Boswood observed that chloride tends to significantly decrease with the administration of treatment [32, 33]. The serum levels of potassium showed a decrease in the H group compared with the S group; however, this variation was not statistically significant.

All of the CKCS included in the study belonging to the S group received furosemide, which might be the reason for the lower potassium levels in the more severely affected dogs [32].

Furosemide could also be considered responsible for the significantly lower levels of serum calcium found in the dogs belonging to group S, as loop diuretics reduce the activity of the sodium-potassium-chloride cotransporter (NKCC2), which stimulates paracellular calcium reabsorption, causing an increase in renal calcium losses and hypocalcemia [34].

In our population, no significant alterations in haemoglobin, red blood cells or haematocrit were found.

Thrombocytopenia and macro thrombocytosis were also considered as a breed-specific idiopathic condition rather than a pathological feature in this study, consistent with other previously published studies [35–37]. Among other differentially expressed proteins, dystrobrevin beta isoform X7 was found to be down-regulated (Table 4) in the M and S groups in comparison to the H group, with a positive correlation with the disease severity. The role of dystrobrevin in hypertrophic cardiomyopathy has already been demonstrated in humans [38]. This evidence demonstrates how the impairment of the α-dystrobrevin gene (which also encodes for the β form) is linked to the development of cardiovascular diseases. Its strong down-regulation in MVD affected CKCS dogs, could suggest a role in the onset of this disease.

Complement factor H isoform 2 and CD5 molecule-like have also been found to be related to the severity of the pathology. The role of these proteins in the pathology still has to be elucidated; proteomic analysis of human plasma in chronic rheumatic mitral stenosis has revealed proteins involved in the complement and coagulation cascades [39]. However, their statistically significant down-regulation both in the M and S groups could suggest a role as molecular markers for this pathology.

This study reports a novel finding on canine MVD from the point of view of protein expression; however, there were several limitations. One of these concern the possibility that the changes in protein patterns, observed in each severity group, might be consistent with disease processes different from MVD. Nowadays the clinical examination and, above all the conventional Echo-Doppler exam represent the diagnostic gold standard of canine MVD. Nevertheless the lacking of post-mortem examination might represents a limitation to take in account [17]. Furthermore the relatively small sample size of each group could have resulted in less significant changes in the electrolyte concentrations compared with other studies, and, also the therapy could have influenced the electrolyte balance in the subjects belonging to the S group.

Another limitation was that the stratification of the patients takes into account the presence (group S) or absence (group M) of symptoms, and the ACVIM classes B1 and B2 CKCS are in the same strata. This limit must be considered in the next study, as the cardiac remodelling process that could be present in ACVIM class B2 and not in B1 could cause different protein expression patterns.

This is a pilot study and clearly further prospective cohort researches are needed to confirm our results, however, finding the same proteins on all groups of dog could be considered a confirmation of their functional importance, and encourage further investigations in studying the protein expression patterns in dogs affected by MVD.

Conclusion

The genetic and the proteomics studies of MVD are important for providing additional information for the comprehension of this pathology and for the evaluation of the outcome of this disease. Obtained results and further studies on these different parameters may contribute to the improvement of the genetic selection of pure breeds to reduce the incidence of this pathology. Moreover, protein identified that were found to be positively or negatively related to the pathology may be helpful in the future for the diagnosis, for choosing the best therapeutic approach and for evaluating the therapeutic response to improve the quality of life and the clinical outcome in dogs affected by MVD.

Abbreviations

ACVIM: American college of veterinary internal medicine; CKCS: Cavalier King Charles Spaniel; EDVI: End diastolic volume index; EF: Ejection fraction; ESVI: End systolic volume index; F: Female; FS: Neutered female; H: Healthy dogs; La/Ao: Left auricle to aorta ratio; LV: Left ventricle; LVIDad: Left ventricular internal dimension in diastole normalized for the body weight based on an allometric equation; LVIDas: Left ventricular internal dimension in systole normalized for the body weight based on an allometric equation; LVIDd: Left ventricular internal dimension in diastole; LVIDs: Left ventricular internal dimension in systole; M: Male; M: Mildly affected; MR: Mitral regurgitation; MVD: Mitral valve disease; S: Severely affected

Acknowledgments

We thank Marco Maria Colombo for his technical artwork in the preparation of the digital format of figures and tables. We thank Prof. Saverio Paltrinieri for the revision of the manuscript.

Funding

Not applicable.

Authors' contributions

CL: was involved in enrolment of the patient and performed the echocardiographic examinations CP: wrote the manuscript, interpretation of data. CL and CP contributed equally to this work. GR: made substantial contributions to conception and design. IA performed proteomics experiments. IS: was involved in enrolment of the patient and performed the echocardiographic examinations. AS: Data interpretation of proteomics, statistics. VG: mass spectrometry experiments, data interoperation. LB: supplementary interpreation of bioinformatic dataset and data analysis. PR: supervised proteomics experiments and contributes in the manuscripts organization and writing. PGB: supervised the research project from the clinical point of view, and has been involved in drafting the manuscript. All authors read and approved the final manuscript.

Competing interests

The authors declare that they have no competing interest.

Consent for publication

Not applicable.

Author details

[1]DIMEVET, Department of Veterinary Medicine, University of Milan, Milan, Italy. [2]Fondazione Santa Lucia -IRCCS, Rome, Italy. [3]Istituto Sperimentale Italiano L. Spallanzani, Milan, Italy.

References

1. Borgarelli M, Crosara S, Lamb K, Savarino P, La Rosa G, Tarducci A, Haggstrom J. Survival characteristics and prognostic variables of dogs with preclinical chronic degenerative mitral valve disease attributable to myxomatous degeneration. J Vet Intern Med. 2012;26:69–75.
2. Lewis T, Swift S, Woolliams JA, Blott S. Heritability of premature mitral valve disease in Cavalier King Charles spaniels. Vet J. 2011;188:73–6.
3. Borgarelli M, Buchanan JW. Historical review, epidemiology and natural history of degenerative mitral valve disease. J Vet Cardiol. 2012;14:93–101.
4. Madsen MB, Olsen LH, Häggström J, Höglund K, Ljungvall I, Falk T, Wess G, Stephenson H, Dukes-McEwan J, Chetboul V, Gouni V, Proschowsky HF, Cirera S, Karlskov-Mortensen P, Fredholm M. Identification of 2 Loci associated with development of myxomatous mitral valve disease in Cavalier King Charles spaniels. J Hered. 2011;102:62–7.
5. Misbach C, Lefebvre HP, Concordet D, Gouni V, Trehiou-Sechi E, Petit AM, Damoiseaux C, Leverrier A, Pouchelon JL, Chetboul V. Echocardiography and conventional Doppler examination in clinically healthy adult Cavalier King Charles Spaniels: effect of body weight, age, and gender, and establishment of reference intervals. J Vet Cardiol. 2014;16:91–100.
6. Parker HG, Kilroy-Glynn P. Myxomatous mitral valve disease in dogs: does size matter? J Vet Cardiol. 2012;14:19–29.
7. Swenson L, Häggström J, Kvart C, Juneja RK. Relationship between parental cardiac status in Cavalier King Charles spaniels and prevalence and severity of chronic valvular disease in offspring. J Am Vet Med Assoc. 1996;208:2009–12.
8. Cui Z, Dewey S, Gomes A. Cardioproteomics: advancing the discovery of signaling mechanisms involved in cardiovascular diseases. Am J Cardiovascular Dis. 2011;10:1274–92.
9. Gao G, Xuan C, Yang Q, Liu XC, Liu ZG, He GW. Identification of altered plasma proteins by proteomic study in valvular heart diseases and the potential clinical significance. PLoS ONE. 2013;8:1–8.
10. Xuan C, Gao G, Yang Q, Wang XL, Liu ZG, Liu XC, He GW. Proteomic study reveals plasma protein changes in congenital heart diseases. Ann Thorac Surg. 2015;97:1414–9.
11. Lacerda CM, Disatian S, Orton EC. Differential protein expression between normal, early-stage, and late-stage myxomatous mitral valves from dogs. Proteomics Clin Appl. 2009;3:1422–9.
12. Tan HT, Ling LH, Dolor-Torres MC, Yip JW, Richards AM, Chung MC. Proteomics discovery of biomarkers for mitral regurgitation caused by mitral valve prolapse. J Proteomics. 2013;94:337–45.
13. Lundin T, Kvart C. Evaluation of the Swedish breeding program for cavalier King Charles spaniels. Acta Vet Scand. 2010;23:52–4.
14. Birkegard AC, Reimann MJ, Martinussen T, Häggström J, Pedersen HD, Olsen LH. Breeding restrictions decrease the prevalence of mixomatous mitral valve disease in Cavalier King Charles Spaniels over an 8- to 10- years period. J Vet Intern Med. 2016;30:63–8.
15. Brown S, Atkins C, Bagley R, Carr A, Cowgill L, Davidson M, Egner B, Elliott J, Henik R, Labato M, Littman M, Polzin D, Ross L, Snyder P, Stepien R. Guidelines for the identification, evaluation, and management of systemic hypertension in dogs and cats. J Vet Intern Med. 2007;21:542–58.
16. Ljungvall I, Hoglund K, Lilliehook I, Oyama MA, Tidholm A, Tvedten H, Häggström J. Serum serotonin concentration is associated with severity of myxomatous mitral valve disease in dogs. J Vet Intern Med. 2013;27:1105–12.
17. Thomas WP, Gaber CE, Jacobs GJ, Kaplan PM, Lombard CW, Moise NS, Moses BL. Recommendations for standards in transthoracic two-dimensional echocardiography in the dog and cat. J Vet Intern Med. 1993;7:247–52.
18. Chetboul V, Tissier R. Echocardiographic assessment of canine degenerative mitral valve disease. J Vet Cardiol. 2012;14:127–48.
19. Hansson K, Häggström J, Kvart C, Lord P. Left atrial to aortic root indices using two-dimensional and M-mode echocardiography in cavalier King Charles spaniels with and without left atrial enlargement. Vet Radiol Ultrasound. 2002;43:568–675.
20. Teichholtz LE, Kreulen T, Herman MV, Gorlin R. Problems in echocardiographic volume determinations: Echocardiographic angiographic correlations in the presence of absence of asynergy. Am J Cardiol. 1976;37:7–11.
21. Cornell CC, Kittleson MD, Della Torre P, Häggström J, Lombard CW, Pedersen HD, Vollmar A, Wey A. Allometric scaling of M-mode cardiac measurements in normal adult dogs. J Vet Intern Med. 2004;18:311–21.
22. Atkins C, Bonagura J, Ettinger S, Fox P, Gordon S, Häggström J, Hamlin R, Keene B, Luis-Fuentes V, Stepien R. Guidelines for the diagnosis and treatment of canine chronic valvular heart disease. J Vet Intern Med. 2009;23:1142–50.
23. Piras C, Soggiu A, Greco V, Cassinotti A, Maconi G, Ardizzone S, Amoresano A, Porro GB, Bonizzi L, Roncada P. Serum protein profiling of early and advanced stage Crohn's disease. EuPA Open Proteomics. 2014;3:48–59.
24. Marco-Ramell A, de Almeida AM, Cristobal S, Rodrigues P, Roncada P, Bassols A. Proteomics and the search for welfare and stress biomarkers in animal production in the one-health context. Mol Biosyst. 2016;12:2024–35.
25. Boon JA. Veterinary Echocardiography. 2nd ed. Denver: Wiley-Blackwell; 2010.
26. Borgarelli M, Tarducci A, Zanatta R, Haggstrom J. Decreased systolic function and inadequate hypertrophy in large and small breed dogs with chronic mitral valve insufficiency. J Vet Intern Med. 2007;21:61–7.
27. Stockham SL, Scott MA. Fundamentals of Veterinary Clinical Phatology. 2nd ed. Victoria: Blackwell Publishing ltd; 2008.
28. De Oliveira MC, Santos KS, Ferreira FM, Teixeira PC, Pomerantzeff PMA, Brandão CMA, Sampaio RO, Spina GS, Kalil J, Guilherme L, Cunha-Neto E. Distinct Mitral Valve Proteomic Profiles in Rheumatic Heart Disease and Myxomatous Degeneration. Clin Med Insights Cardiol. 2014;8:79–86.
29. Krikken JA, Lely AT, Bakker SJ, Borghuis T, Faas MM, van Goor H, Navis G, Bakker WW. Hemopexin activity is associated with angiotensin II responsiveness in humans. J Hypertens. 2013;31:537–41.
30. Bakker WW, Spaans F, el Bakkali L, Borghuis T, van Goor H, van Dijk E, Buijnink J, Faas MM. Plasma hemopexin as a potential regulator of vascular responsiveness to angiotensin II. Reprod Sci. 2013;20:234–7.
31. Porter KE, Turner NA. Cardiac fibroblasts: At the heart of myocardial remodeling. Pharmacol Ther. 2009;123:255–78.
32. Pat B, Chen Y, Killingsworth C, Gladden JD, Shi K, Zheng J, Powell PC, Walcott G, Ahmed MI, Gupta H, Desai R, Wei C, Hase N, Kobayashi T, Sabri A, Granzier H, Denney T, Tillson M, Dillon AR, Husain A, Dell'Italia LJ. Chymase inhibition prevents fibronectin and myofibrillar loss and improves cardiomyocyte function and LV torsion angle in dogs with isolated mitral regurgitation. Circulation. 2010;122:1488–95.
33. Boswood A, Murphy A. The effect of heart disease, heart failure and diuresis on selected laboratory and electrocardiographic parameters in dogs. J Vet Cardiol. 2006;8:1–9.
34. Schrier RW, Abraham WT. Hormones and hemodynamics in heart failure. N Engl J Med. 1999;341:577–85.
35. Ruppe MD. Medications that affect calcium. Endocr Pract. 2011;17:26–30.
36. Bertazzolo W, Comazzi S, Sesso L, Scarpa P, Ruz G, Paltrinieri S. Comparison of methods for determining platelet numbers and volume in Cavalier King Charles spaniels. J Small Anim Pract. 2007;48:556–61.
37. Cowan SM, Bartges JW, Gompf RE, Hayes JR, Moyers TD, Snider CC, Gerard DA, Craft RM, Muenchen RA, Carroll RC. Giant platelet disorder in the Cavalier King Charles Spaniel. Exp Hematol. 2004;32:344–50.
38. Pedersen HD, Häggström J, Olsen LH, Christensen K, Selin A, Burmeister ML, Larsen H. Idiopathic asymptomatic thrombocytopenia in Cavalier King Charles spaniels is an autosomal recessive trait. J Vet Intern Med. 2002;16:169–73.
39. Ichida F, Tsubata S, Bowles KR, Noriyuki N, Uese K, Miyawaki T, Dreyer WJ, Messina J, Li H, Bowles NE, Towbin JA. Novel gene mutations in patients with left ventricular noncompaction or Barth syndrome. Circulation. 2001;103:1256–63.

Evaluation of a species-specific C-reactive protein assay for the dog on the ABX Pentra 400 clinical chemistry analyzer

Sarah Hindenberg[1*], Stefanie Klenner-Gastreich[2], Nicole Kneier[2], Sabine Zielinsky[1], Kris Gommeren[3], Natali Bauer[1] and Andreas Moritz[1]

Abstract

Background: A canine-specific immunoturbidimetric CRP assay, Gentian Canine CRP Immunoassay) with species-specific controls and calibrators was introduced and recently evaluated on the clinical chemistry analyzer Abbott Architect c4000 as well as on the Olympus AU600.
Aims of our study were 1) to independently evaluate the canine-specific CRP assay on the ABX Pentra 400 clinical chemistry analyzer in comparison to the previously validated human-based immunoturbidimetric assay (Randox Canine CRP assay) and 2) to assess the impact of different sample types (serum versus heparinized plasma) on the results. Imprecision, accuracy, interference and the prozone effect were determined using samples from healthy and diseased dogs ($n = 278$). The Randox Canine CRP assay calibrated with canine specific control calibration material served as a reference method. Additionally, the impact of the sample type (serum and lithium heparin) was evaluated based on samples of healthy and diseased dogs ($n = 49$) in a second part of the study.

Results: Linearity was present for CRP concentrations ranging from 4 to 281 mg/l. For clinically relevant CRP concentrations of 7–281 mg/l, recovery ranged between 90 and 105% and intra- and inter-assay CVs ranged between 0.68% - 12.12% and 0.88% - 7.84%, respectively. CV was thus lower than 12.16%, i.e. the desired CV% based on biological variation. Interference was not present up to a concentration of 5 g/l hemoglobin, 800 mg/l bilirubin and 10 g/l triglycerides. No prozone effect occurred up to 676 mg/l CRP. Method comparison study revealed a Spearman's rank correlation coefficient of $r_s = 0.98$ and a mean constant bias of 5.2%. The sample type had a significant ($P = 0.008$) but clinically not relevant impact on the results (median CRP of 30.9 mg/l in lithium heparin plasma versus 31.4 mg/l in serum).

Conclusions: The species-specific Gentian Canine CRP Immunoassay reliably detects canine CRP on the ABX Pentra 400 clinical chemistry analyzer whereby both serum and heparin plasma can be used. The quality criteria reached on the Abbott Architect c4000 and Olympus AU600 could be met.

Keywords: Acute phase protein, Canine, Method validation, Analyzer, Repeatability, Linearity, Total allowable error, Heparin plasma, Interference

* Correspondence: sarah.hindenberg@vetmed.uni-giessen.de
[1]Department of Veterinary Clinical Sciences, Clinical Pathology and Clinical Pathophysiology, Justus-Liebig-University Giessen, 35392 Giessen, Germany
Full list of author information is available at the end of the article

Background

C-reactive protein (CRP) is a major acute phase protein (APP) in the dog. As a part of innate immune response, APPs change their serum concentration in response to a systemic inflammation [1–4]. In contrast to classic inflammatory markers such as the white blood cell count, APPs react more rapidly and with a shorter half-life period [1, 5]. According to their kinetics in response to a pathological stimulus, positive APPs are classified as major, moderate and minor APPs. While major APPs show a 100- to 1000-fold increase within 24–48 h and decrease rapidly, moderate APPs react with a 5- to 10-fold increase within a period of 2–3 days and a slow decrease. In contrast, minor APPs react with a mild 1.5- to 2-fold increase [3]. Due to their marked, rapid increase, especially major APPs are sensitive diagnostic and prognostic measurands [6, 7] to monitor systemic inflammation. In dogs, an increase of CRP was shown in several conditions including infectious diseases [8–11], immune mediated diseases [12–14], neoplasias [12, 15, 16], and surgery [17].

A canine species-specific enzyme-linked immunosorbent assay (ELISA) [18] proved to be sensitive but too time-consuming to be used for routine measurements of canine CRP. First evaluation of immunoturbidimetric assays designed for the detection of human CRP showed unsatisfactory interspecies cross-reactivity between canine CRP and human CRP-antibodies [19], which was mainly attributed to a species-specific pattern of glycosylation of the CRP molecule [20, 21]. Later, an immunoturbidimetric assay with a reasonable cross-reactivity was evaluated [22].

In 2010, our group investigated three human-based immunoturbidimetric test systems in comparison to a species-specific ELISA [23]. However, application of human CRP reagents and heterologous control and calibration material may lead to unpredictable results with false low values in dog samples [22, 24]. The growing interest in standardizing and communicating the range of methods of APP measurement in veterinary species [2, 24, 25] led to the development of canine-specific assays with specific calibrators and controls. Meanwhile, purified canine CRP became commercially available and was used as calibrator in human CRP assays [24]. Canine specific controls as internal quality material still had to be prepared out of serum pools of healthy and diseased patients.

Recently, a species-specific immunoturbidimetric assay for canine CRP (Gentian Canine CRP Immunoassay, Gentian AS, Moss, Norway) became available and had been validated by Hillström et al. 2014 on the Abbott Architect c4000 (Abbott Park, IL, USA) in comparison to the Randox Canine CRP assay [26]. However, quality performance differences between various clinical chemistry analyzers have been demonstrated previously [27] making it difficult to both generalize results and compare studies. Muñoz-Prieto et al. investigated the same assay run on an Olympus AU600 analyzer but used the heterologous Olympus CRP assay as a reference method [28]. Apart from the analyzer, the sample material might also have an impact on assay performance. Acute phase proteins are commonly measured in serum, however, sometimes only either serum or lithium heparin plasma samples are submitted, when a clinical chemistry profile including CRP is requested. Unfortunately it is not always possible to collect a further comparable sample. It is therefore important to determine if both sample materials can be used interchangeably.

To the authors′ knowledge, the impact of the ABX Pentra 400 as a different analyzer on the performance of the Gentian CRP test as well as the effect of the sample material (serum versus heparin plasma) has not been evaluated so far. The aim of our study was thus to validate this assay with a different analyzer (i.e, Pentra 400 analyzer compared to the Abbott Architect c4000 and Olympus AU600 analyzer, respectively) using a similar methodology as the previous studies.

Our hypothesis was that the automated analyzer used has only a minor impact on the test performance; however, the sample material (heparin plasma versus serum) cannot be used interchangeably.

Methods

Study design

The present validation study was conducted between April 2013 and March 2016.

The study was structured into two parts: First, method validation was performed, including the evaluation of accuracy, recovery, precision, interference, prozone effect, and method comparison. The method comparison study was conducted according to recent recommendations [29], whereby the previously validated human-based immunoturbidimetric Randox Canine CRP assay (Randox Laboratories Ltd., Crumlin, UK) [23] served as the reference method. In the second part comparative measurements between lithium heparin plasma and serum samples were conducted to assess potential influence of an anticoagulant in order to simplify future routine diagnostics by allowing the application of both serum and heparin plasma samples.

Measurement of C-reactive protein

Both the Gentian Canine CRP Immunoassay and the Randox Canine CRP assay were run on the ABX Pentra 400 clinical chemistry analyzer (Horiba ABX SAS, Montpellier, France).

Gentian canine CRP immunoassay

The canine-specific CRP assay (Gentian Canine CRP Immunoassay, Gentian AS, Moss, Norway) designed to be run on an automated analyzer is a quantitative immunoturbidimetric in-vitro diagnostic test using polyclonal chicken-derived canine-specific anti-CRP antibodies. The anti-CRP-immunoparticles aggregate with canine CRP and form complexes that can be measured with turbidimetric methods and are correlated with canine CRP concentrations by interpolation on a calibration curve. Calibration (Gentian Canine CRP Calibrator Kit, Gentian AS, Moss, Norway) and the measurement of canine-specific control material serving as internal quality control (Gentian Canine CRP Control Kit, Gentian AS, Moss, Norway) were performed daily.

Randox canine CRP assay

In our study, LOT 1303404 of Randox Canine CRP assay and - in contrast to the previous validation study [23] but in accordance with the previous validation study for the Gentian Canine CRP assay using the Randox Canine CRP assay as the reference method - a canine calibrator (Canine CRP Life Diagnostics, Inc., West Chester, USA) was used. Using canine calibration material for the human-based Randox Canine CRP assay, intra-assay CV ranged between 0.7% - 2.1% (unpublished data).

Measurements were performed as batch analysis at one day. Canine-specific calibration (Canine CRP Life Diagnostics, Inc., West Chester, USA) was done before the analyses were started while canine-specific control measurements (Canine CRP Reference Standard Biozol Diagnostica Vertrieb GmbH, Eching, Germany) were performed prior to the analyses and after each measurement of 60 samples.

Method validation

To avoid preanalytical error due to numerous dilution steps, as it may occur by serially diluting a sample with very high CRP concentration to achieve a very low CRP concentration, linearity was evaluated in two dilution experiments with a partially overlapping CRP range: Linearity was first assessed by manual dilution of a canine serum specimen with markedly increased CRP concentration of 281.3 mg/l, achieving samples with 1.0, 0.8, 0.6, 0.4, 0.2, 0.1, 0.05, and 0.025 of the original CRP concentration. In addition, the diluted samples were used to calculate the recovery rate at eight different CRP levels.

To gain more information about the test performance at low CRP concentrations, linearity was also assessed by manual, stepwise dilution of pooled canine quality control material, whereby a normal and an abnormal control were mixed in equal parts (Gentian Canine CRP Control Kit, Gentian AS, Moss, Norway) so that a pooled sample with a mean CRP concentration of 66.5 mg/l was obtained that was then serially diluted to assess linearity at low CRP concentrations. For all dilution steps, double-distilled water was used as diluent to achieve samples with 1.0, 0.8, 0.6, 0.4, 0.2, 0.1, 0.05, 0.025 and 0.0125 of the original CRP concentration of the pooled samples. All samples were analyzed in triplicates in a single run. Intra-assay and inter-assay repeatability including between-run and between-day CV were determined by measurement of four canine serum samples with different CRP concentrations (A: 7.2 mg/l, B: 58.4 mg/l, C: 103.9 mg/l, D: 272.1 mg/l). Sample analysis was carried out in duplicates twice daily (morning and evening to assess between-run CV) over 5 days without recalibration. Sample order was changed randomly every run.As recommended for a verification of the limit of quantification [30], additional measurements were performed to evaluate intra-assay precision specifically for CRP values close to zero (A1: 2.3 mg/l, A2: 3.8 mg/l). Here, samples were analyzed 20 times in a single run without recalibration.

Interference was investigated by spiking aliquots of a canine serum sample of 35.5 mg/l CRP with 800 mg/l bilirubin (Bilirubin, Sigma-Aldrich Co. LLC., St. Louis, Missouri, USA), 5 g/l hemoglobin (Hemoglobin human, Sigma-Aldrich Co. LLC., St. Louis, Missouri, USA) or 10 g/l 20% soy bean emulsion (Intralipid 20%, Fresenius Kabi Canada, Ontario, Canada) before analyzing them in triplicates in random order.

A stock solution containing bilirubin in a concentration of 20 g/l was prepared by diluting 20 mg bilirubin in 1 ml of 0.1 M NaOH. Then, 0.1 ml of the product was added to 2.4 ml non-spiked serum sample to achieve a bilirubin level of 800 mg/l.Lyophilized human hemoglobin was dissolved in 0.09% NaCl (1 part in 10 parts of NaCl) so that a stock solution containing 100 g/l hemoglobin was obtained and 0.125 ml of the solution were added to 2.375 ml non-spiked serum sample to receive a hemoglobin concentration of 5 g/l.To assess the impact of lipemia on results, 0.125 ml of Intralipid were added to 2.375 ml of non-spiked serum sample resulting in concentration of soya bean oil of 10 g/l.

The samples were compared to serum aliquots spiked with an equal volume of either 100 mM NaOH (in case of bilirubin), 0.09% NaCl (hemoglobin) or pure water (in case of Intralipid). Antigen overload may provoke falsely low CRP measurements. This so called prozone effect was evaluated by spiking a serum sample containing a very low CRP concentration with purified canine CRP (Dog C-Reactive Protein, Life Diagnostics, Inc., West-Chester, USA) until a CRP concentration of 1069.5 mg/l was obtained. The spiked sample was subsequently diluted with 0.9% NaCl so that final concentrations of 455 mg/l, 676 mg/l, and 890 mg/l were achieved. Samples were measured in duplicates in a single run.

Method comparison study

In the method comparison study, the Gentian Canine CRP Immunoassay was compared to the previously validated human-based immunoturbidimetric Randox Canine CRP assay.

Overall, 278 serum samples of healthy and diseased dogs presented at the Department of Clinical Sciences, School of Veterinary Medicine, University of Liège, Liège, Belgium, were analyzed with both immunoturbidimetric assays. The samples have already been used for a previous study in which inflammatory cytokines and CRP were investigated in canine systemic inflammatory response syndrome patients [31]. In our study, residual sample material was used.

Samples were collected between January and August 2010, stored at −80 °C and shipped frozen to the Department of Veterinary Clinical Sciences, Clinical Pathology and Clinical Pathophysiology, Justus-Liebig-University Giessen, Germany, and stored again at −80 °C for 4 weeks until batch-analysis was performed.

Effect of sample material

To assess the impact of an anticoagulant (lithium heparin plasma versus serum sample) on the CRP measurements, blood samples of 49 healthy and diseased dogs presented at the Clinic for Small Animals, Faculty of Veterinary Medicine, Justus-Liebig University, Giessen, Germany, were obtained simultaneously by venipuncture with a sterile disposable cannula into tubes (1.3 ml) containing lithium heparin as anticoagulant and tubes without additives.

Inclusion criterion was that both a heparinized blood sample and a serum sample were taken for diagnostic purposes. Between March and April 2014, samples were analyzed in matched pairs within the first hour after blood collection. Lithium heparin anticoagulated samples were centrifuged for 1 min with 8944 g without delay, while samples without additives were allowed to clot for at least 10 min after receipt in the laboratory. Intra-assay repeatability for measurement of CRP in heparinized plasma was first assessed for ten consecutive measurements with samples from three dogs with low, moderate and high CRP values (10, 53, 77 mg/l respectively). Additionally, the LoQ of the CRP assay determined for serum (A1, A2, Table 1) was verified for heparinized plasma as well, whereby both the heparinized and the serum samples were taken from the same dogs with CRP values close to zero and analyzed 20 times.

Statistical analysis

Statistical analyses were carried out using statistical software packages (MedCalc, software version 16.2.1; Ostend, Belgium and GraphPad Prism 6 Software, GraphPad Software, Inc., La Jolla, USA).

Method validation study

Limits of acceptance were set according to Total allowable error (TE) guidelines of the American college of Veterinary Clinical Pathology (ASVCP) [32]. Although no definite TE for CRP was recommended by the workgroup, an optimal and desired coefficient of variation (CV), bias, and TE based on biologic variation was given in the addendum of the ASVCP guidelines: The optimal / desired allowable imprecision (CV_{opt}/CV_{des}) were reported to be 6.08% and 12.16% respectively, the optimal and desired allowable bias ($bias_{opt}/bias_{des}$) were 4.76% / 9.52% and the optimal / desired total allowable error (TE_{opt}/TE_{des}) were 14.79% / 29.58%, respectively [32]. Here, numbers rounded to one decimal place are used.

Descriptive statistics were performed to calculate arithmetic means, standard deviations (SD), and CV. All data were evaluated for normal distribution using the Shapiro-Wilk Test.

To evaluate the linearity under dilution of the assay, mean results of measured values were plotted against

Table 1 Precision of CRP determination in pooled serum samples with CRP concentrations below a clinical decision limit (A1 - A2) as well as pooled serum samples with clinically relevant CRP concentrations

		Intra-assay CV		Inter-assay CV			
				Between run CV		Between day CV	
Level	Mean CRP concentration (mg/l)	SD (mg/l)	CV%	SD (mg/l)	CV%	SD (mg/l)	CV%
A1	2.3	0.72	**31.1**	n.d.	n.d.	n.d.	n.d.
A2	3.8	0.35	9.3	n.d.	n.d.	n.d.	n.d.
A	7.2	0.87	12.1	0.56	7.8	0.44	6.1
B	58.4	1.08	1.9	1.25	2.1	2.7	4.6
C	103.9	0.88	0.9	0.91	0.9	1.9	1.8
D	272.1	1.85	0.7	4.98	1.8	2.8	1.1

A1, A2: CVs for intra-assay imprecision of two canine serum pools analyzed 20 times in a single run without recalibration.
A – D: Inter- and intra-assay CVs of 6 canine serum pools analyzed in duplicates twice daily over 5 days.
CVs not fulfilling the quality specifications i.e., are higher than 12.2% [32] are marked in bold letters.Abbreviations: n.d. = not done, SD = standard deviation; CV = coefficient of variation.

theoretical CRP concentration. The 'best fit' line was visually inspected for linearity. In addition, recovery after dilution was calculated by subtracting the measured CRP result from the calculated (expected) CRP concentration according to the following formula:

$$\text{Recovery } \% = \frac{measuredconcentration - expectedconcentration}{expectedconcentration} x100.$$

Acceptance criteria for recovery rates were set at 80–120% for samples as recommended previously for validation of immunoassays [33, 34]. The intra-assay CVs were calculated as follows based on mean and standard deviation (SD):

$$CV\ \% = \frac{SD}{Mean} x100$$

For the interference study, non-spiked samples (control) and samples spiked with the interfering substances (test) were measured in triplicates. Observed interference effect (d_{obs}) was computed as the % bias between the means of the test and control specimens:

$$d_{obs}\ \% = \frac{meantest - meancontrol}{meancontrol} x100$$

In accordance with the literature, bias between control and test sample was considered acceptable if the bias for the interfering substance (i.e., d_{obs} %) was smaller than the allowable TE [35], i.e. 29.6% (TE_{des}), and 14.8% (TE_{opt}) for canine CRP [32].

Method comparison study

Data of the method comparison experiment were analyzed with Spearman's rank correlation and Passing & Bablok regression analysis. Bland-Altman difference plot was performed to investigate % bias. In addition, the total observed error TE_{obs} was calculated to judge acceptability according to the quality specifications recommended by the American Society for Veterinary Clinical Pathology (ASVCP) [32]. TE_{obs} was calculated using following formula:

$$TE_{obs} = \text{bias } \% + 2CV\%.$$

Effect of sample material

Comparative measurements of plasma samples: Normality was assessed with a Shapiro Wilk test. Since data were not normally distributed, Wilcoxon signed-rank test was performed to assess potential differences between the methods. For method validation, Spearman's rank correlation as well as Passing-Bablok regression and Bland-Altman analysis were performed.

Results

Method validation study

Results of the precision study are shown in Table 1. For clinically relevant CRP concentrations ranging between 7.2 and 272.1 mg/l (concentrations A-D), both intra- and inter-assay CVs fulfilled the quality specifications, i.e., the CVs did not exceed 12.2% [32]. Intra-assay imprecision <2% was present for clinically relevant CRP-ranges >40 mg/l. Only for CRP concentrations of 2.5 mg/l, a CV markedly exceeding the desired CV was noted, so that the LoQ was set above the lowest concentrations still fulfilling the quality specifications i.e., 3.8 mg/l (≈ 4 mg/l). Evaluation of inter-assay precision showed slightly higher inter-assay CVs of 0.88–7.84% than intra-assay CVs.

The results of the linearity study for higher and lower concentration ranges are demonstrated in Fig. 1, Table 2, and Table 3. As shown in Fig. 1, there was an excellent correlation between expected and measured values for both concentrations ranges. Considering the LoQ, linearity under dilution of the Gentian Canine CRP Immunoassay was present in a range of 4–281 mg/l for serially diluted canine specimens (Figure 1). Recovery rate ranged between 88.9–105.4% at expected CRP values of 7.0–281.3 mg/l (Table 2) and thus fulfilling the quality requirements. For CRP concentrations ranging between 0.8 mg/l and 66.5 mg/l (Table 3), however, quality requirements were not fulfilled for the lowest CRP concentrations of 0.8 mg/l and 1.7 mg/l, respectively.

Overall, no interference was detectable up to a concentration of 5 g/l hemoglobin, 800 mg/l bilirubin and 10 g/l soy bean oil (Table 4). Mean absolute bias between control and spiked test samples was 0.1 mg/l, 0.6 mg/l and 1.6 mg/l respectively. At a clinically relevant CRP concentration of about 30 mg/l, the systematic errors are lower than TE_{opt} for all interfering substances. No prozone effect was present up to a concentration of 676 mg/l CRP as CRP values were measured correctly: The recovery rates for high CRP concentrations were 130% for 455 mg/l, 121% for 676 mg/l and 28% for 890 mg/l, respectively.

Method comparison study

As demonstrated in Fig. 2, there was an excellent correlation (r_s = 0.98) between the results obtained with the species specific canine CRP test and the reference method. Passing-Bablok regression equation revealed small constant and proportional errors reflected by an intercept of −1.18 (with 95% confidence intervals (CI) of −2.07 to −0.43 mg/l) and a slope of 0.99 (95% CI 0.97 to 1.08) (Figure 2). Bland-Altman analysis revealed a mean constant bias of 5.2% (Figure 3). Taking the bias and the inter-assay CV at the 4 different CRP concentrations (A-D, Table 1) under consideration, TE_{obs} was calculated and results are shown in Table 5. TE_{obs} ranged from 20.9% at low levels to 7.0–9.5% at higher levels B-D (table 5). Overall, TE_{obs} was < TE_{des} of 29.6% for all CRP concentration levels and even < TE_{opt} of 14.8% for the clinically relevant concentration levels B-D [32].

Effect of sample material

Spearman's rank correlation coefficient revealed an excellent correlation between CRP measurements obtained

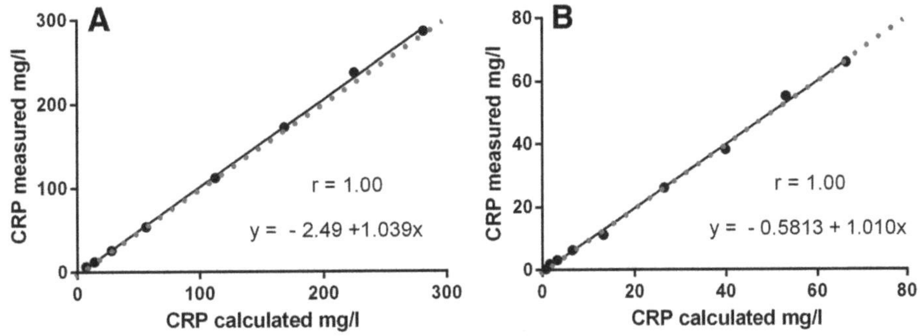

Fig. 1 Linearity of CRP determination at a high (**a**) and low concentration range (**b**). (**a**) Linearity under dilution for measurement of a canine serum sample originally containing 281.3 mg/l CRP. A serial dilution was performed to achieve 8 different CRP concentrations, i.e., 1.0, 0.8, 0.6, 0.4, 0.2, 0.1, 0.05, 0.025 parts of the original concentration (**b**) Linearity range of CRP determination for a canine serum sample containing 66.5 mg/l CRP. A serial dilution was performed to achieve 9 different CRP concentrations i.e., 1.0, 0.8, 0.6, 0.4, 0.2, 0.1, 0.05, 0.025, 0.0125 parts of the original concentration

in serum and heparin plasma samples (r_s = 0.995). There was a significant (*P* = 0.008), but clinically not relevant difference between the median CRP results obtained for both sample types (30.9 mg/l for lithium heparin plasma versus 31.4 mg/l for serum samples).Passing-Bablok regression equation showed a small constant error with an intercept of 0.29 and a small proportional error with a slope of 0.97 (Figure 4). Bland-Altman difference plot (Figure 5) revealed a mean bias of 4.3% between results obtained with both sample types.

Discussion

Overall, the Gentian Canine CRP Immunoassay accurately and precisely detects canine CRP similar to the previously used human-based immunoturbidimetric method on the ABX Pentra 400 clinical chemistry analyzer.

Comparisons of results of the current and previous studies evaluating the Gentian CRP test for different analyzers are shown in Table 6. As seen in the table, comparable results have been obtained for the majority of quality parameters demonstrated on the Abbott Architect c4000 [26] so that performance quality could be also confirmed for the ABX Pentra 400. There are some small differences that have the potential to be clinically relevant including a different CRP concentration at which a prozone effect occurs, a slightly different LoQ and a different linearity range (table 6). The evaluation on the Olympus AU600 revealed a LoQ lying between the values of the other two studies (table 6). Linearity and prozone effect were not investigated in comparably high ranges as performed in the other studies. It remains unclear if the differences between the studies are due to pre-analytic or analytic factors. As such, evaluation of these discrepant quality parameters for different types of analyzer across laboratories is recommended. The main discrepancy between the current and the study by Hillström et al. is the CRP concentration at which a prozone effect is seen which is markedly higher (1200 mg/l) in the previous than in the current study (676 mg/l). Muñoz-Prieto et al. mentioned the prozone effect to occur above a CRP level of 400 mg/l but did not

Table 2 Linearity and recovery rates of CRP measurements in a clinically relevant range of 7.0–281.3 mg/l after serial dilution of a canine serum sample containing 281.3 mg/l CRP

Dilution Factor	Expected concentration [mg/l]	Mean measured concentration[mg/l]	Recovery [%]	Bias[%]	% bias < TE_{des} (29.6%)	% bias < TE_{opt} (14.8%)
0.025	7.0	6.9	97.6	−2.4	Yes	Yes
0.05	14.1	12.5	88.9	−11.1	Yes	Yes
0.1	28.1	26.1	92.9	−7.1	Yes	Yes
0.2	56.3	54.1	96.1	−3.9	Yes	Yes
0.4	112.5	112.3	99.8	−0.2	Yes	Yes
0.6	168.8	172.3	102.1	2.2	Yes	Yes
0.8	225.0	237.3	105.4	5.4	Yes	Yes
1	281.3	286.2	101.7	1.7	Yes	Yes

Recovery rates not fulfilling the quality specifications of 80–120% are marked in bold letters as well as % bias between expected and measured mean CRP concentration exceeding the desired (TE_{des}) and optimal total allowable error (TE_{opt}) reported previously [32].

Table 3 Linearity and recovery rates of CRP measurements at a lower concentration range of 0.8–66.5 mg/l obtained after serial dilution of a canine serum sample containing 66.5 mg/l CRP

Dilution Factor	Expected concentration [mg/l]	Mean measured concentration[mg/l]	Recovery [%]	Bias[%]	% bias < TE_{des} (29.6%)	% bias < TE_{opt} (14.8%)
0.0125	0.8	0.3	**36.1**	**−63.9**	**No**	**No**
0.025	1.7	2.0	**122.5**	22.5	Yes	**No**
0.05	3.3	3.3	98.4	−1.6	Yes	Yes
0.1	6.7	6.4	95.7	−4.3	Yes	Yes
0.2	13.3	11.2	84.3	−15.7	Yes	Yes
0.4	26.6	26.2	98.6	−1.4	Yes	Yes
0.6	39.9	38.1	95.6	−4.4	Yes	Yes
0.8	53.2	55.3	103.9	3.9	Yes	Yes
1	66.5	65.9	99.2	−0.8	Yes	Yes

For quality specifications regarding recovery rate and % bias, see Table 2.

evaluate higher levels [28]. The term prozone effect describes the event of false low values of the analyte in immunoassays due to an excess of the analyte and is based on the saturation curve of the antibody binding capacity for antigen. The high number of analyte particles inhibits the formation of antigen-antibody complexes as all binding sites of the antibody are already occupied by antigen. This mechanism can lead to a false low signal detected by turbidimetry [36]. Regarding the origin of the markedly different prozone effect observed here and in the previous study, pre-analytic factors such as pipetting errors are considered an unlikely cause. However, analytical factors including analyzer performance, variations in test application or differences between variable batches of the test are a likely explanation for the discrepant prozone effect between the studies. Marked batch-specific differences in test performance due to manufacturing tolerances have been previously observed for the human Randox CRP assay when applied for canine specimens [23, 24]. However, the marked variation between different batches of the CRP assay was mainly caused by the highly variable cross-reactivity between anti-human-CRP antibodies applied in the test and canine CRP. In a canine species-specific CRP test, such high variation is unlikely, however, differences between various batches have to be evaluated in future studies. Another possible explanation would be a variation between different batches of calibrators which could influence the calibration curve in detail and therefore cause small differences in CRP values reported. It is a limitation of this study that it was not possible to directly compare the performance of both analyzers using the same batch of test reagents, calibrators and samples to exclude batch related variances. The instrument settings of the different analyzers used may contribute to a variation of the CRP-concentration causing a prozone effect. If the recommended standard instrument settings [37] are used, however, no major differences between the settings can be found. There is no pre-dilution of the sample by both analyzers which could potentially influence a prozone effect. Moreover, minor differences between the analyzers such as a minimally different measuring wave length (600 nm for the ABX Pentra 400, 604 nm for Abbott Architect c4000) are unlikely to have a major impact on the occurrence of a prozone effect.

The use of latex particles reduces prozone effects [36] as well as an endpoint measurement instead of a kinetic analysis, but both factors were constant here as the same assay was used on both analyzers.

In contrast, a different reagent volume and ratio of reagent to sample volume (270 μl of reagent 1, 75 μl of reagent 2, 3 μl sample volume for the ABX Pentra 400; 270 μl of reagent 1, 70 μl of reagent 2, 2 μl sample volume for Abbott Architect c4000) may be a possible explanation for different CRP concentrations at which a prozone effect occurs but it remains questionable if it is

Table 4 Interference effects of hemoglobin, bilirubin and lipid (soya bean oil) on CRP measurement performed with the new automated species-specific immunoturbidimetric assay

Interferent	$CRP_{control}$ [mg/l] ± SD	CRP_{test} [mg/l] ± SD	Mean bias [mg/l]	% bias	% bias < TE_{des} (29.6%)	% bias < TE_{opt} (14.8%)
Hemoglobin 5 g/l	33.7 ± 0.7	34.3 ± 1	0.57	1.7	Yes	Yes
Bilirubin 800 mg/l	34.8 ± 0.6	34.9 ± 1	0.13	0.37	Yes	Yes
Soy bean emulsion 10 g/l	32.7 ± 0.2	34.4 ± 1	1.63	5.0	Yes	Yes

Test samples (CRP_{test}) with a mean CRP value of 35.5 mg/l spiked with the interfering substances were measured in triplicates and compared to control samples ($CRP_{control}$) spiked with equal amounts of the diluent used in the test sample. %Bias for the interfering substance was considered acceptable when it was < desired total allowable error (TE_{des}) and excellent when it was < optimal total allowable error (TE_{opt}) reported previously [32].

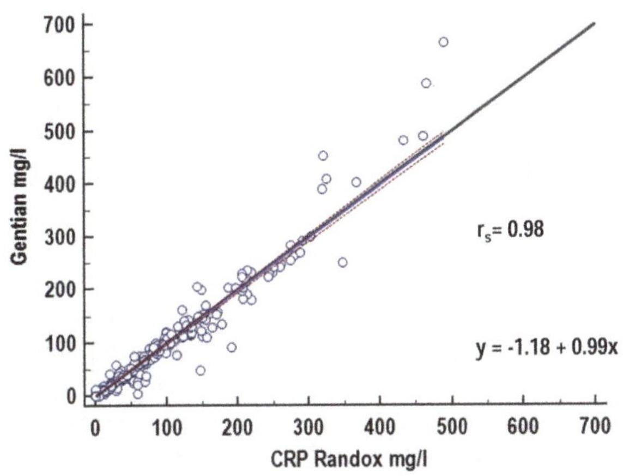

Fig. 2 Passing-Bablok regression analysis for canine C-reactive protein determined in canine serum samples by use of a species-specific immunoturbidimetric assay (Gentian Canine CRP Immunoassay) in comparison to a previously validated human based immunoturbidimetric test system (Randox Canine CRP assay) run with a dog calibrator. The solid blue line illustrates the regression equation with its 95%-confidence intervals (brown dotted line). The thin solid grey line represents the identity line consistent with a perfect correlation of the two methods

the only explanation for the major differences between prozone effects observed in the different studies. Although CRP concentrations >680 mg/l are extremely rare, septic dogs have been occasionally shown to have high CRP ranges of up to 632 mg/l [6] and in dogs with

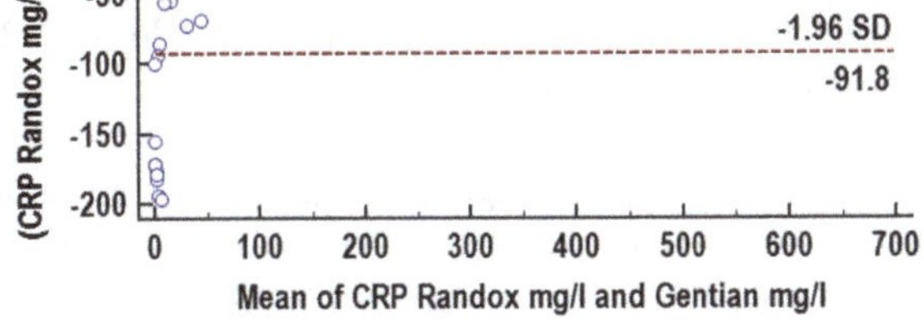

Fig. 3 Bland-Altman difference plot for canine C-reactive protein measured in canine serum samples with a new species-specific immunoturbidimetric assay (Gentian Canine CRP Immunoassay) in comparison to a validated human based test system (Randox Canine CRP assay). The solid blue line demonstrates the mean % bias, the thin solid grey line is consistent with the identity line. The dashed brown lines show the limits of agreement, which are defined as the mean difference plus and minus 1.96 times the standard deviation (SD). The solid red line indicates the desired total allowable error (TE_{des}) of 29.6% [32]. A small bias of 5.2% with a confidence interval of 95% (green dotted lines) is present

Table 5 Observed total allowable error (TE_{obs} %) calculated at four different CRP levels taking the coefficient of variation (CV) and the bias of 5.2% derived from the method validation study under consideration

Level	A	B	C	D
CRP concentration mg/l	7.2	58.8	103.9	272.1
$CV_{Between\text{-}run}$ %	7.84	2.14	0.88	1.83
TE_{obs} %	**20.9**	9.5	7.0	8.9
$TE_{obs} < TE_{des}$	Yes	Yes	Yes	Yes
$TE_{obs} < TE_{opt}$	**No**	Yes	Yes	Yes

TE_{obs} was < desired total error (TE_{des}) of 29.6% [32] for all CRP concentration levels. TE_{obs} % results exceeding the optimal TE (TE_{opt}) of 14.8% [32] are marked in bold letters.

snake envenomation even CRP concentrations above 900 mg/l were detected [38].As the prozone effect was shown to occur above a CRP concentration of 680 mg/l, the issue of false low results in patients with these rarely occurring extremely high CRP values is a consideration. A correlation with other clinical and laboratory parameters is therefore mandatory to detect samples needing a pre-dilution before measurement.

The LoQ determined in the current study was slightly lower than the LoQ determined in previous validation studies [26, 28] (Table 6). In the current study, the LoQ was derived solely from the replication experiment, i.e. the quality goal was based on the CV_{des} published in the addendum of the allowable total error guidelines of the ASVCP [32] that had to be <12.16%. Muñoz-Prieto et al. used a higher CV of <20% as decision criterion [28]. The LoQ in the previous study by Hillström et al. was obtained from the linearity experiment taking both the CV and the bias between expected and measured values into consideration, i.e. the quality goal was based on the

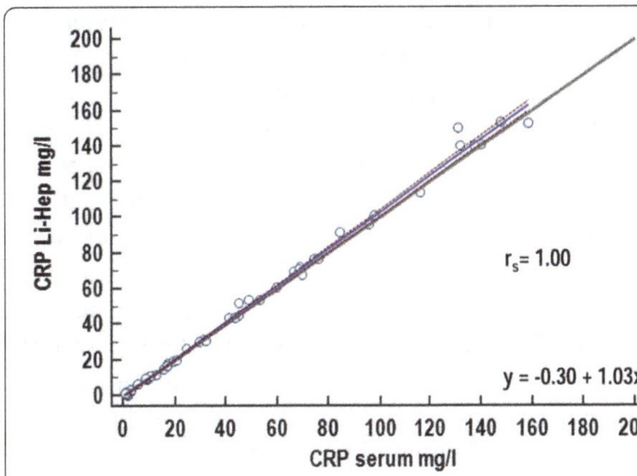

Fig. 4 Passing-Bablok regression analysis detailing the comparison between results of canine C-reactive protein (CRP) determined in either serum samples or lithium heparin samples (Li-Hep) with the Gentian Canine CRP Immunoassay. The solid blue line illustrates the regression with its 95%-confidence intervals (brown dotted line). The diagonal grey line is consistent with the identity line

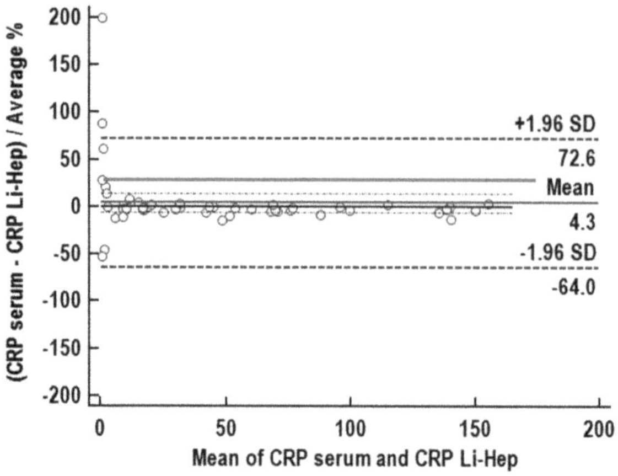

Fig. 5 Bland-Altman difference plot for canine C-reactive protein (CRP) measured in canine serum samples and canine lithium heparin (Li-Hep) samples with a Gentian Canine CRP Immunoassay. The black line is consistent with the zero line. The blue line indicates the mean bias and its 95%-confidence interval (green dotted line). The dotted brown line is consistent with the ±1.96 standard deviation (SD) of the mean absolute bias indicating the limits of agreement. The red line indicates the desired maximum total allowable error (TE_{des}) of 29.6% [32] for measurement of canine CRP

TE_{des} also published in the ACVCP guidelines. While both approaches are justified, it has to be considered that using the TE_{des} - and thus both bias and CV - is a more stringent approach than just applying CV_{des} and is therefore the most likely explanation for the LoQ set at a higher CRP concentration than in the current study (6.8 mg/l and 4.0 mg/l, Table 6). When regarding the results published previously, a SD of 0.39 mg/l was observed at a CRP concentration of 6.8 mg/l, consistent with a CV of 5.5% which would have fulfilled the quality goal of the current study. While a similar study design would have been preferable to allow an exact comparison between both analyzers and thus the true analyzer-dependent effect, both studies have been planned independently from each other in overlapping periods of time.

Possible contributing factors to differences between the studies might be also pre-analytical errors, especially due to pipetting as well as the impact of the analyzer. Also the LoQ determined by Muñoz-Prieto et al. is slightly higher (Table 6) which may be due to preanalytical or analyzer dependent conditions or influenced by the exact CRP levels used to evaluate the limit. However, the differences in LoQs observed in all three studies are rather academic in nature than of true clinical relevance as the clinical decision limit to differentiate between healthy dogs or dogs with and without systemic inflammation was 16.8 mg/l [38] and thus well above the LoQs found here and in the previous investigation.

For CRP concentrations above the LoQ of 4 mg/l, intra-assay and inter-assay CVs ranging between 0.68–12.2% and 0.88–7.84% respectively were comparable to or lower than CVs reported in previous studies evaluating human assays for canine specimens. Evaluated human assays included the Bayer CRP assay (Bayer CRP TIA' Bayer plc, Newbury, Berkshire, United Kingdom: inter- and intra-assay CVs 5.2% - 10.8% and 3% - 10.2% [22]; the Randox CRP assay with human calibrator, Randox Laboratories Ltd., Crumlin, United Kingdom: inter- and intra-assay CVs with human calibrator: 1% - 10% and 18% [23]; the Randox CRP assay with canine calibrator, Randox Laboratories Ltd., Crumlin, United Kingdom: intra-assay CV: 0.7% - 2.1% (own unpublished data); and the Olympus CRP assay, CRP OSR 6147, Olympus Life and Material Science Europe GmbH, Lismeehan, O'Callaghan's Mills, Ireland 6147: inter- and intra-assay CVs: both <10% [39]). When regarding solely canine species specific CRP assays, inter- and intra-assay CVs obtained for the Gentian CRP test here and in the previous investigation by Hillström et al. (Table 6) were markedly lower than for a commercially available canine CRP ELISA test kit and this can be attributed to the higher variation observed in manual methods (Phase Range canine CRP, Tridelta Development Ltd., Kildare, Republic of Ireland: inter- and intra-assay CVs: 6.9% - 10.1% and 7.5% - 29%) [18]. Muñoz-Prieto et al. showed a similarly low intra-assay CV of 1.0–1.3% for the Gentian CRP test at CRP ranges ≥50 mg/l and an only slightly higher inter-assay CV of 4.1–4.7% (Table 6) still lying below the data of the ELISA test. For a previously developed automated immunoturbidimetric canine CRP assay, intra- and inter-assay CVs <5% and ≤11%, respectively [40] were reported which are comparable to the CVs found in the current and previous studies. The drawback of the previous canine CRP assay, however, was that it was never commercially available. For CRP concentrations >26.5 mg/l, the CVs reported in the previous study evaluating the Gentian Canine CRP Immunoassay on the Abbott Architect c4000 were comparable to our results obtained for the clinically relevant concentration levels B-D) (Table 6). For lower CRP concentrations, intra-assay CVs were not calculated in the previous method validation study by Hillström et al. However, an SD of 0.39 mg/l was obtained for a sample with a CRP concentration of 6.8 mg/l which was consistent with a CV of 5.7% and thus comparable to the inter-assay CV observed here for a similar CRP concentration level. The CV of 5.8% observed by Muñoz-Prieto et al. for a low CRP concentration of ~10 mg/l was also comparable to our and the previous results. Excellent correlation for the Gentian CRP test with the compared assay was shown in the current and both previous studies (Table 6).

When regarding the rationale behind the method validation study performed here, assessment of TE_{obs} is an essential point of each method comparison experiment

Table 6 Comparison of observed quality parameters for the Gentian Canine CRP Immunoassay run on three different analyzers

Quality parameters Gentian CRP	ABX Pentra 400	Abbott Architect c4000[a]	Olympus AU600[b]
Limit of quantification (mg/l)	4.0[c]	6,8[d]	5.4[e]
Linearity (mg/l)	4–281	6.8–1201	~5–100
Recovery (%)	90–105	116–123	105–118
No prozone effect (mg/l)	≤ 676	≤ 1200	≤ 400
Precision			
CRP range (mg/l):	< 270; > 25	< 270; > 25	≤ 100, ≥ 50
Intra-assay CV (%)	0.7–1.9	0.5–1.7	1.0–1.3
Inter-assay CV (%)			
- Between run CV (%)	0.9–2.1	0.0–0.3	n.d.
- Between day CV (%)	1.1–4.6	1.1–1.9	4.1–4.7
No Interference up to			
- Hemoglobin (g/l)	5	10	n.d.
- Bilirubin (mg/l)	800	n.d.	n.d.
- Triglycerides (g/l)	10	10	n.d.
Method comparison			
Reference method	Randox Canine CRP assay	Randox Canine CRP assay	Olympus CRP
- r_s	0.98	0.995	0.96
- intercept	-1.18	7.3	n.d.
- slope	0.99	0.92	n.d.
- mean constant bias (%)	5.2	n.d.	41.0–70.5[f]
- TE_{obs} (%) (~CRP 7–60 mg/l)	9.5–20.9	n.d.	50.4–82.6 [f]
(~CRP > 100 mg/l)	7.0–8.9	n.d.	n.d
Sample type comparison	small impact	n.d.	n.d.

The assay was evaluated independently on the ABX Pentra 400 and compared to the data of the previous validation on the Abbott Architect c4000 and on the Olympus AU600.
Abbreviations: *n.d.* not done, *CV* coefficient of variation, TE_{obs} observed total allowable error
[a](Hillström et al. 2014) [b](Muñoz-Prieto et al.2017)[c]based on the desirable CV < 12.16%, [d]based on desirable TE < 29.58%; both published in the addendum of the Total allowable error (TE) guidelines of the American College of Veterinary Clinical Pathology [32], [e]based on CV < 20% (Escribano et al. 2012). [f] calculated based on the data of healthy and diseased dogs evaluated by Muñoz-Prieto et al.: healthy dogs: $bias\% = \frac{median\ control - median\ test}{mean\ of\ the\ medians} = \frac{2.82\frac{mg}{l} - 1.35\frac{mg}{l}}{(2.82-1.35):2} x100\% \approx 70.5\%$;
$TE_{obs} = \text{bias } \% + 2CV\% = 70.5\% + 2 \times 6.05\% = 82.6\%$
dogs with inflammatory conditions: $bias\% = \frac{73.7\frac{mg}{l} - 48.6\frac{mg}{l}}{(73.7+48.6):2} x100\% \approx 41.0\%$; $TE_{obs} = 41.0\% + 2 \times 4.70\% = 50.4\%$

[29]. In our study, observed CVs and TEs were lower than recommended desirable quality specification published in the addendum of the allowable total error guidelines of the ASVCP [32]. As the quality specifications published by the ASVCP are based on biological variation, they have been considered too stringent for method validation studies [32]. Nevertheless, they were used in this study as no other quality specifications are available for dogs. Even in human studies, quality specifications for CRP are based on biological variation. Interestingly, TE_{des} for CRP reported for people is 56.6% [41] and thus markedly higher than the recommended desirable TE_{des} given for dogs of 29.58% and even slightly higher than the recommended minimally acceptable TE for dogs of 44.37% [32]. Moreover, national recommendations are available for people such as the German Rili-BÄK quality specifications (i.e., Guidelines (= RichtLinie "Rili") of the German Federal Medical Council (= Bundesärztekammer "BÄK") [42], for which unofficial translations [43] have been performed to allow an international use. Overall, German RiliBÄK quality specifications are most stringent as only deviations of 13.5% are allowed. Interestingly, they are comparable with the recommended TE_{opt} for canine CRP of 14.79% published in the ASVCP guidelines [32]. TE_{opt} being comparable with German RiliBÄK quality specifications has been also observed previously for hematology measurands [44]. For CRP concentrations >58 mg/dl, TE_{obs} was even below these most stringent quality specifications. For lower CRP concentrations close to physiologic values, TE_{obs} was higher which was mainly based on a higher CV. Despite all advantages of the calculation of TE_{obs} (encompassing various sources of error by the inclusion of imprecision and bias) [45], it has to be considered

that also the TE_{obs} is not a perfectly objective quality parameter as it is dependent on the reference method used to calculate the bias as was shown before for hematology analyzers [44]. At the moment, there is no consensus about the methodology for bias determination for quality assessments. A high bias does not necessarily indicate a poor assay performance but might be solely induced by differences in the test protocol [46]. Only if the reference method can be considered as a current gold standard, a high bias has to be interpreted as a deficient quality performance. If the quality data of the current study are compared to the bias and TE_{obs} calculated based on data of the previous method comparison with another human based CRP assay [28] at for clinical decisions relevant CRP levels, major differences can be detected which may mainly be due to the different reference method applied (Table 6). Hillström et al. [26] used the same reference assay as was used in our study but did not provide data for an estimation of the TE_{obs}. At the moment there is no superior alternative to the assessment of TE_{obs}. Even the use of the TE as quality standard is not without limitations as there are several methods of its determination (i.e, derived on experts′ opinion, human quality specifications or biological variation [44]) which might come to different results. For the canine CRP, only a TE derived from biological variation is available, however, it has to be considered that the analytical method and the analyzer initially used for its determination have an impact on the results. Analysis of possible interferences of hemolysis, hyperbilirubinemia and lipemia on the assay performance revealed no interferences in clinically relevant concentrations up to 5 g/l hemoglobin, 800 mg/l bilirubin and 10 g/l soy bean oil (Intralipid). The absence of interference of lipemia and hemolysis with the CRP measurement was also confirmed in the previous study evaluating the species-specific Gentian Canine CRP Immunoassay [26] (Table 6), however, the potential interfering effect of bilirubin was not assessed previously. To the author's knowledge, this is the first time effects of hyperbilirubinemia are investigated on the Gentian Canine CRP Immunoassay. The lack of interference effects has to be claimed as a major advantage in CRP analysis as associated metabolic states frequently occur in patients with inflammatory and infectious diseases [26]. In contrast, significant interferences for all three substances were noted for a commercial solid phase sandwich immunoassay (Tridelta Phase Range Canine C-reactive Protein Assay; Tridelta Development, Bray, Ireland) although the low magnitude of the differences did not appear of relevance for clinical interpretation of the test [47].

To the authors′ knowledge, the effect of the sample type (heparinized plasma as an alternative to serum) has not been evaluated before for the Gentian Canine CRP Immunoassay. However, there are data available for the dog-specific CRP ELISA (Tridelta Phase Range Canine C-reactive Protein Assay, Tridelta Development, Bray, Ireland). As in our study, there was no major difference (P = 0.008) in CRP results measured in heparin plasma or serum, although in contrast to our findings, the results tended to be slightly but insignificantly higher in heparin plasma than in serum [47]. As CRP measurements in heparin plasma showed a similar CV than those performed in serum samples, it can be concluded that both heparin plasma and serum can be used. Due to the small bias, however, follow-up examinations should be ideally performed in the same sample type.

Conclusion

The results of this study are comparable to the findings observed during the previous evaluation of the canine species-specific CRP test run on different analyzers [26, 28]. The good performance of the test enables its application to several types of large bench top analyzers. However the discrepant findings between the current and previous studies such as the CRP concentration at which a prozone effect occurs, linearity range and LoQ should be specifically evaluated for each analyzer and laboratory performing the test.

Acknowledgements

We thank Julia Klotz (scil animal care company GmbH, Viernheim, Germany) for her contribution in sample measurements.

Ethics approval

The study was conducted in accordance with the German Animal Welfare Act (Article 8) and the competent authority was informed. According to the information of our ethics committee (Regierungspräsidium Giessen, Dezernat 54, Wetzlar, Germany, ethics committee number: GI 17/18), a particular approval for the study was not needed, because the study itself was not the indication of blood sampling and did not require taking an additional amount of blood. The healthy dogs included in this study where presented in the Department of Veterinary Clinical Sciences in Giessen, Germany, either for annual health checks or blood donation. For the diseased dogs the measurement of CRP was part of the routine clinical chemical profile, whereby a 1.2 cm^3 serum tube for measurement of CRP and a 1.2 cm^3 heparin tube for measurement of the remainder clinical chemical measurands was required. In case of the samples obtained from the School of Veterinary Medicine, University of Liège, Liège, Belgium, only residual sample material was used.

Funding

The authors received the following financial support for the research, authorship, and/or publication of this article: Assay development was sponsored by the German Federal Ministry of Education and Research (promotional reference 01QE1110).

The Gentian Canine CRP Immunoassay including species-specific controls and calibrators was provided by Gentian AS, Moss, Norway.

Competing interests

SK and NK are working for scil animal care company GmbH, Viernheim, Germany which owns the distribution rights of the Gentian Canine CRP Immunoassay. The commercial interests of scil animal care company GmbH did not influence the presentation or interpretation of the results of the current study.SH, SZ, KG, NB and AM declare that they have no competing interests.

Consent for publication
Not applicable.

Author details
[1]Department of Veterinary Clinical Sciences, Clinical Pathology and Clinical Pathophysiology, Justus-Liebig-University Giessen, 35392 Giessen, Germany. [2]Scil animal care company GmbH, 68519 Viernheim, Germany. [3]Department of Clinical Sciences, School of Veterinary Medicine, University of Liège, 4000 Liège, Belgium.

References

1. Higgins MA, Berridge BR, Mills BJ, Schultze AE, Gao H, Searfoss GH, et al. Gene expression analysis of the acute phase response using a canine microarray. Toxicol Sci. 2003;74:470–84.
2. Cerón JJ, Eckersall PD, Martínez-Subiela S. Acute phase proteins in dogs and cats: current knowledge and future perspectives. Vet Clin Pathol. 2005;34: 85–99.
3. Eckersall PD, Bell R. Acute phase proteins: biomarkers of infection and inflammation in veterinary medicine. Vet J. 2010;185:23–7.
4. Torrente C, Manzanilla EG, Bosch L, Fresno L, Rivera Del Alamo M, Andaluz A, et al. Plasma iron, C-reactive protein, albumin, and plasma fibrinogen concentrations in dogs with systemic inflammatory response syndrome. J Vet Emerg Crit Care (San Antonio). 2015;25:611–9.
5. Burton SA, Honor DJ, Mackenzie AL, Eckersall PD, Markham RJ, Horney BS. C-reactive protein concentration in dogs with inflammatory leukograms. Am J Vet Res. 1994;1994
6. Gebhardt C, Hirschberger J, Rau S, Arndt G, Krainer K, Schweigert FJ, et al. Use of C-reactive protein to predict outcome in dogs with systemic inflammatory response syndrome or sepsis. J Vet Emerg Crit Care (San Antonio). 2009;19:450–8.
7. McClure V, van Schoor M, Thompson PN, Kjelgaard-Hansen M, Goddard A. Evaluation of the use of serum C-reactive protein concentration to predict outcome in puppies infected with canine parvovirus. JAVMA (Journal of the American Veterinary Medical Association). 2013;243:361–6.
8. Martínez-Subiela S, Tecles F, Eckersall PD, Cerón JJ. Serum concentrations of acute phase proteins in dogs with leishmaniasis. Vet Rec. 2002;150:241–4.
9. Ulutas B, Bayramli G, Ulutas PA, Karagenc T. Serum concentration of some acute phase proteins in naturally occurring canine babesiosis: a preliminary study. Vet Clin Pathol. 2005;34:144–7.
10. K-w S, Lee J-b, Ahn J-O, Lee H-w, C-y H, H-y Y, et al. C-reactive protein as an indicator of inflammatory responses to experimentally induced cystitis in dogs. J Vet Sci. 2012;13:179–85.
11. Viitanen SJ, Laurila HP, Lilja-Maula LI, Melamies MA, Rantala M, Rajamäki MM. Serum C-reactive protein as a diagnostic biomarker in dogs with bacterial respiratory diseases. J Vet Intern Med. 2014;28:84–91.
12. Tecles F, Spiranelli E, Bonfanti U, Cerón JJ, Paltrinieri S. Preliminary studies of serum acute-phase protein concentrations in hematologic and neoplastic diseases of the dog. J Vet Intern Med. 2005;19:865–70.
13. Kjelgaard-Hansen M, Jensen AL, Houser GA, Jessen LR, Kristensen AT. Use of serum C-reactive protein as an early marker of inflammatory activity in canine type II immune-mediated polyarthritis: case report. Acta Vet Scand. 2006;48:9.
14. Bathen-Noethen A, Carlson R, Menzel D, Mischke R, Tipold A. Concentrations of acute-phase proteins in dogs with steroid responsive meningitis-arteritis. J Vet Intern Med. 2008;22:1149–56.
15. Nielsen L, Toft N, Eckersall PD, Mellor DJ, Morris JS. Serum C-reactive protein concentration as an indicator of remission status in dogs with multicentric lymphoma. J Vet Intern Med. 2007;21:1231–6.
16. Nakamura M, Takahashi M, Ohno K, Koshino A, Nakashima K, Setoguchi A, et al. C-reactive protein concentration in dogs with various diseases. J Vet Med Sci. 2008;70:127–31.
17. Dabrowski R, Wawron W, Kostro K. Changes in CRP, SAA and haptoglobin produced in response to ovariohysterectomy in healthy bitches and those with pyometra. Theriogenology. 2007;67:321–7.
18. Kjelgaard-Hansen M, Kristensen AT, Jensen AL. Evaluation of a commercially available enzyme-linked immunosorbent assay (ELISA) for the determination of C-reactive protein in canine serum. J Vet Med Series A. 2003;50:164–8.
19. Fransson BA, Bergström A, Wardrop KJ, Hagman R. Assessment of three automated assays for C-reactive protein determination in dogs. Am J Vet Res. 2007;68:1281–6.
20. Caspi D, Baltz ML, Snel F, Gruys E, Niv D, Batt RM, et al. Isolation and characterization of C-reactive protein from the dog. Immunology. 1984;53:307–13.
21. Yamamoto S, Miyaji S, Abe N, Otabe K, Furukawa E, NAIKI M. Canine C-reactive protein (CRP) does not share common antigenicity with human CRP. Vet Res Commun. 1993;17:259–66.
22. Kjelgaard-Hansen M, Jensen AL, Kristensen AT. Evaluation of a commercially available human C-reactive protein (CRP) turbidometric immunoassay for determination of canine serum CRP concentration. Vet Clin Pathol. 2003;32:81–7.
23. Klenner S, Bauer N, Moritz A. Evaluation of three automated human immunoturbidimetric assays for the detection of C-reactive protein in dogs. J Vet Diagn Invest (Journal of Veterinary Diagnostic Investigation). 2010;22:544–52.
24. Kjelgaard-Hansen M. Comments on measurement of C-reactive protein in dogs. Vet Clin Pathol. 2010;39:402.
25. Skinner JG. International standardization of acute phase proteins. Vet Clin Pathol. 2001;30:2–7.
26. Hillström A, Hagman R, Tvedten H, Kjelgaard-Hansen M. Validation of a commercially available automated canine-specific immunoturbidimetric method for measuring canine C-reactive protein. Vet Clin Pathol. 2014;43:235–43.
27. Farr AJ, Freeman KP. Quality control validation, application of sigma metrics, and performance comparison between two biochemistry analyzers in a commercial veterinary laboratory. J Vet Diagn Investig. 2008;20:536–44.
28. Munoz-Prieto A, Tvarijonaviciute A, Escribano D, Martinez-Subiela S, Ceron JJ. Use of heterologous immunoassays for quantification of serum proteins: the case of canine C-reactive protein. PLoS One. 2017;12:1–14/14.
29. Jensen AL, Kjelgaard-Hansen M. Method comparison in the clinical laboratory. Vet Clin Pathol. 2006;35:276–86.
30. Armbruster DA, Pry T. Limit of blank, limit of detection and limit of quantitation. Clin Biochem Rev. 2008:49–52.
31. Gommeren K, Desmas I, Garcia A, Bauer N, Moritz A, Roth, J, Peeters, D. Inflammatory cytokines and C-reactive protein in canine systemic inflammatory response syndrome. J Vet Emerg Crit Care (San Antonio). in press.
32. Harr KE, Flatland B, Nabity M, Freeman KP. ASVCP guidelines: allowable total error guidelines for biochemistry. Vet Clin Pathol. 2013;42:424–36.
33. Jensen AL, Kjelgaard-Hansen M. Diagnostic test validation. In: Weiss DJ, Wardrop KJ, editors. Schalm's veterinary hematology. 6th ed. Ames: Wiley-Blackwell; 2010. p. 1027–33.
34. Andreasson U, Perret-Liaudet A, van Waalwijk van Doorn, Linda JC, Blennow K, Chiasserini D, Engelborghs S, et al. A practical guide to immunoassay method validation. Front Neurol. 2015;6:179.
35. American Society for Veterinary Clinical Pathology (ASVCP). Principles of quality assurance and standards for veterinary clinical pathology. 2009. [http://www.asvcp.org/pubs/pdf/ASVCPQualityControlGuidelines.pdf]. Accessed 25 May 2017.
36. Dodig S. Interferences in quantitative immunochemical methods. Biochem Med. 2009:50–62.
37. Gentian. Application Notes. http://gentian.no/products/canine-crp/application-notes/ . Accessed 25 May 2017.
38. Christensen MB, Langhorn R, Goddard A, Andreasen EB, Moldal E, Tvarijonaviciute A, et al. Comparison of serum amyloid a and C-reactive protein as diagnostic markers of systemic inflammation in dogs. Can Vet J. 2014;55:161–8.
39. Caldin M, Tasca S, Carli E, Bianchini S, Furlanello T, Martinez-Subiela S, et al. Serum acute phase protein concentrations in dogs with hyperadrenocorticism with and without concurrent inflammatory conditions. Vet Clin Pathol. 2009;38:63–8.
40. Eckersall PD, Conner JG, Harvie J. An immunoturbidimetric assay for canine C-reactive protein. Vet Res Commun. 1991;15:17–24.
41. Ricos C, Alvarez V, Cava F, Garcia-Lario J, Hernandez A, Jimenez C, et al. Desirable biological variation database specifications - Westgard. 2014. [https://www.westgard.com/biodatabase1.htm]. Accessed 25 May 2017.
42. Bundesärztekammer. Neufassung der „Richtlinie der Bundesärztekammer zur Qualitätssicherung laboratoriumsmedizinischer Untersuchungen – Rili-BÄK". Dtsch Arztebl. 2014;111.
43. Westgard S. Rilibak - German guidelines for quality - Westgard. 2015. [https://www.westgard.com/rilibak.htm]. Accessed 25 May 2017.

44. Cook AM, Moritz A, Freeman KP, Bauer N. Quality requirements for veterinary hematology analyzers in small animals-a survey about veterinary experts' requirements and objective evaluation of analyzer performance based on a meta-analysis of method validation studies: bench top hematology analyzer. Vet Clin Pathol. 2016;
45. Lester S, Harr KE, Rishniw M, Pion P. Current quality assurance concepts and considerations for quality control of in-clinic biochemistry testing. J Am Vet Med Assoc. 2013;242:182–92.
46. Krouwer JS. Setting performance goals and evaluating Total analytical error for diagnostic assays. Clin Chem. 2002:919–27.
47. Martìnez-Subiela S, Ceron JJ. Effects of hemolysis, lipemia, hyperbilirubinemia, and anticoagulants in canine c-reactive protein, serum amyloid a, and ceruloplasmin assays. Can Vet J. 2005:625–9.

10

Non-invasive assessment of adrenocortical activity as a measure of stress in giraffe (*Giraffa camelopardalis*)

Meredith J. Bashaw[1,2*], Florian Sicks[3], Rupert Palme[4], Franz Schwarzenberger[4], Adrian S. W. Tordiffe[5,6] and Andre Ganswindt[6,7]

Abstract

Background: Numbers of giraffes are declining rapidly in their native habitat. As giraffe research and conservation efforts increase, the demand for more complete measures of the impact of conservation interventions and the effects of captive environments on animal health and welfare have risen. We compared the ability of six different enzyme immunoassays to quantify changes in fecal glucocorticoid metabolites (FGM) resulting from three sources: adrenocorticotropic hormone stimulation test, transport, and time of day that samples were collected.

Results: Two male giraffes underwent ACTH injections; all six assays detected FGM increases following injection for Giraffe 1, while only three assays detected FGM increases following injection for Giraffe 2. Consistent with other ruminant species, the two 11-oxoetiocholanolone assays (one for 11,17-dioxoandrostanes and the other for 3α,11-oxo metabolites) measured the most pronounced and prolonged elevation of FGM, while an assay for 3β,11β-diol detected peaks of smaller magnitude and duration. Both of the 11-oxoetiocholanolone assays detected significant FGM increases after transport in Giraffes 3–7, and preliminary data suggest FGM detected by the assay for 11,17-dioxoandrostanes may differ across time of day.

Conclusions: We conclude the assay for 11,17-dioxoandrostanes is the most sensitive assay tested for FGM in giraffes and the assay for FGM with a 5β-3α-ol-11-one structure is also effective. 11-oxoetiocholanolone enzyme immunoassays have now been demonstrated to be successful in a wide variety of ruminant species, providing indirect evidence that 5β-reduction may be a common metabolic pathway for glucocorticoids in ruminants. As FGM peaks were detected in at least some giraffes using all assays tested, giraffes appear to excrete a wide variety of different FGM. The assays validated here will provide a valuable tool for research on the health, welfare, and conservation of giraffes.

Keywords: ACTH challenge, Validation, Ungulate, Ruminant, Zoo, Endocrine, Adrenal physiology, Glucocorticoid, Health

Background

Giraffes (*Giraffa camelopardalis*) are currently listed as a species of least concern by the International Union for Conservation of Nature (IUCN) [1]. However, wild populations have recently suffered major declines, from an estimated 140,000 individuals to an estimated 80,000 individuals over the course of a decade, and two subspecies (*G. c. peralta* [2] and *G. c. rothschildi* [3]) are now recognized as endangered by IUCN. Against this backdrop, efforts to study and conserve wild giraffes and to ensure optimal health and welfare for captive giraffes have intensified.

Studies of wild populations are revealing that giraffes have complex social structures and habitat dynamics with implications for conservation strategies [4–7]. Giraffes' habitat preferences are shaped by energetically costly reproductive strategies, resulting in sex segregation and female habitat preferences that change during

* Correspondence: mbashaw@fandm.edu
[1]Wildlife Reproductive Centre, Taronga Conservation Society of Australia, Dubbo, NSW, Australia
[2]Department of Psychology, Franklin & Marshall College, Lancaster, PA, USA
Full list of author information is available at the end of the article

lactation [8, 9]. Zoos maintain a population of captive giraffes that could be used as a hedge against extinction, but at the turn of the century some captive giraffes exhibited poor health [10–12] and behavioral problems [13–15]. Zoos have worked successfully to improve giraffe health and reduce abnormal repetitive behaviors [15–17], but these problems still persist at low rates so it is unclear whether captive environments are yet optimal for housing giraffes. The adrenal system plays a role in energy regulation [18], reproduction [19], immune function [20], and physiological responses to disturbance [21], so an efficient and ideally noninvasive measure of adrenal responses in giraffes could shed important light on population dynamics, conservation efforts, health, and welfare in both *in* and *ex situ* populations. To the best of our knowledge no data are currently available on hypothalamic-pituitary-adrenal (HPA) axis functioning in giraffes.

Measuring an individual's physiological arousal provides a window into how that individual animal is coping with its environment, whether in the wild or captivity. As Webster [22] describes, arousal produced by exciting or stressful stimuli results in an activation of the HPA axis, which results in the release of glucocorticoid hormones (GC), amongst others. GC produce a negative feedback such that once the animal is no longer excited or stressed, the HPA axis response ends and GC return to baseline levels. If the organism is unable to resolve or escape the situation, HPA axis activation continues and negative feedback systems are disrupted, resulting in prolonged elevations of GC concentrations with negative consequences for the animals' behaviour, health, and ability to respond to future events [23, 24]. In addition to within-animal changes, differences in GC levels between animals have been linked to behavioral differences that may contribute to or reflect different life history strategies [25, 26].

Fecal glucocorticoid metabolites (FGM) have become a popular measure of physiological function and welfare in a variety of species [27, 28] because they reflect adrenocortical activity over a certain time period [29] and can therefore be used to answer a wide variety of research questions. Technically, animals are not disturbed during fecal sample collection, and sampling is therefore feedback-free due to the absence of capture and handling. This is particularly beneficial for field studies, where capture and handling may be logistically challenging or cause long-term health consequences [30]. However, species-specific differences in the composition of excreted FGM and the different affinities of the antibodies used in each assay for specific FGM [31–33] require the measurement of FGM to be validated for each species [21, 29] and ideally each sex [34]. Validation is accomplished by experimentally stimulating the HPA axis using e.g., an injection of adrenocorticotrophic hormone (an ACTH challenge) or by subjecting the animal to a putative stressor (e.g., transport or aggressive interaction). These two validation techniques reveal two aspects of measurement effectiveness. Because an ACTH challenge provides direct physiological stimulation of the adrenal glands, it measures how well an assay detects an increase in GC concentrations. Subjecting an animal to a putative stressor, on the other hand, targets the degree to which the assay is sensitive enough to detect biologically-relevant changes in GC. If an assay detects increased FGM levels following the event, one can conclude both that the event was indeed stressful and that the assay is sensitive enough to detect an environmental stress of that magnitude. When using feces as a hormone matrix, these techniques allow researchers to verify that FGM measured with a particular assay reflect both increased GC concentrations and perceived stress [29].

This study aimed to demonstrate that measurement of FGM in giraffes provides a feasible and noninvasive way to assess the physiological function and affective state of individual giraffes. More specifically, this study: a) compared the ability of six different enzyme immunoassays (EIAs) to quantify changes in FGM produced by an adrenocorticotropic hormone stimulation test (ACTH challenge test) at two different sampling rates, b) measured changes in FGM concentrations in daily samples as a result of transport, a putative stressor, and c) preliminarily investigated the influence of time of day samples were collected on FGM results.

Methods

Study animals

A total of 7 giraffes were monitored in this study. Giraffe 1 was a 6-year old male South African (*Giraffa camelopardalis giraffa*) singly housed in a 4000 m^2 enclosure at the National Zoological Gardens of South Africa (NZG), Pretoria, South Africa. Giraffe 2 was a 17-year-old male hybrid-subspecies *G. camelopardalis* housed in a 10-ha exhibit with two other adult male giraffes and zebra (*Equus burchellii*), eland (*Taurotragus oryx*), forest buffalo (*Syncerus caffer nanus*), and ostrich (*Struthio camelus*) at Taronga Western Plains Zoo, Dubbo, NSW, Australia. Giraffes 3–7 were a juvenile male (3), two juvenile females (4 and 5), and two adult females (6 and 7) transported among seven German zoos (see Table 1). The study of Giraffes 3–7 consisted solely of opportunistic non-invasive collection of feces during and after transfers that were occurring for management reasons.

ACTH challenge tests

Giraffe 1 was remotely injected into the caudal thigh muscle with Synacthen Depot (Novartis) loaded into a

Table 1 Demographic and transport information for focal animals 3–7

Giraffe	Sex	Subspecies	Age at Transport (years)	Transport Type	Transport Duration[a] (h)	Samples Collected[b]	No. of Samples
3	M	*G. c. rothschildi*	1	Within-zoo	0.33	−10 to +30 d	$n = 38$
4	F	*G. c. reticulata*	3	Between-zoo	4	−38 to +41 d	$n = 37$
5	F	*G. c. reticulata*	2.5	Between-zoo	4.5	−3 to +14 d	$n = 18$
6	F	*G. c. angolensis*	10	Between-zoo	6	−8 to +38 d	$n = 38$
7	F	*G. c. angolensis*	11	Between-zoo	6	−5 to +38 d	$n = 38$

[a]The reported transport duration is the amount of time the animal was actually moving in the transport vehicle; the time to load, secure and unload the animal is not included
[b]Date range for sample collection relative to the date of transport, followed by number of samples collected. - indicates the number of days before transport and + indicates the number of days after transport

10 ml dart syringe with a 60 mm × 2 mm standard needle (Dan-Inject, Denmark) at an estimated dose 1 IU/kg at 18:00 on day 1 (21 October 2012). The animal was continuously monitored and a fecal sample (3–4 pellets) collected from each defecation beginning 12 h before the ACTH injection and continuing until 72 h post-injection. Fecal samples were frozen within 1 h of collection.

Giraffe 2 was injected with approximately 0.7 IU/kg of Synacthen Depot using two darts delivered 2 min. apart into the shoulder beginning at 12:18 on day 6 (21 May 2013). To facilitate identification of the feces, the animal was fed glitter beginning 1 week before the injection. Fecal samples were collected daily between 08:00 and 10:00 for 5 days before and 4 days after injection and transferred to a −20 °C freezer within 30 min. Fecal samples from each defecation between 20 and 28 h post-injection were also collected; these samples were placed on ice after collection and transferred to a −20 °C freezer when animal care staff were available to let the researcher out of the exhibit. All samples were frozen within 1 h of defecation except two: one was on ice for 64 min and a second for 110 min before freezing.

Transport

Giraffes 3–7 were monitored opportunistically during management-necessitated transfers between zoos or between exhibits within a zoo. Transports occurred in winter (Giraffes 3 and 5), summer (Giraffe 4), and autumn (Giraffes 6 and 7). For each transport, giraffes were loaded onto a vehicle, driven for at least 20 min (individual transport lengths given in Table 1), and unloaded into an unfamiliar location. Fecal samples were collected daily at approximately 11:00 for at least 3 days before and 14 days after transport (sampling details given in Table 1). Fecal samples were collected within 1 h after defecation and directly transferred to a −20 °C freezer.

Effects of collection time

To assess the effect of time of day on FGM concentration, samples were collected from Giraffe 1 immediately following every defecation over a 48-h period. A total of 32 samples were collected beginning at 06:00 on 17 October 2012 and ending at 06:00 on 19 October 2012. Fecal samples were frozen within 1 h of collection.

Sample processing and extraction procedures

Samples collected during the ACTH challenge trials as well as for determining effects of collection time were pulverized, mixed, and 0.1 - 0.11 g extracted by adding 3 ml 80 % methanol and vortexed for 15 min. Feces were then pelleted by centrifuging at 2000 g for 15 min and the supernatant decanted into polypropylene tubes for storage. For shipping or storage at room temperature, 0.5 ml of each fecal sample's extract were transferred into Eppendorf tubes and air-dried [35]. Subsequent steroid analyses were conducted at the Wildlife Reproductive Centre, Taronga Conservation Society, Dubbo, NSW Australia.

Samples collected for monitoring the effect of transport were extracted by weighing 0.495–0.505 g of wet feces, adding 5 ml 80 % methanol, vortexing for 30 min, and centrifuging at 2500 g for 15 min [35]. Sample processing and assays were performed at the University of Veterinary Medicine, Vienna, Austria.

Assay procedures

Fecal extracts resulting from the ACTH challenge test samples were measured for immunoreactive FGM concentrations using six different enzyme immunoassays (EIAs), namely a cortisol, corticosterone, 11-oxoetiocholanolone I (detecting 11,17-dioxoandrostanes; 11,17-DOA), 11-oxoetiocholanolone II (detecting FGM with a 5β-3α-ol-11-one structure; 3α,11-oxo-CM), 5α-pregnane-3β,11β,21-triol-20-one (measuring 3β,11β-diol-CM), and an 11β-hydroxyetiocholanolone EIA (measuring 3α,11β-diol-CM). Detailed assay characteristics, including references providing full descriptions of the assay components and cross-reactivities, are provided in Table 2. Samples collected for monitoring the effect of transport and collection time were assessed using only the two 11-oxoetiocholanolone EIAs, which most effectively identified FGM peaks following ACTH administration (Fig. 2).

Table 2 Details of the enzyme immunoassays (EIAs) used

EIA (source laboratory, abbrev.)	Sensitivity (ng/g feces)	Intra-assay CV[a]	Inter-assay CV[b]	References
Cortisol (Munro, R4866)	2.3	4.9 %	3.7 %, $n = 4$	[77, 78]
Corticosterone (Munro, CJM06)	17.6	8.1 %	8.1 %, $n = 4$	[79, 80]
11-oxoetiocholanolone I (Palme, 72a, 11,17-DOA)	7.2	4.8 %	12.3 %, $n = 5$	[63, 81]
11-oxoetiocholanolone II (Palme, 72T, 3α,11-oxo-CM)	9.6	8.8 %	13.8 %, $n = 4$	[61, 67]
5α-pregnane-3β,11β,21-triol-20-one (Palme, 37e, 3β,11β-diol-CM)	9.6	6.1 %	9.5 %, $n = 4$	[34]
11ß-hydroxyetiocholanolone (Palme, 69a, 3α,11β-diol-CM)	48.0	9.1 %	9.7 %, $n = 4$	[54, 82]

[a]Intra-assay CV = SD/mean percent binding for 10 wells each of high- and low-concentrated pool samples, averaged across concentrations
[b]Inter-assay CV = SD/mean percent binding for standards (72T, 69a) or high- and low-concentrated pool samples (other assays), averaged across concentrations, n indicates number of plates used

To determine whether giraffe fecal extracts contained FGM that would bind to the antibody in each EIA in a way comparable to its standard, we first created a fecal extract pool consisting of equal volumes of 10 samples collected for the ACTH challenge experiment: 2 pre-injection, 2 at the expected peak (12–48 h post-injection), and 1 post-peak sample from each giraffe. For all assays, parallelism was then demonstrated by comparing serial dilutions of a fecal extract pool to serial dilutions of the steroid standard against which the antibody was raised [36]. Parallelism was acceptable for all assays but best for the two 11-oxoetiocholanolone assays; the correlation between percent binding for standards and samples within each assay was at least $r = 0.96$ ($Mean_r = 0.98$, Fig. 1). Using these data, appropriate dilution for samples in each assay was identified by determining what dilution produced close to 50 % sample binding for the pool.

Data analysis

For data from both the ACTH challenges and the transport events, the range of baseline FGM for each individual as measured by each assay was determined by iteratively calculating a mean + 2SD threshold of concentration based on all samples collected from that individual [33, 37, 38]. At each step, samples that fell above the threshold were excluded and the mean and SD were recalculated until all remaining samples fell below the threshold and could be considered baseline values. After the baseline range was established, the post-injection peak was defined as the longest series of consecutive post-injection samples above the final mean + 2SD threshold. Data are available in Additional file 1.

Once the post-injection peak had been identified, three measures of assay effectiveness were computed. First, we found the duration of the peak by computing the difference between the times the first and last peak samples were collected. This allowed us to assess how useful the assay would be in identifying FGM peaks under field or zoo conditions with limited sampling frequency. Second, we calculated the fold difference by taking the concentration of the highest sample in the peak and dividing it by the mean concentration of the baseline samples. Third, we determined Z_{peak}, the height of the peak as measured by the number of standard deviations away from the baseline mean, by taking the concentration of the highest sample in the peak, subtracting the mean concentration of the baseline samples, and dividing the result by the standard deviation of the baseline samples.

To assess the effects of time of day, we conducted a simple linear regression in which time since sunrise was used to predict FGM, and then a hierarchical linear regression in which time since sunrise was used to predict FGM after controlling for the day on which the samples were collected. Assays for which the addition of time since sunrise significantly increased R^2 after the effect of collection day was accounted for were considered to detect a diurnal pattern. Data are available in Additional file 1 (see Giraffe 1).

Results

ACTH challenge test

All EIAs showed acceptable performance characteristics with giraffe samples (Table 2). Results of the assay comparison for ACTH samples are shown in Table 3 and Fig. 2. For both giraffes, the two antibodies raised against 11-oxoetiocholanolone (measuring 11,17-DOA and 3α,11-oxo-CM) performed best by all measures, identifying elevations in FGM levels above individual baseline for longer periods of time with respective peak values being comparatively higher than those determined by other assays (Fig. 2). The 3β,11β-diol-CM assay also performed acceptably for both individuals, though respective peak values were not as distinct from baseline as the ones determined by the 11-oxoetiocholanolone assays (Fig. 2). The cortisol, corticosterone, and 3α,11β-diol-CM EIAs detected peaks in Giraffe 1 but not Giraffe 2, and the peaks detected were substantially shorter in duration and differed less from baseline values (Table 3). One sample from Giraffe 2 was stored on ice for almost 2 h, which could have affected FGM [29, 39], but

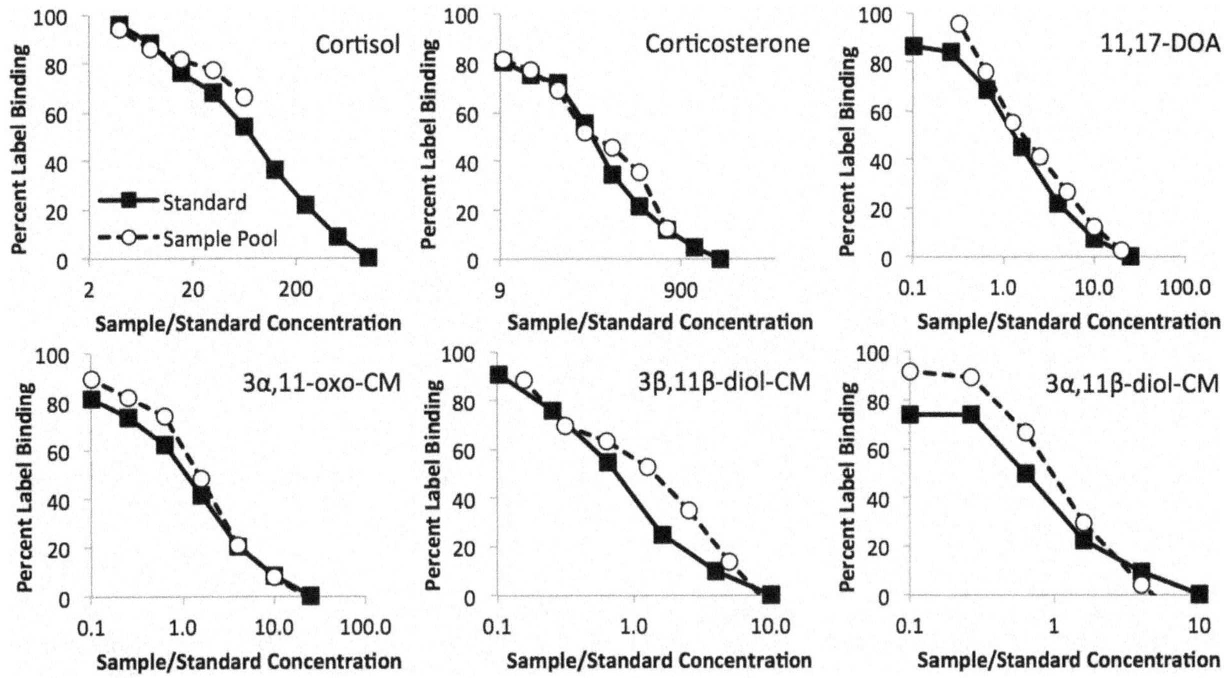

Fig. 1 Parallelism of serial dilutions of a fecal extract pool with standards for each of the six EIAs. Correlations between percent binding for standards and samples within each assay were at least $r = 0.96$

patterns of change over time were smooth, peaks detected in 11,17-DOA, 3α,11-oxo-CM, and 3β,11β-diol-CM included both samples held on ice and those frozen immediately, and this sample did not have the highest or lowest FGM for any assay.

Transport

As samples from the transported giraffes were collected once per day and only the two 11-oxoetiocholanolone EIAs identified peaks lasting more than 24 h following ACTH challenge, we selected these two EIAs to assess the influence of transportation on FGM levels. Post-transport peaks were identified in both 11,17-DOA and 3α,11-oxo-CM in all 5 giraffes tested, regardless of the sex of the giraffe (Fig. 3).

The responses of individual giraffe as measured by both 11-oxoetiocholanolone EIAs are presented in Table 4. Three of the five giraffes showed peak 11,17-DOA concentrations the day after transport and the longest delay to peak values was 2 days. Peak duration averaged 4.2 days (range: 2–6 days) and intensity was comparable to the ACTH challenge (Fold difference:

Table 3 Assay comparison for the ACTH challenge tests

		Enzyme immunoassay targeting					
Animal	Measure	Cortisol	Cortico-sterone	11,17- DOA	3α,11-oxo-CM	3β,11β-diol-CM	3α,11β-diol-CM
Giraffe 1[a]	Latency to Peak	13.5 h	50.5 h	13.5 h	11.5 h	13.5 h	30.0 h
	Peak Duration (no. of peak samples)	6 h $n=4$	<2 h $n=1$	37 h $n=24$	39 h $n=25$	22 h $n=12$	5 h $n=3$
	Fold Increase ($X_{peak}/M_{baseline}$)	2.6	1.6	33.4	18.2	4.1	2.6
	Z_{peak}	7.4 sd	2.2 sd	64.4 sd	79.6 sd	13.6 sd	3.4 sd
Giraffe 2[b]	Latency to Peak	no peak	no peak	20.5 h	24.0 h	23.2 h	no peak
	Peak Duration (no. of peak samples)			7 h $n=4$	<5 h $n=1$	5 h $n=3$	
	Fold Increase ($X_{peak}/M_{baseline}$)			9.6	2.9	2.9	
	Z_{peak}			17.1 sd	3.3 sd	11.3 sd	

[a]For Giraffe 1, fecal samples collected from every defecation from 12 h pre-injection to 72 h post-injection

[b]For Giraffe 2, fecal samples collected daily (between 8 am and 10 am) for 5 days before and 4 days after injection, as well as from every defecation between 20 h and 28 h post-injection

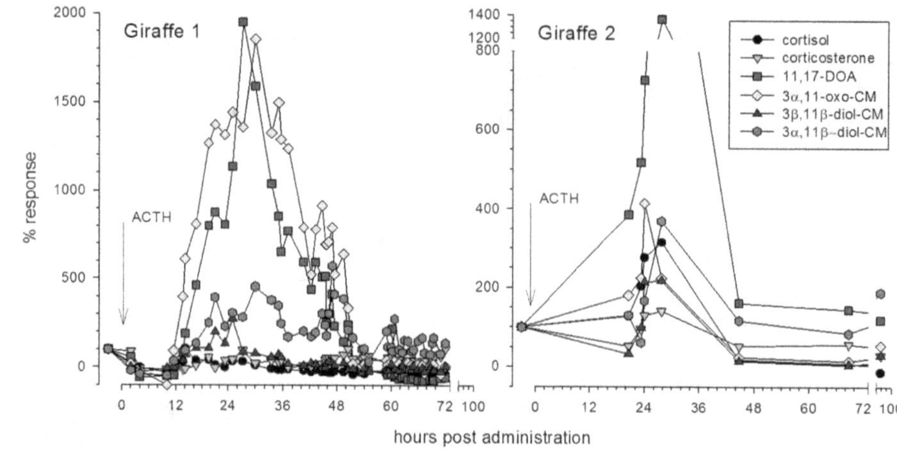

Fig. 2 ACTH response of the two giraffes as measured by each of the six EIAs. Percent response was calculated by setting the individual median FGM value for pre-injection samples from each giraffe at 100 % and calculating the change in FGM levels for each post-injection sample. Vertical arrow marks injection time

Median = 5.99, range: 2.33–8.00; Z_{peak}: Median = 12.24, range: 4.74–20.10). As in the ACTH challenge, 11,17-DOA varied less within the baseline than 3α,11-oxo-CM. Peak 3α,11-oxo-CM occurred at a longer delay; only two of the five giraffes showed peaks the day after transport and the longest delay to peak was 6 days. Peaks in 3α,11-oxo-CM were less prolonged (Mean = 2.4 days, range: 1–3 days) but of similar overall intensity (Fold difference: Median = 2.78, range: 2.48–5.19; Z_{peak}: Median = 4.37, range: 3.26–16.87). The two juvenile females (Giraffes 4 and 5) had exceptionally high 3α,11-oxo-CM concentrations in the three days following transport.

Effects of collection time

11,17-DOA and 3α,11-oxo-CM were affected by collection time. With the 11,17-DOA EIA, time since sunrise significantly predicted higher FGM concentrations (R^2 = 0.38, $F_{1,30} = 18.05$, $p < 0.001$, $\beta = 0.61$, t = 4.25, Fig. 4), and this relationship was still significant even when collection day was controlled ($\Delta R^2 = 0.37$, $F_{1,29} = 26.49$, $p < 0.001$, $\beta = 0.61$, t = 5.15). 3α,11-oxo-CM revealed a pulsatile excretion pattern, but it was not significantly predicted by time since sunrise (without controlling collection day: $p = 0.364$; controlling collection day: $p = 0.345$, Fig. 4).

Discussion

Assay selection

We demonstrated that FGM changes produced by both physiological stimulation (ACTH) and an environmental event (transport) could be reliably measured in daily fecal samples from giraffes using two 11-oxoetiocholanolone EIAs (measuring FGM with a 3α,11-oxo and 11,17-DOA structure, respectively). 11-oxoetiocholanolone EIAs best identified FGM peaks under field or zoo conditions where sampling frequency is limited. These assays found more samples with significant FGM elevation, better discriminated peak samples from baseline samples, identified a transport response with once-daily sampling, and were effective for both males and females. The other four EIAs we tested detected an increase in FGM following the ACTH challenge in at least one animal, but did not provide as clear and reliable peak detection and so were not as sensitive or consistent as the 11-oxoetiocholanolone EIAs.

For the ACTH challenge with more frequent sampling and larger dose (Giraffe 1: 1 IU/kg), both 11-oxoetiocholanolone EIAs had peaks of similar duration and intensity as measured by fold difference. However, the Z_{peak} for 3α,11-oxo-CM was larger because there was less variability among baseline samples. With less frequent sampling and lower ACTH dose (Giraffe 2: 0.7 IU/kg), peak duration and intensity were reduced for both assays; in fact, the peak in 3α,11-oxo-CM was identified in only a single sample. We did not collect blood samples following ACTH administration to verify an increase in serum GC because it would have required anesthetizing the giraffe. We therefore cannot rule out the possibility that Giraffe 2's ACTH challenge did not sufficiently increase circulating GC, resulting in the failure of the Cortisol, Corticosterone, and 11ß-hydroxyetiocholanolone EIAs to detect a FGM peak. However, given that the other three assays did detect a peak it is unlikely the ACTH challenge failed entirely. ACTH injections produce a dose-dependent increase in GC that affects both serum GC concentration and clearance time [40, 41]. As the dose of ACTH used in these challenges was on the low end of the range used in other published

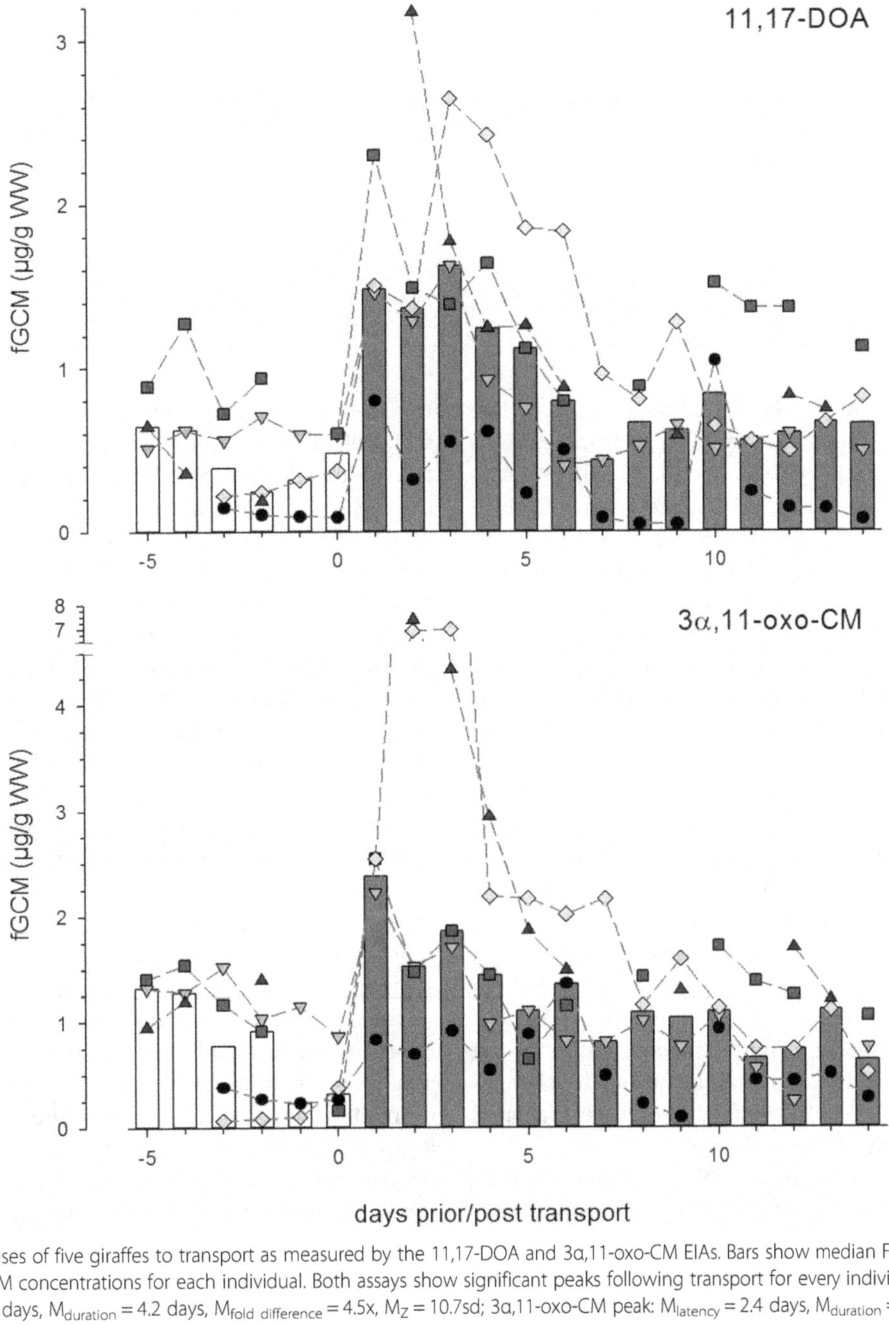

Fig. 3 FGM responses of five giraffes to transport as measured by the 11,17-DOA and 3α,11-oxo-CM EIAs. Bars show median FGM values, points and lines show FGM concentrations for each individual. Both assays show significant peaks following transport for every individual (11,17-DOA peak: $M_{latency}$ = 1.6 days, $M_{duration}$ = 4.2 days, $M_{fold\ difference}$ = 4.5x, M_Z = 10.7sd; 3α,11-oxo-CM peak: $M_{latency}$ = 2.4 days, $M_{duration}$ = 2.4 days, $M_{fold\ difference}$ = 3.8x, M_Z = 7.4sd)

challenges (1 and 0.7 IU/kg here; 0.5 to 12.5 IU/kg in [42]; 0.5 to 31 IU/kg in [43]), and ACTH was administered over a span of less than 2 min, the resulting increase in GC would be expected to be of shorter duration and perhaps lower intensity than those seen in other ACTH challenge studies. In contrast to the acute GC increase produced by the ACTH challenge, transport to a new environment is a longer-duration, more substantial environmental stressor [44]. Under these conditions, both 11-oxoetiocholanolone EIAs reliably detected a peak in all animals, but 11,17-DOA peaks had more rapid onset and greater duration.

The 11-oxoetiocholanolone I and II EIAs appear to robustly measure giraffe FGM. Our experiments relied on opportunistic access to zoo-housed giraffes, so there was considerable variability in the management of and procedures applied to each individual animal. We noted possible effects of differences in ACTH dose and sampling frequency above. In addition, the two animals subjected to ACTH challenges also differed in age, housing,

Table 4 Individual giraffe's responses to transport as measured by 11-oxoetiocholanolone EIAs

EIA	Measure	Giraffe 3	Giraffe 4	Giraffe 5	Giraffe 6	Giraffe 7
11-oxoetiocholanolone I, targets 11,17- DOA	Latency to Peak	1 d	2 d	2 d	1 d	1 d
	Peak Duration	6 d	4 d	2 d	4 d	5 d
	Fold Increase ($X_{peak}/M_{baseline}$)	8.00	6.00	5.99	2.33	3.11
	Z_{peak}	20.10	12.24	6.88	4.74	13.14
11-oxoetiocholanolone II, targets 3α,11-oxo-CM	Latency to Peak	6 d	2 d	3 d	1 d	1 d
	Peak Duration	1 d	3 d	2 d	3 d	3 d
	Fold Increase ($X_{peak}/M_{baseline}$)	2.78	5.19	3.04	2.48	2.66
	Z_{peak}	3.62	16.87	3.26	4.37	5.42

climate, diet, and time of ACTH administration. While these factors likely increased variability in FGM patterns between the individuals [21, 29, 36, 45, 46], three assays (measuring 3α,11-oxo-CM, 11,17-DOA, and 3β,11β-diol-CM) reliably detected post-injection FGM increases despite these differences. Similarly, demographic factors, management, season of transport, and length of transport differed among giraffes in the transport study. This study also used a somewhat different extraction protocol than the ACTH challenge. Despite these differences, the 11-oxoetiocholanolone I and II EIAs still detected significant FGM increases as a result of transport in every animal. We noted differences in the shape of the FGM response to transport among individuals, which could be explained by differences in demographic effects, management, season, transport variables, or individual differences in reactivity to the same event [47]. The contributions of each of these factors to variation in FGM in giraffes should be studied in more detail. In addition, published experiments of domestic ruminant feces stored at room temperature suggest results of the 11-oxoetiocholanolone EIAs may be prone to changes during storage [48, 49]; these effects should be evaluated for exotic ruminants.

11,17-DOA also showed diurnal variation in giraffe feces similar to those found in African buffalo (*Syncerus caffer*) [45]. With only a single subject and no serum hormone data, it is not possible to determine whether the observed pattern reflects a circadian rhythm in circulating hormones; blood samples have shown circadian secretion rhythms for cortisol are present in some ruminants [50] but are weak [51, 52] or absent [53] in others. The diurnal variations in 11,17-DOA may be idiosyncratic to this individual or to the days samples were collected. However, the more substantial 11,17-DOA peaks in response to both ACTH and transport and a consistent diurnal pattern suggests that the 11-oxoetiocholanolone I EIA is the most biologically sensitive assay we tested for giraffes.

Though the 11-oxoetiocholanolone I EIA (for 11,17-DOA) is more sensitive, there may be situations where the 11-oxoetiocholanolone II EIA (for 3α,11-oxo-CM) is still preferable. First, for the two juvenile female giraffes, the 11-oxoetiocholanolone II EIA detected a greater change in FGM following transport than the 11-oxoetiocholanolone I EIA. Cross-reactivity with gonadal hormones could be responsible for the difference [54]. However, cross-reactivity should increase FGM concentrations independent of the transport event, and these two individuals only had higher FGM concentrations in the post-transfer peak, not in baseline. Instead, immunoreactive 3α,11-oxo-CM may be more prevalent in the metabolite profiles of these two giraffes, perhaps as a result of age- of sex-specific differences in metabolism [34, 55]. Our data support using 3α,11-oxo-CM in studies of juvenile female giraffes. Second, we found systematic changes in 11,17-DOA concentrations across time of day, so studies using this assay must control for the time of day during either sampling or statistical analysis. If such control is not possible, assessing 3α,11-oxo-CM using the 11-oxoetiocholanolone II EIA is advised. Finally, if the aim of one's study is to identify husbandry or environmental events that are perceived as very stressful, as in [56, 57], the less biologically sensitive 11-oxoetiocholanolone II EIA may set a higher criterion for identifying peaks and so identify a smaller number of events.

Ruminant FGM measurement

Consistent with other studies of ruminants, we found that group-specific assays designed to target GC metabolites were more effective at measuring FGM than assays using antibodies raised against circulating GC. Circulating GC are metabolized extensively in the liver and additionally by gut microbes before excretion, so the types and ratios of specific FGM differ across sex and species (for review, see [21]). While cortisol or corticosterone EIAs effectively measure FGM in many species including some ruminants [42, 58–60], native GC are absent from the feces of most vertebrates [21, 42, 61] so this measurement depends on having a sufficient

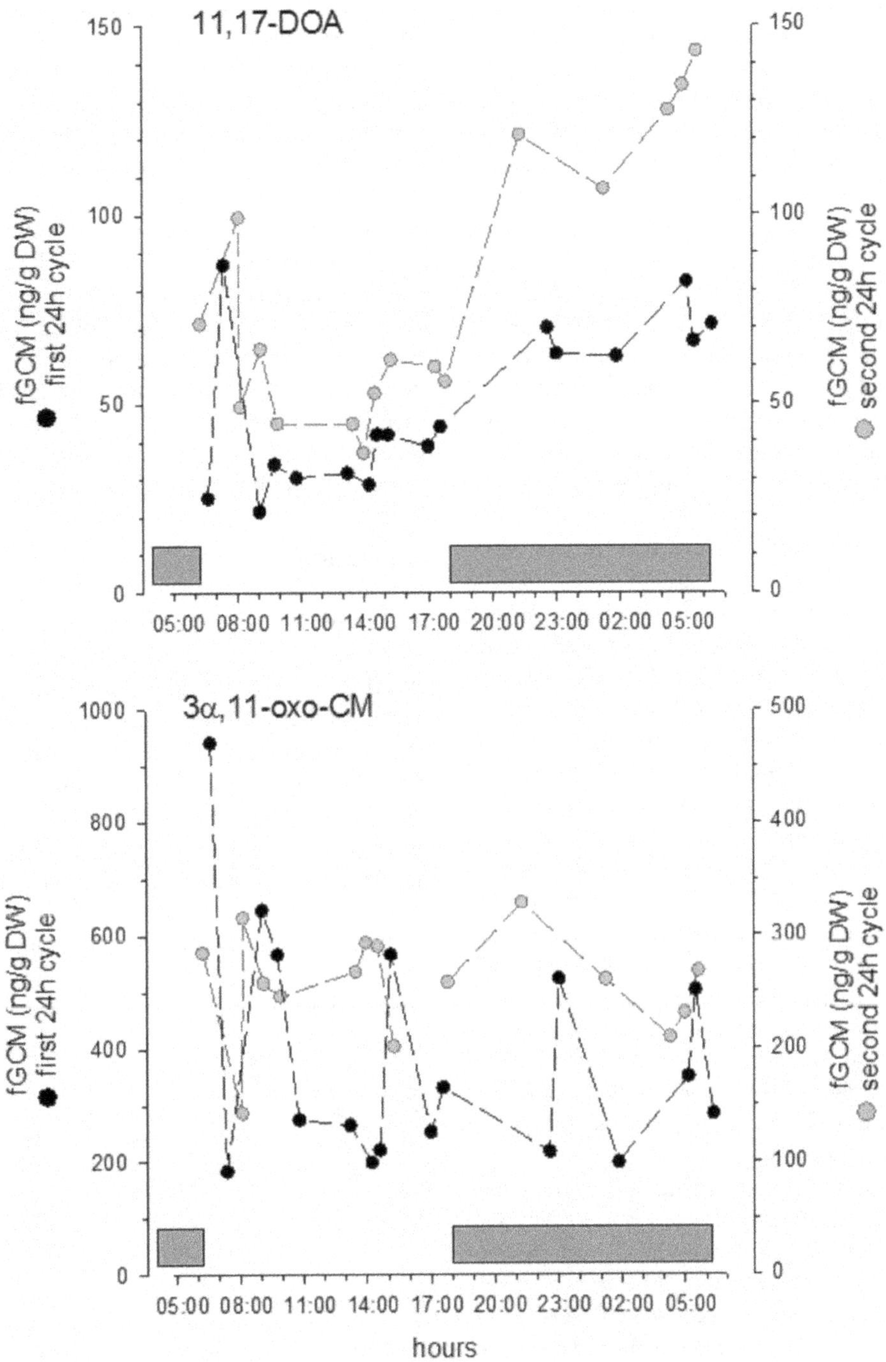

Fig. 4 24 h patterns in baseline FGM levels in one male captive giraffe. 11,17-DOA (*top*) 3α,11-oxo-CM (*bottom*)

concentration of FGM that have retained the characteristic of GC structure recognized by the particular antibody. A radiometabolism study could be used to identify exactly which FGM are present in a particular species and allow targeting of assays based on metabolite profiles [61, 62], but it is difficult to conduct such a study in wildlife species the size of a giraffe. Instead, comparing assays that target different metabolite structures can be used to infer some information about metabolite profiles [43].

So-called group-specific assays targeting GC metabolites [32] have been effectively used to measure FGM in ruminant species for which GC-specific assays have failed (e.g., sheep, cattle [63, 64]). Our study adds giraffes to the list of ruminant species for which one of the 11-oxoetiocholanolone EIAs is most effective in measuring

FGM (dromedary camels: *Camelus dromedarius* [65], cattle: *Bos primigenius f. taurus* [64], sheep: *Ovis ammon f. aries* [61, 64], goats: *Capra aegagrus f. hircus* [66], red deer: *Cervus elaphus* [67], roe deer: *Capreolus capreolus* [68], pampas deer: *Ozotoceros bezoarticus* [69], llama: *Lama guanicoe f. glama*, alpaca: *Vicugna vicugna f. pacos*, and vicuña: *Vicugna vicugna* [70]). The success of the 11-oxoetiocholanolone EIAs in such a large number of ruminant species suggests 5β-reduction may be a common metabolic pathway for GC in ruminants. However, all assays we used detected some post-event FGM peaks, which may indicate giraffes excrete a great variety of measurable metabolites like other ruminants. While FGM assays should still be validated for each species, we suggest FGM validation studies in other ruminants should begin by trying a group-specific 11-oxoetiocholanolone EIA.

Applications for giraffe health, welfare, and conservation

Our validation of multiple assays to measure FGM in giraffes provides a tool that can be applied in monitoring health and welfare, as well as conservation research. Zoos are particularly interested in generating data that will allow them to assess and improve giraffe health and management. The adrenal system responds similarly to exciting and stressful events, so FGM changes are best interpreted in the context of information about the animal's environment and behavior [22]. Adding FGM measurement to behavior data in other species has allowed animal managers unique insights into animals' perceptions of captive environments. For example, captive wombats showed behavioral habituation to interaction with humans, but their FGM response to these interactions remained unchanged, suggesting they may have developed learned helplessness [56]. Physiological measures of giraffe health and perceived stress will help supplement behavioral welfare indicators and may reveal critical aspects of the relationship between captive management and welfare.

As giraffes can be individually identified by their natural markings [71], validation of FGM assays will also allow researchers to obtain longitudinal measures of adrenal activity from individual wild giraffes. Non-invasive longitudinal adrenal assessment will aid in determining the effects of environmental degradation and conservation efforts on giraffe health, reproduction, diet, and life history strategies [31, 72]. Giraffes in captivity might reasonably be expected to have different baseline levels of GC and/or respond differently to stressors than wild giraffes [72], so field studies should seek within-individual patterns of FGM that can be attributed to particular events. Recent studies have used FGM to evaluate how primates perceive conservation-related stressors, from ecotourism (orangutans: *Pongo pygmaeus morio* [73], gorillas: *Gorilla gorilla gorilla* [74]) to long-term changes in food distribution and disease prevalence (red colobus: *Procolobus rufomitratus* [75]); similar studies could now be undertaken in giraffes. Across species, Dantzer and colleagues' [76] meta-analysis found that anthropogenic disturbances are consistently associated with increased FGM, but argue that these FGM changes may enhance survival in disturbed populations. However, there are well-described negative health consequences of chronic exposure to elevated GC [22], so the relationship between FGM and fitness in disturbed populations is ripe for research. Giraffes live in a diverse array of habitats with varying degrees of human disturbance; in some areas giraffe populations are increasing, while in most of the range populations are crashing. Giraffes are therefore an ideal species in which to use FGM measures to investigate questions of captive health, welfare, physiology, ecology, and conservation.

Conclusions

We conclude the assay for 11,17-dioxoandrostanes is the most sensitive assay tested for FGM in giraffes and the assay for FGM with a 5β-3α-ol-11-one structure is also effective. 11-oxoetiocholanolone enzyme immunoassays have now been demonstrated to be successful in a wide variety of ruminant species, providing indirect evidence that 5β-reduction may be a common metabolic pathway for glucocorticoids in ruminants. As FGM peaks were detected in at least some giraffes using all assays tested, giraffes appear to excrete a wide variety of different FGM. The assays validated here will provide a valuable tool for research on the health, welfare, and conservation of giraffes.

Abbreviations

ACTH: Adrenocorticotropic hormone; EIAs: Enzyme immunoassays; FGM: Fecal glucocorticoid metabolites; GC: Glucocorticoids; HPA: Hypothalamic-pituitary-adrenal; IUCN: International Union for Conservation of Nature; NZG: National Zoological Gardens of South Africa

Acknowledgements

We thank Pascale Benoit, Kevin Milton, and Jackie Stuart, as well as Frankfurt Zoo, Dortmund Zoo, Neunkirchen Zoo, Cologne Zoo, Allwetterzoo Münster, Karlsruhe Zoo and Opel-Zoo for help with animal care and sample collection. We thank Günther Fleissner for his assistance with the transport study.

Funding

The Association of Friends and Supporters of Goethe University Frankfurt provided financial support for F. Sicks to travel to Vienna to analyze fecal samples and von Opel Hessische Zoostiftung supported a studentship for F. Sicks. One commercial funder [Tierpark Berlin] provided support in the form of salary for F. Sicks during data analysis and preparation of this manuscript. The specific role of this author is articulated in the 'Author Contributions' section. No funders had any role in the study design, data collection and analysis, decision to publish, or preparation of the manuscript.

Authors' contributions
MJB and AG designed the study of Giraffes 1 and 2. AG and ASWT conducted the study of Giraffe 1 and MJB conducted the study of Giraffe 2. F. Sicks acquired funding for, designed, and conducted the study of Giraffes 3–7. MJB and F. Sicks assayed fecal samples with assistance from RP and F. Schwarzenberger. MJB and AG analysed the data. MJB drafted and revised the manuscript with assistance from AG and RP. All authors critically revised the manuscript and approved the final version.

Competing interests
One of the authors [F. Sicks] was employed by Tierpark Berlin during the completion of this study. There are no patents, products in development or marketed products to declare. This does not alter our adherence to editorial policies on sharing data and materials, nor does Tierpark Berlin benefit financially from publication of these data.

Consent for publication
Not applicable.

Ethics approval and consent to participate
The study of Giraffe 1 complied with relevant ethical guidelines in South Africa and was conducted with permission of the Animal Use and Care Committee (#EC074-12) of the University of Pretoria, South Africa and with permission of the NZG, which owned the animal. The study of Giraffe 2 complied with relevant ethical guidelines in Australia and was conducted with permission of the Animal Ethics Committee (#4a/12/12) of Taronga Conservation Society of Australia and with permission of the Taronga Western Plains Zoo, which owned the animal. The study of giraffes 3–7 complied with relevant ethical guidelines in Germany and was performed as a normal part of animal management with the permission of the zoos that owned the animals (Frankfurt Zoo, Dortmund Zoo, Neunkirchen Zoo, Cologne Zoo, Allwetterzoo Münster, Karlsruhe Zoo, and Opel-Zoo). The participating zoos specifically approved all sampling procedures and no experimental manipulations were conducted on these giraffes; opportunistic sampling of this type requires no additional specific permission under the German Animal Welfare Act.

Author details
[1]Wildlife Reproductive Centre, Taronga Conservation Society of Australia, Dubbo, NSW, Australia. [2]Department of Psychology, Franklin & Marshall College, Lancaster, PA, USA. [3]Tierpark Berlin, Berlin, Germany. [4]Department of Biomedical Sciences, University of Veterinary Medicine, Vienna, Austria. [5]Department of Paraclinical Sciences, Faculty of Veterinary Science, University of Pretoria, Onderstepoort, Pretoria, South Africa. [6]National Zoological Gardens of South Africa, Pretoria, South Africa. [7]Department of Anatomy and Physiology, Endocrine Research Laboratory, Faculty of Veterinary Science, University of Pretoria, Onderstepoort, Pretoria, South Africa.

References

1. Fennessy J, Brown D. *Giraffa camelopardalis* [Internet]. The IUCN Red List of Threatened Species. Version. 2010. Available from: iucnredlist.org/details/9194/0. [Accessed 17 July 2015].
2. Fennessy J, Brown D. *Giraffa camelopardalis ssp. peralta* [Internet]. The IUCN Red List of Threatened Species. Version. 2008. Available from: http://www.iucnredlist.org/details/136913/0. [Accessed 17 July 2015].
3. Fennessy J, Brenneman R. *Giraffa camelopardalis ssp. rothschildi* [Internet]. The IUCN Red List of Threatened Species. Version. 2010. Available from: http://www.iucnredlist.org/details/174469/0. [Accessed 17 July 2015].
4. Shorrocks B, Croft DP. Necks and networks: a preliminary study of population structure in the reticulated giraffe (*Giraffa camelopardalis reticulatade Winston*). Afr J Ecol. 2009;47:374–81.
5. Bercovitch FB, Berry PSM. Age proximity influences herd composition in wild giraffe. J Zool. 2013;290:281–6.
6. Carter KD, Seddon JM, Frère CH, Carter JK, Goldizen AW. Fission–fusion dynamics in wild giraffes may be driven by kinship, spatial overlap and individual social preferences. Anim Behav. 2013;85:385–94.
7. Bercovitch FB, Berry PSM. Herd composition, kinship and fission-fusion social dynamics among wild giraffe. Afr J Ecol. 2013;51:206–16.
8. Caister LE, Shields WM, Gosser A. Female tannin avoidance: a possible explanation for habitat and dietary segregation of giraffes (*Giraffa camelopardalis peralta*) in niger. Afr J Ecol. 2003;41:201–10.
9. Seeber PA, Duncan P, Fritz H, Ganswindt A. Androgen changes and flexible rutting behaviour in male giraffes. Biol Lett. 2013;9:20130396.
10. Clauss M, Franz-Odendaal TA, Brasch J, Castell JC, Kaiser T. Tooth wear in captive giraffes (*Giraffa camelopardalis*): mesowear analysis classifies free-ranging specimens as browsers but captive ones as grazers. J Zoo Wild Med. 2007;38:433–45.
11. Muneza AB, Montgomery RA, Fennessy JT, Dickman AJ, Roloff GJ, Macdonald DW. Regional variation of the manifestation, prevalence, and severity of giraffe skin disease: a review of an emerging disease in wild and captive giraffe populations. Biol Cons. 2016;198:145–56.
12. Potter JS, Clauss M. Mortality of captive giraffe (*Giraffa camelopardalis*) associated with serous fat atrophy: a review of five cases at Auckland Zoo. J Zoo Wildl Med. 2005;36:301–7.
13. Bashaw MJ, Tarou LR, Maki TS, Maple TL. A survey assessment of variables related to stereotypy in captive giraffe and okapi. Appl Anim Behav Sci. 2001;73:235–47.
14. del Castillo SM, Bashaw MJ, Patton ML, Rieches RR, Bercovitch FB. Fecal steroid analysis of female giraffe (*Giraffa camelopardalis*) reproductive condition and the impact of endocrine status on daily time budgets. Gen Comp Endocrinol. 2005;141:271–81.
15. Koene P. When feeding is just eating: How do farm and zoo animals use their spare time? In: van der Huide D, Huisman EA, Kanis E, Osse J, Verstegen M, editors. Regulation of Feed Intake. New York: CABI. 1999. p. 13–20.
16. Fernandez LT, Bashaw MJ, Sartor RL, Bouwens NR, Maki TS. Tongue twisters: feeding enrichment to reduce oral stereotypy in giraffe. Zoo Biol. 2008;27:200–12.
17. Baxter E, Plowman AB. The effect of increasing dietary fibre on feeding, rumination, and oral stereotypies in captive giraffes (*Giraffa camelopardalis*). Anim Welf. 2001;10:281–90.
18. Sapolsky RM, Romero LM, Munck AU. How do glucocorticoids influence stress responses? Integrating permissive, suppressive, stimulatory, and preparative actions. Endocr Rev. 2000;21:55–89.
19. Whirledge S, Cidlowski JA. A role for glucocorticoids in stress-impaired reproduction: beyond the hypothalamus and pituitary. Endocrinol. 2013; 154:4450–68.
20. Padgett DA, Glaser R. How stress influences the immune response. Trends Immunol. 2003;24:444–8.
21. Palme R, Rettenbacher S, Touma C, El-Bahr SM, Möstl E. Stress hormones in mammals and birds: comparative aspects regarding metabolism, excretion, and noninvasive measurement in fecal samples. Ann N Y Acad Sci. 2005; 1040:162–71.
22. Webster J. Animal Welfare: Limping Towards Eden. Oxford, UK: Blackwell Publishing Ltd; 2005.
23. McEwen BS. Protective and damaging effects of stress mediators. N Engl J Med. 1998;338:171–9.
24. Sapolsky RM. Endocrinology of the stress response. In: Becker JB, Breedlove SM, Crews D, McCarthy MM, editors. Behavioral Endocrinology. 2nd ed. Cambridge: MIT Press. 2002. p. 409–50.
25. Koolhaas JM, de Boer SF, Coppens CM, Buwalda B. Neuroendocrinology of coping styles: towards understanding the biology of individual variation. Front Neuroendocrinol. 2010;31:307–21.
26. Carere C, Caramaschi D, Fawcett TW. Covariation between personalities and individual differences in coping with stress: converging evidence and hypotheses. Curr Zool. 2010;56:728–40.
27. Sheriff MJ, Dantzer B, Delehanty B, Palme R, Boonstra R. Measuring stress in wildlife: techniques for quantifying glucocorticoids. Oecologia. 2011;166:869–87.
28. Palme R. Monitoring stress hormone metabolites as a useful, non-invasive tool for welfare assessment in farm animals. Anim Welf. 2012;21:331–7.
29. Touma C, Palme R. Measuring fecal glucocorticoid metabolites in mammals and birds: the importance of validation. Ann N Y Acad Sci. 2005;1046:54–74.
30. Cattet M, Boulanger J, Stenhouse G, Powell RA, Reynolds-Hogland MJ. An evaluation of long-term capture effects in ursids: implications for wildlife welfare and research. J Mammal. 2008;89:973–90.
31. Möstl E, Palme R. Hormones as indicators of stress. Domest Anim Endocrinol. 2002;23:67–74.

32. Möstl E, Rettenbacher S, Palme R. Measurement of corticosterone metabolites in birds' droppings: an analytical approach. Ann N Y Acad Sci. 2005;1046:17–34.
33. Fanson KV, Best EC, Bunce A, Fanson BG, Hogan LA, Keeley T, et al. One size does not fit all: Monitoring faecal glucocorticoid metabolites in marsupials. Gen Comp Endocrinol. 2016; Epub ahead of print. doi:10.1016/j.ygcen.2015.10.011.
34. Touma C, Sachser N, Möstl E, Palme R. Effects of sex and time of day on metabolism and excretion of corticosterone in urine and feces of mice. Gen Comp Endocrinol. 2003;130:267–78.
35. Palme R, Touma C, Arias N, Dominchin MF, Lepschy M. Steroid extraction: Get the best out of faecal samples. Wien Tierärztl Mschr. 2013;100:238–46.
36. Keay JM, Singh J, Gaunt MC, Kaur T. Fecal glucocorticoids and their metabolites as indicators of stress in various mammalian species: a literature review. J Zoo Wildl Med. 2006;37:234–44.
37. Brown JL, Citino SB, Shaw J, Miller C. Endocrine profiles during the estrous cycle and pregnancy in the Baird's tapir (*Tapirus bairdii*). Zoo Biol. 1994;13:107–17.
38. Wielebnowski NC, Fletchall N, Carlstead K, Busso JM, Brown JL. Noninvasive assessment of adrenal activity associated with husbandry and behavioral factors in the North American clouded leopard population. Zoo Biol. 2002;21:77–98.
39. Morrow CJ, Kolver ES, Verkerk GA, Matthews LR. Fecal glucocorticoid metabolites as a measure of adrenal activity in dairy cattle. Gen Comp Endocrinol. 2002;126:229–41.
40. Lay Jr DC, Friend TH, Randel RD, Jenkins OC, Neuendorff DA, Kapp GM, et al. Adrenocorticotropic hormone dose response and some physiological effects of transportation on pregnant Brahman cattle. J Anim Sci. 1996;74: 1806–11.
41. Palme R, Robia C, Messmann S, Hofer J, Möstl E. Measurement of faecal cortisol metabolites in ruminants: a non-invasive parameter of adrenocortical function. Wien Tierärztl Mschr. 1999;86:237–41.
42. Wasser SK, Hunt KE, Brown JL, Cooper K, Crockett CM, Bechert U, et al. A generalized fecal glucocorticoid assay for use in a diverse array of nondomestic mammalian and avian species. Gen Comp Endocrinol. 2000;120:260–75.
43. Heistermann M, Palme R, Ganswindt A. Comparison of different enzymeimmunoassays for assessment of adrenocortical activity in primates based on fecal analysis. Am J Primatol. 2006;68:257–73.
44. Palme R, Robia C, Baumgartner W, Möstl E. Transport stress in cattle as reflected by an increase in faecal cortisol metabolite concentrations. Vet Rec. 2000;146:108–9.
45. Ganswindt A, Tordiffe ASW, Stam E, Howitt MJ, Jori F. Determining adrenocortical activity as a measure of stress in African buffalo (*Syncerus caffer*) based on faecal analysis. Afr Zool. 2012;47:261–9.
46. Goymann W. On the use of non-invasive hormone research in uncontrolled, natural environments: the problem with sex, diet, metabolic rate and the individual. Methods Ecol Evol. 2012;3:757–65.
47. Grandin T. Assessment of stress during handling and transport. J Anim Sci. 1997;75:249–57.
48. Möstl E, Messman S, Bagu E, Robia C, Palme R. Measurement of glucocorticoid metabolite concentrations in faeces of domestic livestock. J Vet Med A. 1999;46:621–31.
49. Lexen E, El-Bahr SM, Sommerfeld-Stur I, Palme R, Möstl E. Monitoring the adrenocortical response to disturbances in sheep by measuring glucocorticoid metabolites in the faeces. Wien Tierärztl Mschr. 2008;95:64–71.
50. Ingram JR, Crockford JN, Matthews LR. Ultradian, circadian and seasonal rhythms in cortisol secretion and adrenal responsiveness to ACTH and yarding in unrestrained red deer (*Cervus elaphus*) stags. J Endocrinol. 1999;162:289–300.
51. Lefcourt AM, Bitman J, Kahl S, Wood DL. Circadian and ultradian rhythms of peripheral cortisol concentrations in lactating dairy cows. J Dairy Sci. 1993;76:2607–12.
52. Fulkerson WJ, Sawyer GJ, Gow CB. Investigations of ultradian and circadian rhythms in the concentration of cortisol and prolactin in the plasma of dairy cattle. Aust J Biol Sci. 1980;33:557–61.
53. Alila-Johansson A, Eriksson L, Soveri T, Laakso M-L. Serum cortisol levels in goats exhibit seasonal but Not daily rhythmicity. Chronobiol Int. 2003;20:65–79.
54. Ganswindt A, Palme R, Heistermann M, Borragan S, Hodges JK. Non-invasive assessment of adrenocortical function in the male African elephant (*Loxodonta africana*) and its relation to musth. Gen Comp Endocrinol. 2003; 134:156–66.
55. Dufty Jr AM, Belthoff JR. Corticosterone and the stress response in young western screech-owls: effects of captivity, gender, and activity period. Physiol Zool. 1997;70:143–9.
56. Hogan LA, Johnston SD, Lisle AT, Keeley T, Wong P, Nicolson V, et al. Behavioural and physiological responses of captive wombats (*Lasiorhinus latifrons*) to regular handling by humans. Appl Anim Behav Sci. 2011;134:217–28.
57. Hogan LA, Lisle AT, Johnston SD, Robertson H. Non-invasive assessment of stress in captive numbats, *Myrmecobius fasciatus* (*Mammalia: Marsupialia*), using faecal cortisol measurement. Gen Comp Endocrinol. 2012;179:376–83.
58. Creel S, Fox JE, Hardy A, Sands J, Garrott B, Peterson RO. Snowmobile activity and glucocorticoid stress responses in wolves and elk. Conserv Biol. 2002;16:809–14.
59. Christofoletti MD, Pereira RJG, Duarte JMB. Influence of husbandry systems on physiological stress reactions of captive brown brocket (*Mazama gouazoubira*) and marsh deer (*Blastocerus dichotomus*)—noninvasive analysis of fecal cortisol metabolites. Eur J Wildl Res. 2010;56:561–8.
60. Millspaugh JJ, Washburn BE, Milanick MA, Beringer J, Hansen LP, Meyer TM. Non-invasive techniques for stress assessment in white-tailed deer. Wildl Soc Bull. 2002;30:899–907.
61. Möstl E, Maggs JL, Schrötter G, Besenfelder U, Palme R. Measurement of cortisol metabolites in faeces of ruminants. Vet Res Commun. 2002;26:127–39.
62. Oates JE, Bradshaw FJ, Bradshaw SD, Stead-Richardson EJ, Philippe DL. Reproduction and embryonic diapause in a marsupial: insights from captive female honey possums, tarsipes rostratus (*tarsipedidae*). Gen Comp Endocrinol. 2007;150:445–61.
63. Palme R, Möstl E. Measurement of cortisol metabolites in faeces of sheep as a parameter of cortisol concentration of blood. Z Saugetierkd. 1997;62 Suppl 2:192–7.
64. Why did Copenhagen Zoo kill its giraffe? - BBC News. 1999;86:237–41. http://www.bbc.com/news/science-environment-26118748.
65. Sid-Ahmed O-E, Sanhouri A, Elwaseela B-E, Fadllalah I, Mohammed G-EE, Möstl E. Assessment of adrenocortical activity by non-invasive measurement of faecal cortisol metabolites in dromedary camels (*Camelus dromedarius*). Trop Anim Health Prod. 2013;45:1453–8.
66. Kleinsasser C, Graml C, Klobetz-Rassam E, Barth K, Waiblinger S, Palme R. Physiological validation of a non-invasive method for measuring adrenocortical activity in goats. Wien Tierärztl Mschr. 2010;97:182–91.
67. Huber S, Palme R, Zenker W, Möstl E. Non-invasive monitoring of the adrenocortical response in red deer. J Wildl Manage. 2003;67:258.
68. Dehnhard M, Clauss M, Lechner-Doll M, Meyer HHD, Palme R. Noninvasive monitoring of adrenocortical activity in roe deer (*Capreolus capreolus*) by measurement of fecal cortisol metabolites. Gen Comp Endocrinol. 2001;123:111–20.
69. Munerato MS, Marques JA, Caulkettt NA, Tomás WM, Zanetti ES, Trovati RG, et al. Hormonal and behavioural stress responses to capture and radio-collar fitting in free-ranging pampas deer (*Ozotoceros bezoarticus*). Anim Welf. 2015;24:437–46.
70. Arias N, Requena M, Palme R. Measuring faecal glucocorticoid metabolites as a non-invasive tool for monitoring adrenocortical activity in South American camelids. Anim Welf. 2013;22:25–31.
71. Pratt DM, Anderson VH. Giraffe social behaviour. J Nat Hist. 1985;19:771–81.
72. Millspaugh JJ, Washburn BE. Use of fecal glucocorticoid metabolite measures in conservation biology research: considerations for application and interpretation. Gen Comp Endocrinol. 2004;138:189–99.
73. Muehlenbein MP, Ancrenaz M, Sakong R, Ambu L, Prall S, Fuller G, et al. Ape conservation physiology: Fecal glucocorticoid responses in wild *Pongo pygmaeus morio* following human visitation. PLoS One. 2012;7:e33357.
74. Shutt K, Heistermann M, Kasim A, Todd A, Kalousova B, Profosouva I, et al. Effects of habituation, research and ecotourism on faecal glucocorticoid metabolites in wild western lowland gorillas: implications for conservation management. Biol Conserv Elsevier Ltd. 2014;172:72–9.
75. Chapman CA, Schoof VAM, Bonnell TR, Gogarten JF, Calme S. Competing pressures on populations: long-term dynamics of food availability, food quality, disease, stress and animal abundance. Philos Trans R Soc Lond B Biol Sci. 2015;370:20140112.
76. Dantzer B, Fletcher QE, Boonstra R, Sheriff MJ. Measures of physiological stress: a transparent or opaque window into the status, management and conservation of species? Conserv Physiol. 2014;2:1–18.
77. Fanson KV, Keeley T, Fanson BG. Cyclic changes in cortisol across the estrous cycle in parous and nulliparous Asian elephants. Endocr Connect. 2014;3:57–66.

78. Munro CJ, Stabenfeldt G. Development of a cortisol enzyme-immunoassay in plasma. Clin Chem. 1985;31:956.
79. Keeley T, O'Brien JK, Fanson BG, Masters K, McGreevy PD. The reproductive cycle of the Tasmanian devil (*Sarcophilus harrisii*) and factors associated with reproductive success in captivity. Gen Comp Endocrinol. 2012;176:182–91.
80. Watson R, Munro CJ, Edwards KL, Norton V, Brown JL, Walker SL. Development of a versatile enzyme immunoassay for non-invasive assessment of glucocorticoid metabolites in a diversity of taxonomic species. Gen Comp Endocrinol. 2013;186:16–24.
81. Schatz S, Palme R. Measurement of faecal cortisol metabolites in cats and dogs: a non-invasive method for evaluating adrenocortical function. Vet Res Commun. 2001;25:271–87.
82. Frigerio D, Dittami J, Möstl E, Kotrschal K. Excreted corticosterone metabolites co-vary with ambient temperature and air pressure in male Greylag geese (*Anser anser*). Gen Comp Endocrinol. 2004;137:29–36.

Measurements of C-reactive protein (CRP) and nerve-growth-factor (NGF) concentrations in serum and urine samples of dogs with neurologic disorders

Ulrike Kordass*, Regina Carlson, Veronika Maria Stein and Andrea Tipold

Abstract

Background: The purpose of this study was to prove the hypothesis that C-reactive protein (CRP) and nerve growth factor (NGF) may be potential biomarkers for lower urinary tract disorders and may be able to distinguish between micturition dysfunctions of different origin in dogs with spinal cord diseases. NGF- and CRP-concentrations were measured in serum and urine samples using specific ELISA-Kits. Results in urine were standardized by urine-creatinine levels.

Results: CRP in serum was detectable in 32/76 and in urine samples in 40/76 patients. NGF could be measured in all serum and in 70/76 urine samples. Urinary CRP concentrations were significantly higher in dogs with micturition dysfunction ($p = 0.0009$) and in dogs with different neurological diseases ($p = 0.0020$) compared to the control group. However, comparing dogs with spinal cord disorders with and without associated micturition dysfunction no significant difference could be detected for NGF and CRP values in urine or serum samples. Additionally, levels did not decrease significantly, when measured at the time when the dogs regained the ability to urinate properly (urinary NGF $p = 0.7962$; urinary CRP $p = 0.078$). Urine samples with bacteria and/or leukocytes had no significant increase in urinary NGF ($p = 0.1112$) or CRP ($p = 0.0534$) concentrations, but higher CRP-levels in urine from dogs with cystitis were found compared to dogs without signs of cystitis.

Conclusions: From these data we conclude that neither CRP nor NGF in urine or serum can be considered as reliable biomarkers for micturition disorders in dogs with spinal cord disorders in a clinical setting, but their production might be part of the pathogenesis of such disorders. Significantly higher levels of CRP could be found in the urine of dogs with micturition dysfunctions compared to control dogs. This phenomenon could potentially be explained by unspecific extrahepatic CRP production by smooth muscle cells in the dilated bladder.

Keywords: Dog, Nerve growth factor, C-reactive protein, Micturition disorders, Spinal cord disease, Cystitis

Background

Complications with the voluntary control of micturition are commonly observed in disorders of the nervous system [1] and can worsen the prognosis in intervertebral disc diseases [2], a common neurological disorder in dogs [3]. Intervertebral disc disease cranial to the lumbosacral level can affect the voluntary voiding process [4] and might result in a detrusor-urethral dyssynergia with an areflectic bladder and urine retention [5]. Micturition disorders may be caused by the neurological disorder itself or an associated cystitis [6] precipitated by bacterial infections [7]. Escherichia coli is the most common isolate from canine urine [8, 9]. The pathogens reach the bladder from either gastrointestinal sources or the skin via the urethra [7]. The clinical signs are either pollakiurie, stranguria, dysuria, hematuria, inappropriate urination or periuria [10] and are difficult to distinguish from a neurogenic induced micturition disorder. Dogs with spinal cord injuries display a high prevalence of

* Correspondence: ulrike.kordass@web.de
Department of Small Animal Medicine and Surgery, University of Veterinary Medicine Hannover, Hannover, Germany

developing urinary tract infections [11, 12] even after recovery of voluntary urination [13].

Therefore, a biomarker helping to distinguish between neurogenic and non-neurogenic micturition disorders might be useful for pathogenesis studies and initiating appropriate treatment.

A biomarker should be an indicator for a specific disease and is supposed to identify the presence, severity, progression and the response to a specific treatment [14, 15]. Specific cells, enzymes, hormones, genes or gene products can be used as biomarkers [16]. The measurement can be performed in different tissues or body fluids [14, 16]. Two of the urinary biomarkers identified in human medicine so far are the nerve growth factor (NGF) and the C-reactive protein (CRP) [16].

NGF being a well-known neurotrophin, plays an important role in conditions of inflammatory and neuropathic pain [17, 18]. It is responsible for the growth, survival and development of neural cells, as well as the regulation of neural plasticity in the micturition pathway [19]. NGF is produced by urethral cells and cells of the detrusor muscle [20]. Different studies show that NGF is involved in the development of neurogenic bladder overactivity at the spinal level following the disruption of supraspinal micturition control after spinal cord injury [19]. Raised NGF levels in serum could be found in bladder dysfunctions [21]. There are several studies in humans on NGF as a urinary biomarker [22] showing increased NGF levels in patients with urinary tract disorders [21, 23, 24].

CRP is an acute-phase protein, mainly produced in the liver and elevated after infection, inflammation or trauma. The CRP concentration rises depending on the tissue damage [25]. In human studies CRP in serum is increased in patients with lower urinary tract disorders and it correlates with the severity of clinical signs [26, 27]. In dogs, CRP in serum can be used as an indicator of inflammatory response to experimentally induced cystitis [28].

Therefore, we hypothesize that CRP and NGF are measurable in serum and urine samples and can be used as biomarkers in either serum or urine to distinguish between micturition disorders caused by neurologic dysfunctions or bacterial cystitis in dogs with spinal cord disease.

Results

76 dogs were included in the study. The patients were categorized into four different groups (Table 1).

Diseases included in the study are summarized in Table 2. Urinary CRP could not be detected in each patient. The highest levels were found in dogs with spinal cord disorders and micturition problems. 80 % of the dogs in the control group, 64 % with different neurological disorders, 41 % with spinal cord disorders with micturition problems and 29 % with spinal cord disorders without micturition problems had detectable CRP values. In detail, urinary CRP was measurable in 16/20 dogs of the control group with a mean concentration of 1.08 ng/ml (range: 0–1.76 ng/ml). After normalizing CRP to creatinine the mean ratio was 0.01 CRP/Crea (range: 0–0.02 CRP/Crea) (Table 3). In 9/14 of the patients within the group of different neurological disorders urinary CRP was measurable with a mean concentration of 2.21 ng/ml (range: 0–11.39 ng/ml) and after normalizing to creatinine the mean ratio accounted for 0.04 CRP/Crea (range: 0–0.26 CRP/Crea) (Table 3). In the group "spinal cord disorders without micturition problems" CRP was measurable in 4/15 dogs with a mean concentration of 1.45 ng/ml (range: 0–14.91 ng/ml) and after normalizing to creatinine the mean ratio was 0.02 CRP/Crea (0–0.17 CRP/Crea) (Table 3). CRP was measurable in 11/27 patients of the group with the spinal cord disorders with micturition problems with a mean concentration of 9.22 ng/ml (0–131 ng/ml) and after normalizing to creatinine a mean ration of 0.12 CRP/Crea (0–1.14 CRP/Crea) was detected (Table 3).

Serum CRP could be detected in 4/20 patients in the control group with a mean of 946 ng/ml (range: 0–6820 ng/ml) (Table 3). The mean level in 7/14 patients with neurological disorders was 22,452 ng/ml (range: 0–208,658 ng/ml) (Table 3). The wide range of

Table 1 Categorization of the dogs into four different groups

	Groups	N
1	Different neurological disorders (ND)	14
2	Spinal cord disorders without micturition problems (SC)	15
3	Spinal cord disorders with micturition problems (SC MD)	27
4	Healthy dogs (control)	20

Table 2 Different diseases included in the study

Disease	N	ND	SC	SCMD
Idiopathic epilepsy	5	5		
Cryptogenic epilepsy	1	1		
Meningoencephalitis	3	3		
Steroid-responsive meningitis-arteritis	1	1		
Vestibular disease	2	2		
Neoplasia intracranial	1	1		
Polyneuropathy	1	1		
Intervertebral disc herniation	39		15	24
Myelitis	1			1
Vertebral dislocation	2			2
Total	56			

Distribution of the diseases in the different groups (*N* = number): neurological disorders (ND), spinal cord disorders without micturition dysfunction (SC), spinal cord disorders with micturition dysfunction (SCMD)

Table 3 C-reactive protein and nerve-growth-factor levels in urine and serum samples

	CRP urine ng/ml	CRP/Crea urine	CRP serum ng/ml	NGF urine	NGF/Crea urine	NGF serumpg/ml
Control	1.08 (0–1.76)	0.01 (0–0.02)	946 (0–6820)	76.60 (7.17-250)	0.50 (0.06-3.01)	179 (104–250)
Neurological Disorders	2.21 (0–11.39)	0.04 (0–0.26)	22452 (0–208658)	31.98 (0–150)	0.61 (0–2.41)	164 (40–250)
SC	01.45 (0–14.91)	0.02 (0–0.1721)	14764 (0–92035)	63.24 (0–198)	1.00 (0–3.43)	166 (24.77-250)
SC MD	9.22 (0–131)	0.12 (0–1.1462)	9235 (0–81719)	58.11 (0–250)	0.73 (0–4.40)	167 (46–250)

C-reactive protein (CRP) and nerve-growth-factor (NGF) levels in urine and serum samples (mean, range in brackets), CRP/Creatinine and NGF/Creatinine ratios in the different groups: control group ($n = 20$), neurological disorders ($n = 14$), spinal cord disorders without micturition dysfunctions (SC) ($n = 15$) and spinal cord disorders with micturition dysfunctions (SC MP) ($n = 27$)

the values was caused by including dogs with inflammatory CNS diseases. One dog suffering from steroid-responsive meningitis-arteritis displayed the highest value (208,658 ng/ml). This sample was additionally used as a positive control [29] to evaluate the ELISA test, since CRP was not measurable in all serum samples. In 9/15 dogs with spinal cord disorders without micturition problems CRP was measurable with a mean concentration of 14,764 ng/ml (range: 0–92,035 ng/ml) and in 12/27 dogs with micturition problems a mean concentration of 9235 ng/ml (range 0–81,719 ng/ml) could be detected (Table 3).

In all of the 20 patients in the control group urinary NGF was measurable and ranged between 7.17-250 pg/ml (mean 76.60 pg/ml). After normalizing to creatinine a mean ratio of 0.50 NGF/Crea (range 0.06 - 3.00 NGF/Crea) could be found (Table 3). In 13/14 patients with different neurological disorders NGF was measurable with a mean concentration of 31.98 pg/ml (range 0–150 pg/ml) and after normalizing to creatinine the mean ratio was 0.61 NGF/Crea (range 0–2.41 NGF/Crea) (Table 3). Urinary NGF mean value was 63.24 pg/ml (range 0–198 pg/ml) in 13/15 patients with spinal cord disorders without micturition problems (Table 3), the mean NGF/Creatinine ratio was 1.00 NGF/Crea (range 0–3.43 NGF/Crea) (Table 3). In 24/27 dogs with micturition problems the mean concentration of NGF was 58.11 pg/ml (range 0–250 pg/ml). The range of the ratio after normalizing to creatinine was 0–4.40 NGF/Crea with a mean of 0.73 NGF/Crea (Table 3).

Serum NGF was detectable in all of the analyzed serum samples. The mean concentration of the control group was 179 pg/ml (range: 104–250 pg/ml), of different neurological disorders 164 pg/ml (range: 40–250 pg/ml), of the spinal cord disorders without micturition problems 166 pg/ml (range: 24.77-250 pg/ml) and the spinal cord disorders with micturition problems showed a mean concentration of 167 pg/ml (range: 46–250 pg/ml) (Table 3).

In the first group including all dogs, significant differences measuring the CRP/Crea-ratio could be found between the spinal cord disorders without micturition problems and the control group ($p = 0.0118$) as well as with different neurological disorders ($p = 0.0445$). No further significant differences could be detected.

The CRP levels in serum were significantly different in the control group and the spinal cord disorders without micturition problems ($p = 0.0181$) (Table 4), no further significant differences could be evaluated (Table 4).

Additionally, we determined the significances between the concentrations of CRP/Crea in the different groups in the urine only within measurable samples (Fig. 1 and Table 4). Significant differences could be detected between the healthy control group and the neurological disorders ($p = 0.0020$) as well as the spinal cord disorders

Table 4 *p*-values of the different concentrations of C-reactive protein and nerve growth factor in serum and urine samples

	CRP/Crea Urine	CRP/Crea Urine all	CRP Serum	NGF/Crea Urine	NGF Serum
Control Group vs Neurological Disorders	*0.0020**	0.2510	0.0670	0.6119	0.6450
Control Group vs SC	0.5391	*0.0118**	*0.0181**	0.4334	0.9591
Control Group vs SC with micturition dysfunction	*0.0009**	0.4010	0.1113	0.8546	0.6484
Neurological Disorders vs SC without micturition dysfunction	0.6997	*0.0445**	0.4503	0.4712	0.7315
Neurological Disorders vs SC with micturition dysfunction	0.4033	0.3369	0.8576	0.7207	0.9778
SC without micturition dysfunction vs SC with micturition dysfunction	0.3961	0.2837	0.3401	0.4620	0.8298
Cystitis vs No cystits		0.0534		0.1112	
Dogs unable to urinate vs Dogs with normal voiding		0.0778		0.7962	

P-values of the different concentrations of C-reactive protein (CRP) and nerve growth factor (NGF) in serum and after normalizing to creatinine (CRP/ Crea; NGF/ Crea) in urine samples for the different groups. Measurements including all CRP/Crea values are shown in the column "CRP/Crea urine all". Calculations of samples only with detectable values are shown in the column "CRP/Crea Urine". *P*-values comparing dogs with spinal cord disorders and associated micturition dysfunction with (cystitis) and without cystitis (no cystitis) and dogs regaining the ability to urinate (dogs with normal voiding) are shown in the last rows. Significances are highlighted with an asterisk (*).Spinal Cord disorders (SC)

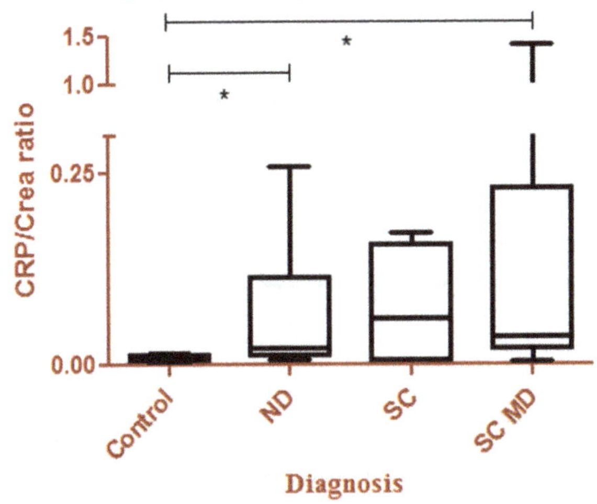

Fig. 1 C-reactive protein/ creatinine ratios in urine. C-reactive protein/ creatinine (CRP/Crea) concentrations: significant differences (*) between the control group (healthy dogs $n = 20$) and different neurological disorders ($n = 14$) (ND) ($p = 0.0020$) as well as spinal cord disorders with micturition dysfunction ($n = 15$) (SC MD) ($p = 0.0009$). The boxplots are indicating minimums and maximums, lower and upper quartiles, and medians

with micturition problems ($p = 0.0009$). No significant difference could be found between spinal cord disorders with and without micturition problems ($p = 0.3961$). However, the highest values of CRP/Crea-ratios occurred in dogs with micturition problems.

No significant differences could be detected in the urine of NGF/Crea ratios and the NGF levels in serum in the four different groups (Fig. 2 and Table 4).

Neither urinary NGF/Crea ($p = 0.7962$) nor CRP/Crea ($p = 0.0778$) showed significantly decreased levels after dogs with micturition disorders regained the ability to urinate (Table 4).

The urine examination revealed leukocytes (8/10) or bacteria and leukocytes (2/10) in 10 samples of the 27 dogs with micturition dysfunction. CRP/Crea and NGF/Crea values of dogs with cystitis were higher than in dogs without bacteria and/or leukocytes in the urine. However, this increase was not statistically significant (NGF/Crea $p = 0.1112$ and CRP/Crea $p = 0.0534$) (Fig. 3 and Table 4).

Discussion

In the current study the hypothesis had to be proven, that CRP or NGF are measurable in urine and serum samples of dogs and that these two proteins may be involved in the pathogenesis of micturition disorders. The aim of the study was to establish CRP and NGF as biomarkers helping to distinguish between neurogenic and non-neurogenic micturition disorders. In this study we concentrated on micturition disorders caused by diseases of the spinal cord and associated bacterial cystitis. Indeed, CRP and NGF are measurable with specific, commercially available ELISA kits in both, urine and serum of dogs as described before [24, 30]. Urine samples were compared to creatinine values of the urine to overcome the different dilutions between the samples [24].

However, the second part of the hypothesis could not be proven. No differences of NGF in serum or urine could be found between the different groups of neurological disorders and the control group.

NGF levels can rise in many different conditions such as neurologic diseases, endocrinological disorders and diseases of the immune system [31]. It is produced by many different cells, including urothelial cells, smooth muscle cells and mast cells [21]. Urinary NGF in particular was examined in lower urinary tract disorders [23]. HT Liu and HC Kuo [21] demonstrated that serum

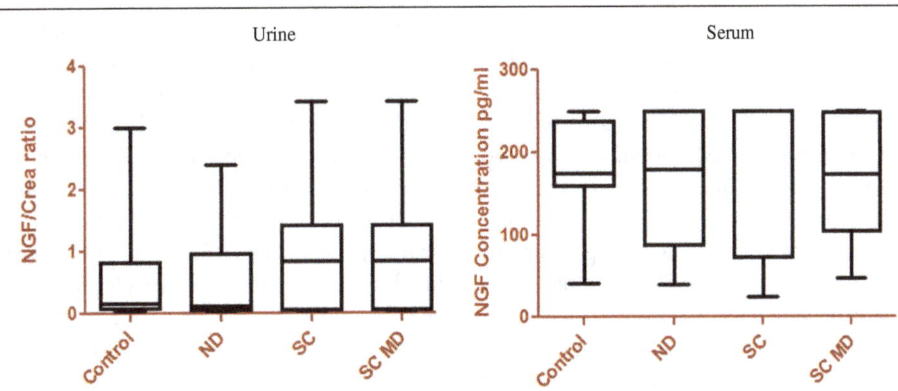

Fig. 2 Ratios of nerve growth factor/ creatinine in urine and nerve growth factor levels in serum in the different groups. Ratios of nerve growth factor/creatinine in urine (NGF/Crea) and nerve growth factor levels in serum (NGF Serum) in the different groups: control group (healthy dogs; $n = 20$), neurological disorders (ND; $n = 14$), spinal cord disorders without micturition dysfunctions (SC; $n = 15$) and spinal cord disorders with micturition dysfunction (SC MD; $n = 27$). No significant differences could be detected. The boxplots are indicating minimums and maximums, lower and upper quartiles and medians

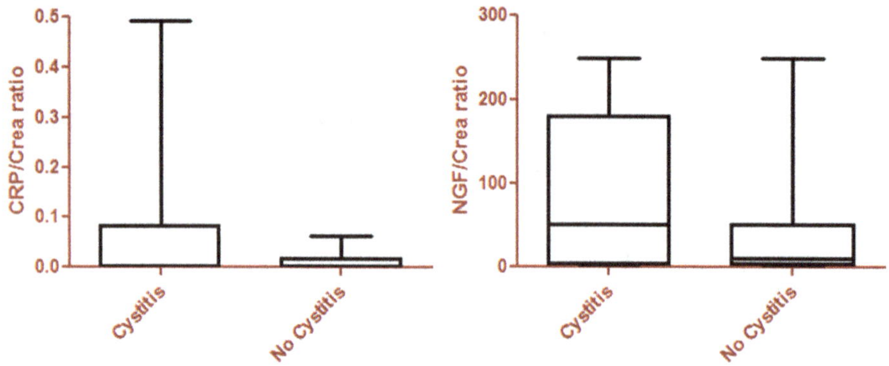

Fig. 3 Spinal cord disorders with micturition dysfunction. Values of C-reactive protein/creatinine ratio (CRP/Crea) and nerve-growth factor/ creatinine ratio (NGF/Crea) of dogs with spinal cord disorders with micturition dysfunction ($n = 27$). No significant difference in CRP/Crea ($p = 0.0534$) or NGF/Crea ($p = 0.1112$) could be detected within the group of dogs with micturition dysfunctions with ($n = 10$) or without cystitis ($n = 17$). However, higher concentrations could be found in dogs with cystitis in the NGF and CRP measurements. The boxplots are indicating minimums and maximums, lower and upper quartiles, and medians

and urine NGF levels were increased in humans suffering from interstitial cystitis and bladder pain syndrome, but no correlation could be found between serum and urinary NGF and the clinical signs. The authors suggest that other systemic disorders are also involved and influence the NGF-levels, especially the levels in serum [21]. In the current study, we tried to rule out other systemic diseases by routine blood examination and different imaging techniques such as ultrasound and radiographs of abdomen and thorax to exclude such an influence.

Urinary NGF levels were also found to be increased in cerebrovascular events and correlate with the severity of neurological impairment but not with urinary tract dysfunctions [32]. In our study dogs with mild and severe spinal cord injury were included leading most probably to the high range of the values and overlap between the groups.

The detected high variability of NGF-levels could be explained by comparing with the following studies. A study with rats experiencing stress showed increased NGF-values in serum [17]. In the current study, dogs with neurological dysfunctions had to be examined in the clinic. It could be expected that these dogs were suffering from stress because of their disease and the medical intervention, which could interfere with the production of NGF.

In human reports urine has been collected, when the bladder was full and the patients had a strong desire to void. NGF in urine increases physiologically while bladder stretching in healthy people [33]. In dogs it is difficult to standardize the urine collection according to those factors. However, urine samples were always taken from a filled bladder either through spontaneous voiding (walking the dog only when the bladder was filled), manual expression or cystocentesis to overcome the influence of heterogenous bladder stretching as much as possible.

NGF in urinary bladder biopsies of rats with spinal cord injuries was found to decrease four days to four weeks after injury, whereas the amount of NGF increased five to six weeks after the injury [34]. The mRNA-levels of total urinary bladder NGF decreased significantly in acute or chronic cyclophosphamide-induced cystitis compared to control animals. In the current study urine and serum collection was performed, when the dogs were presented in the clinic, therefore standardization according to the onset of the clinical signs was not feasible. The dogs had been suffering from neurological signs and/or micturition disorder for a variable amount of time. This well-known shortcoming of clinical studies could be a reason for measuring a wide range of NGF-values.

In conclusion, NGF cannot be developed to serve as a specific biomarker for severity of micturition disorders in a clinical setting shown by the results of the current study and the fact that NGF secretion in urine and especially serum can be influenced by many different factors.

CRP is an acute-phase protein, which is mainly produced by the liver and is raised in conditions of inflammation and tissue damage [25].

In a study performed by Chuang et al. (2010) the authors demonstrated higher serum levels in humans with lower urinary tract disorders (overactive bladder syndrome), but urinary CRP and mRNA expression of CRP in bladder biopsies were barely detectable. Detection of elevated urinary CRP has been reported before in dogs with renal disease caused by leishmaniasis [35], babesiosis [36] and pyometra [37]. A time-resolved immunofluorimetic assay was used to determine the urinary CRP concentration in dogs with leishmaniasis [35], whereas urine samples of dogs with babesiosis and pyometra were analyzed using an ELISA-system as in the current study [36] .

In our study CRP could not be detected in each urine sample, even the study design, control probes and the above mentioned measurements are proof that CRP is measurable in urine of dogs using an ELISA. Evaluating detectable urine samples only a significant higher concentration of CRP/Crea-levels could be found comparing the control group and different neurological disorders and the control group with spinal cord disorders with micturition problems. Measurements in the group spinal cord disorders without micturition problems displayed the widest range. In this group the severity of neurological/motor dysfunction varied the most. Additionally, CRP/Crea levels in dogs suffering from spinal cord disorders with micturition dysfunction with cystitis were higher than in dogs without cystitis. In a study done by KW Seo, JB Lee, JO Ahn, HW Lee, CY Hwang, HY Youn and CW Lee [28], dogs with experimentally induced cystitis showed higher CRP values in serum than the control group. Since no significances could be detected in dogs with spinal cord disorders with and without cystitis, a comparison with a control group of dogs without neurological dysfunction and cystitis was abandoned. Such dogs suffered also from systemic diseases, which would have influenced additionally CRP and NGF concentrations (data not shown).

It is anticipated that many tissues of the body can produce CRP as a part of their own immune system defense [38]. Extrahepatic syntheses have been reported in neuron, atherosclerotic plaques, monocytes and lymphocytes. The mechanisms underlying the extrahepatic synthesis are unknown [38, 39]. In humans CRP can be produced by coronary artery smooth muscle cells [40]. Therefore, a production of CRP by smooth muscle cells of the bladder might be involved in the pathogenesis of micturition disorders.

The highest concentrations can be measured two to four days after the onset of the disease [41]. The individual CRP concentrations can vary significantly between different dogs [42]. S Yamamoto, T Shida, S Miyaji, H Santsuka, H Fujise, K Mukawa, E Furukawa, T Nagae and M Naiki [41] reported increased and decreased CRP serum values in dogs with different disorders such as enteritis, eye diseases and nephritis. Some of the dogs whose medical condition had improved after the treatment had increased, others decreased CRP levels [41]. Levels of CRP in serum can increase after surgery. Moreover, the degree to which the levels rise, corresponds to the surgical trauma [43]. In our study some patients underwent surgical treatment and others did not. This could be a reason for different serum CRP values specifically the high range of the CRP levels. However, a diagnostic biomarker for use in a clinical setting should overcome such differences in treatment of individual patients with spinal cord disorders.

Conclusions

In conclusion, CRP and NGF are measureable in both urine and serum of dogs. Levels of CRP in the urine of dogs with spinal cord disorders with micturition problems were elevated. However, not all dogs with micturition disorders had detectable CRP values. No significant differences of CRP and NGF in serum or urine in the diseased groups could be detected. Therefore, it cannot be recommended to develop CRP and NGF as reliable biomarkers in micturition disorders in a clinical setting. However, these proteins could be valuable for pathogenesis studies or for control examinations of single patients in treatment studies.

Methods

Study design and animals

Paired urine and serum samples were collected from 76 dogs with different neurological disorders and from control dogs at the Department of Small Animal Medicine and Surgery, University of Veterinary Medicine Hannover, Germany. The study was performed according to the ethical rules of the Lower Saxony State Office for Consumer Protection and Food Safety, Germany, animal experiment number: 33.4-42502-04-13A374. An owners' permission was granted for all dogs. The following breeds were included: mixed breed ($n = 17$), Dachshund ($n = 10$), Beagle ($n = 8$), Bernese Mountain Dog ($n = 6$), Labrador ($n = 5$), French bulldog ($n = 4$), Golden Retriever ($n = 3$), Jack Russell Terrier ($n = 2$), Shepherd ($n = 3$), Giant Schnauzer ($n = 2$), Small Münsterländer ($n = 1$), Boxer ($n = 1$), Bolonka Zwetna ($n = 1$), Miniature Schnauzer ($n = 1$), Weimaraner ($n = 1$), Saint Bernard dog ($n = 1$), Old English Sheepdog ($n = 1$), Swiss Mountain Dog ($n = 1$), Pekingese dog ($n = 1$), Chihuahua ($n = 1$), Shi Tzu ($n = 1$), Bracke ($n = 1$), German wirehaired pointer ($n = 1$). The mean age of the dogs was 5.6 years (+/− 2.8 years) and the average weight was 19.8 kg (+/−13 kg). 29 dogs were male, 21 castrated-male, 7 female and 19 spayed female.

Paired urine and serum samples were collected from patients with different neurological disorders and from the control dogs. The clinical diagnosis was established using a combination of clinical examination, neurological examination, blood and urine analysis, magnetic resonance imaging (52/76) and evaluation of cerebrospinal fluid samples (48/72). In all dogs regular clinical and laboratory control examinations were performed to rule out concurrent diseases.

The patients were categorized in 4 different groups (Table 1): healthy dogs ($n = 20$); different neurological disorders except spinal cord disorders (Table 2) ($n = 14$); spinal cord disorders with normal micturition ($n = 15$); spinal cord disorders with micturition problems ($n = 27$) (Table 5); [44] out of the 27 dogs with micturition

Table 5 Number (N) of dogs with different severity of spinal cord dysfunction (grading according to Sharp and Wheeler 2005)

	N
Grade I	2
Grade II	6
Grade III	7
Grade IV	11
Grade V	16

problems, 10 urine samples were taken in a follow up study, when the dogs regained the ability to void. "Normal" micturition was assumed, when dogs with spinal cord disorders had spontaneous voiding when the bladder was filled and they could walk outdoors. Dogs were considered to be healthy, when clinical and neurological examinations were normal and no abnormalities in blood and urine analysis were observed.

Sample collection

Urine samples were collected after spontaneous voiding, manual expression or cystocentesis and immediately analyzed. All urine samples of dogs with normal micturition were taken after spontaneous voiding, urine samples of dogs with micturition disorders were taken after manual expression (n = 12) or cystocentesis (n = 15). To rule out or to diagnose cystitis all urine samples were analyzed with a colorimetric urine analysis reagent test stripe (Urine stripes, Roche Diagnostics GmbH, Mannheim, Germany). Samples with leukocytes and/or bacteria in urine sediment analysis were considered dogs with cystitis. The specific gravity was measured with a refractometer (Manual Handrefractometer, A.KRÜSS Optronic GmbH, Hamburg, Germany). The urine creatinine level was measured to normalize CRP and NGF levels using Cobas C311 Analyzer (Roche Diagnostics GmbH, Mannheim, Germany). Urine and serum samples were centrifuged at 1000 rpm for 10 min and frozen at −20 °C until analyzed.

Analysis of NGF

Urinary and serum NGF concentrations were determined using an immunosorbent assay system (NGF EMAX ®ImmunoAssay System- ELISA Test Kit, Madison, WI, USA). This assay was evaluated for the use of canine samples [24, 30]. The assay had a minimum sensitivity of 7.8 pg/ml, values above 250 pg/ml cannot be quantified and was performed according to the manufacturer's instructions. Serum samples were diluted 1:50, urine samples were not diluted. Values that were above 250 pg/ml were counted as 250 pg/ml, values lower than the detection range as zero. All samples were run in duplicates and the mean of these two values was used for further evaluation.

Analysis of CRP

CRP levels in urinary and serum samples were measured using a commercially available dog specific immunosorbent assay system (dog high- Sensitive CRP ELISA Kit, Kamiya Medical Company, Seattle, WA, USA), which can be applied for several biological fluids such as urine. The detection range was between 3,125 ng/ml and 200 ng/ml. The assays were conducted according to the manufactures instructions. The serum samples were diluted 1:1000, urine samples were diluted 1:2. Results below the detection limit were counted as zero. None of the samples were above the detection limit. All samples were run in duplicates and the mean of these two values was used for further evaluation.

Statistical analysis

After testing for normal distribution, the Wilcoxon-Mann-Whitney-Test was used to evaluate potential significant differences between the four different groups. To distinguish between healthy dogs and dogs with cystitis a t-test was performed. In order to differentiate between dogs with abnormal micturition and dogs that regained ability of normal micturition a f-test was performed. To analyze the number of samples with detectable CRP and NGF values a Fisher-Yate was used. All data analyses were conducted with the statistic program package SAS®, version 9.2 (SAS Institute, Cary, NC, USA). For all statistical tests an error probability of $p < 0.05$ as significance level was chosen. Statistical calculations were performed twice: using all data including the patients without measurable CRP values (counted as zero) and a calculation including only patients with measurable values. Data of calculated p-values are summarized in (Table 4).

Abbreviations

Crea: Creatinin; CRP: C-Reactive Protein; CRP/Crea: C-Reactive Protein/ Creatinin Ratio; ELISA: Enzyme Linked Immunosorbent Assay; ND: Neurological Disorders; NGF: Nerve Growth Factor; NGF/Crea: Nerve Growth Factor/ Creatinin Ratio; SC: Spinal cord disorders; SC MD: Spinal Cord disorders with micturition dysfunction.

Competing interest

None of the authors of this paper has a financial or personal relationship with other people or organizations that could inappropriately influence or bias the content of the paper.

Authors' contributions

UK performed the study and wrote the manuscript. RC helped with the Enzyme Linked Immunosorbent Assays. VS participated in the coordination of the study and helped to draft the manuscript. AT participated in the study design and coordination and helped to draft the manuscript. All authors read and approved the final manuscript.

Acknowledgements

This paper was mainly funded by grant (TI 309/4-2) from the Deutsche Forschungs-gemeinschaft (DFG; Bonn, Germany) within the DFG Research Unit (FOR) 1103. The author wishes to thank Hanna Amendt for her general support and Dr. Karl Rohn (Department of Epidemiology and Information Processing University of Veterinary Medicine Hannover, Germany) for helping with statistical analysis.

References

1. Granger N, Chew D, Fairhurst P, Fawcett JW, Lacour SP, Craggs M, et al. Use of an implanted sacral nerve stimulator to restore urine voiding in chronically paraplegic dogs. J vetintern med/American college of veterinary internal medicine. 2013;27(1):99–105.
2. Ross JC. Management of the bladder in spinal injuries. Br Med J. 1951; 1(4707):616–9.
3. Fluehmann G, Doherr MG, Jaggy A. Canine neurological diseases in a referral hospital population between 1989 and 2000 in Switzerland. J Small Anim Pract. 2006;47(10):582–7.
4. de Groat WC, Yoshimura N. Plasticity in reflex pathways to the lower urinary tract following spinal cord injury. Exp Neurol. 2012;235(1):123–32.
5. Yoshimura N, Ogawa T, Miyazato M, Kitta T, Furuta A, Chancellor MB, et al. Neural mechanisms underlying lower urinary tract dysfunction. Korean journal of urology. 2014;55(2):81–90.
6. Arnold S, Steffen F, Jaggy A. Blasenstörungen. In: *Atlas und Lehrbuch der Kleintierneurologie*. 2nd ed. Hannover: Schlütersche Verlagsgesellschaft mbH & Co; 2007. p. 333–68.
7. Smee N, Loyd K, Grauer G. UTIs in small animal patients: part 1: etiology and pathogenesis. J Am Anim Hosp Assoc. 2013;49(1):1–7.
8. Norris CR, Williams BJ, Ling GV, Franti Johnson CE, Ruby AL. Recurrent and persistent urinary tract infections in dogs: 383 cases (1969–1995). J Am Anim Hosp Assoc. 2000;36(6):484–92.
9. Wooley RE, Blue JL. Quantitative and bacteriological studies of urine specimens from canine and feline urinary tract infections. J Clin Microbiol. 1976;4(4):326–9.
10. Smee N, Loyd K, Grauer GF. UTIs in small animal patients: part 2: diagnosis, treatment, and complications. J Am Anim Hosp Assoc. 2013;49(2):83–94.
11. Stiffler KS, Stevenson MA, Sanchez S, Barsanti JA, Hofmeister E, Budsberg SC. Prevalence and characterization of urinary tract infections in dogs with surgically treated type 1 thoracolumbar intervertebral disc extrusion. Vet Surg. 2006;35(4):330–6.
12. Bubenik L, Hosgood G. Urinary tract infection in dogs with thoracolumbar intervertebral disc herniation and urinary bladder dysfunction managed by manual expression, indwelling catheterization or intermittent catheterization. Vet Surg. 2008;37(8):791–800.
13. Olby NJ, MacKillop E, Cerda-Gonzalez S, Moore S, Munana KR, Grafinger M, et al. Prevalence of urinary tract infection in dogs after surgery for thoracolumbar intervertebral disc extrusion. J vet intern med / American college of veterinary internal medicine. 2010;24(5):1106–11.
14. Fry CH, Sahai A, Vahabi B, Kanai AJ, Birder LA. What is the role for biomarkers for lower urinary tract disorders? Neurourol urodyn. 2014; 33(5):602–5.
15. Schoeman JP, Goddard A, Leisewitz AL. Biomarkers in canine parvovirus enteritis. N Z Vet J. 2013;61(4):217–22.
16. Bhide AA, Cartwright R, Khullar V, Digesu GA. Biomarkers in overactive bladder. Internat urogynecol j. 2013;24(7):1065–72.
17. Levi-Montalcini R, Skaper SD, Dal Toso R, Petrelli L, Leon A. Nerve growth factor: from neurotrophin to neurokine. Trends Neurosci. 1996;19(11):514–20.
18. Pezet S, McMahon SB. Neurotrophins: mediators and modulators of pain. Annu Rev Neurosci. 2006;29:507–38.
19. Ochodnicky P, Cruz CD, Yoshimura N, Michel MC. Nerve growth factor in bladder dysfunction: contributing factor, biomarker, and therapeutic target. NeurourolUrodyn. 2011;30(7):1227–41.
20. Steers WD, Kolbeck S, Creedon D, Tuttle JB. Nerve growth factor in the urinary bladder of the adult regulates neuronal form and function. J Clin Invest. 1991;88(5):1709–15.
21. Liu HT, Kuo HC. Increased urine and serum nerve growth factor levels in interstitial cystitis suggest chronic inflammation is involved in the pathogenesis of disease. PLoS One. 2012;7(9), e44687.
22. Cruz CD. Neurotrophins in bladder function: what do we know and where do we go from here? NeurourolUrodyn. 2014;33(1):39–45.
23. Rachaneni S, Arya P, Latthe P. Urinary nerve growth factor: a biomarker of detrusor overactivity? A systematic review. Int urogynecol j. 2013; 24(10):1603–9.
24. Seth JH, Sahai A, Khan MS, van der Aa F, de Ridder D, Panicker JN, et al. Nerve growth factor (NGF): a potential urinary biomarker for overactive bladder syndrome (OAB)? BJU Int. 2013;111(3):372–80.
25. Ceron JJ, Eckersall PD, Martynez-Subiela S. Acute phase proteins in dogs and cats: current knowledge and future perspectives. Vet clin pathol/ American society for veterinary clinical pathology. 2005;34(2):85–99.
26. Chuang Y-C, Tyagi V, Liu R-T, Chancellor MB, Tyagi P. Urine and serum c-reactive protein levels as potential biomarkers of lower urinary tract symptoms. Urological science (previously Journal of Taiwan urological association). 2010; 21(3):132–6.
27. Hsiao SM, Lin HH, Kuo HC. The role of serum c-reactive protein in women with lower urinary tract symptoms. Int urogynecol j. 2012;23(7):935–40.
28. Seo KW, Lee JB, Ahn JO, Lee HW, Hwang CY, Youn HY, et al. C-reactive protein as an indicator of inflammatory responses to experimentally induced cystitis in dogs. J Vet Sci. 2012;13(2):179–85.
29. Bathen-Noethen A, Carlson R, Menzel D, Mischke R, Tipold A. Concentrations of acute-phase proteins in dogs with steroid responsive meningitis-arteritis. J vet int med / American college of veterinary internal medicine. 2008;22(5):1149–56.
30. Isola M, Ferrari V, Miolo A, Stabile F, Bernardini D, Carnier P, et al. Nerve growth factor concentrations in the synovial fluid from healthy dogs and dogs with secondary osteoarthritis. Vet Comp Orthop Traumatol. 2011;24(4):279–84.
31. Aloe L, Bracci-Laudiero L, Bonini S, Manni L, Aloe L. The expanding role of nerve growth factor: from neurotrophic activity to immunologic diseases. Allergy. 1997;52(9):883–994.
32. Liu H-T, Liu A-B, Chancellor MB, Kuo H-C. Urinary nerve growth factor level is correlated with the severity of neurological impairment in patients with cerebrovascular accident. BJU Int. 2009;104(8):1158–62.
33. Liu H-T, Kuo H-C. Urinary nerve growth factor levels are elevated in patients with overactive bladder and do not significantly increase with bladder distention. NeurourolUrodyn. 2009;28(1):78–81.
34. Vizzard MA. Changes in urinary bladder neurotrophic factor mRNA and NGF protein following urinary bladder dysfunction. Exp Neurol. 2000; 161(1):273–84.
35. Martinez-Subiela S, Garcia-Martinez JD, Tvarijonaviciute A, Tecles F, Caldin M, Bernal LJ, et al. Urinary C reactive protein levels in dogs with leishmaniasis at different stages of renal damage. Res Vet Sci. 2013;95(3):924–9.
36. Defauw P, Schoeman JP, Smets P, Goddard A, Meyer E, Liebenberg C, et al. Assessment of renal dysfunction using urinary markers in canine babesiosis caused by Babesia rossi. Vet Parasitol. 2012;190(3–4):326–32.
37. Maddens B, Heiene R, Smets P, Svensson M, Aresu L, van der Lugt J, et al. Evaluation of kidney injury in dogs with pyometra based on proteinuria, renal histomorphology, and urinary biomarkers. J vet int med / American college of veterinary internal medicine. 2011;25(5):1075–83.
38. Yasojima K, Schwab C, McGeer EG, McGeer PL. Human neurons generate c-reactive protein and amyloid P: upregulation in Alzheimer's disease. Brain Res. 2000;887(1):80–9.
39. Black S, Kushner I, Samols D. C-reactive Protein. J Biol Chem. 2004;279(47): 48487–90.
40. Calabro P, Willerson JT, Yeh ET. Inflammatory cytokines stimulated c-reactive protein production by human coronary artery smooth muscle cells. Circulation. 2003;108(16):1930–2.
41. Yamamoto S, Shida T, Miyaji S, Santsuka H, Fujise H, Mukawa K, et al. Changes in serum c-reactive protein levels in dogs with various disorders and surgical traumas. Vet Res Commun. 1993;17(2):85–93.
42. Otabe K, Sugimoto T, Jinbo T, Honda M, Kitao S, Hayashi S, et al. Physiological levels of C-reactive protein in normal canine sera. Vet Res Commun. 1998;22(2):77–85.
43. Kjelgaard-Hansen M, Strom H, Mikkelsen LF, Eriksen T, Jensen AL, Luntang-Jensen M. Canine serum C-reactive protein as a quantitative marker of the inflammatory stimulus of aseptic elective soft tissue surgery. Vet clin pathol/ American society for veterinary clinical pathology. 2013;42(3):342–5.
44. Sharp NJH, Wheeler SJ. Small animal spinal disorders. 2nd ed. Edinburgh, London: Elsevier Mosby; 2005. p. 41–159.

12

Stimulating collaboration between human and veterinary health care professionals

Björn G.M. Eussen*, Jaap Schaveling, Maria J. Dragt and Robert Jan Blomme

Abstract

Background: Despite the need to control outbreaks of (emerging) zoonotic diseases and the need for added value in comparative/translational medicine, jointly addressed in the One Health approach [One health Initiative (n.d.a). *About the One Health Initiative.* http://www.onehealthinitiative.com/about.php. Accessed 13 September 2016], collaboration between human and veterinary health care professionals is limited. This study focuses on the social dilemma experienced by health care professionals and ways in which an interdisciplinary approach could be developed.

Results: Based on Gaertner and Dovidio's Common Ingroup Identity Model, a number of questionnaires were designed and tested; with PROGRESS, the relation between collaboration and common goal was assessed, mediated by decategorization, recategorization, mutual differentiation and knowledge sharing. This study confirms the Common Ingroup Identity Model stating that common goals stimulate collaboration. Decategorization and mutual differentiation proved to be significant in this relationship; recategorization and knowledge sharing mediate this relation.

Conclusions: It can be concluded that the Common Ingroup Identity Model theory helps us to understand how health care professionals perceive the One Health initiative and how they can intervene in this process. In the One Health approach, professional associations could adopt a facilitating role.

Keywords: One health, Social dilemma, Collaboration, Veterinarians, Physicians, Knowledge sharing, Common Ingroup Identity Model

Background

To control outbreaks of (emerging) diseases at an early stage, effective collaboration between human and veterinary healthcare professionals is essential [1]. However, to date, collaboration has taken place only on a very limited scale [1–6]. For this reason, One Health, an interdisciplinary approach addressing the connections between health care for humans, animals and the environment and focused on the elements biomedical research, enhanced public health efficacy, an expanded scientific knowledge base and improved medical educational and clinical care in which human and veterinary healthcare and other stakeholders work together [7], is placed high on the agendas of organizations such as the WHO, the European Commission's Directorate-General for Health and Consumers, USA Centers for Disease Control and Prevention [CDCP] and Worldbank [1, 8–10].

Because more than three-quarters of all the infections seen in humans originate in animals [1], there is great and widespread interest in the effective collaboration between human and veterinary healthcare professionals as a means to halt outbreaks of infections at an early stage. The outbreak of Severe Acute Respiratory Syndrome (SARS), for instance, which was not even known to be an animal-transmitted infection when it first occurred, is estimated to have caused a loss of as much as US$40 billion in terms of Gross Domestic Product (GDP) worldwide [11]. Other examples include the recent outbreaks of avian influenza and Q fever in the Netherlands, which have shown that serious outbreaks can have major consequences for human and animal health [12]. Areas where close cooperation would be fruitful because they share the same goals include combatting and controlling zoonoses and emerging zoonoses; here, the interdependence of the two fields requires an integrated approach. In efforts to reach mutual goals, an interdisciplinary exchange of knowledge between the two

* Correspondence: B.Eussen@nyenrode.nl
Center for Leadership and Management Development, Nyenrode Business University, P.O. Box 1303620 AC Breukelen, Netherlands

professional groups can lead to a sharing of domain-specific expertise and experience, thus enabling experts to identify possible zoonotic infections and to fight them with the help of appropriate control measures at earlier stages [2]. Another advantage of collaboration between these two groups of healthcare professionals, besides the more adequate fight against infectious diseases, is the exchange of knowledge on the treatment of diseases [2] leading to major healthcare cost savings [6, 11] and to new scientific insights [7]. In order to better understand the mental motivation of health care professionals with respect to the One Health approach, this study used psychosocial concepts such as social dilemma, (group) identification and category thinking.

Collaboration as a social dilemma

Collaboration can be defined as "any action which is intended to benefit others, regardless of whether the actor also benefits in the process" [13]. However, collaboration can also fail to take place: in human and veterinary healthcare, cooperation between professionals can fail to materialize because there is a social dilemma, for instance. To illustrate, there are situations in which a non-cooperative course of action is (at times) tempting for each individual in that it yields superior (often short-term) outcomes for the individual himself or herself [13]. For example, it is commonly accepted that professionals have a constant and permanent responsibility for their patients, who expect care and action in the short term. A healthcare professional may therefore view collaboration, which may (at times) exceed or influence his own day-to-day operations, as not sufficiently important, at least for the short term. But if everyone pursues this non-cooperative course of action, then everyone will ultimately be worse off (often in the longer term) than would have been the case if everyone had collaborated.

Collaboration between human and veterinary healthcare professionals can be characterized as a social dilemma. It is often thought that a lack of time is the main reason why healthcare professionals feel they have so little psychological room for greater collaboration. Fleuren, Wieferink and Paulussen [14], however, show that healthcare professionals actually have other reasons than time; what lies at the heart of their limited cooperation is a lack of clarity as to why collaboration should be organized in the first place. The individuals concerned do not always have a sufficiently well-defined idea of the benefits offered by increased contact and collaboration, even though collaboration is highly desirable both for the sector itself and for society as a whole [2]. In this regard and in any event, the (long-term) awareness of sharing a common goal is of crucial importance.

Collaboration is stimulated if the (perceived) benefits outweigh the individual arguments or circumstances of the healthcare professionals concerned. This type of calculation, or dilemma, can lead to cooperation 'for the public good'. Considering its objectives, One Health can be seen as a public good dilemma, because "public good dilemmas require individuals to make an active contribution to establish or maintain a collective good, such as building a local bridge or joining a social movement" [13]. However, in terms of making room for the bigger collective goal alongside their responsibilities related to the day-to-day care of their own patients, human and veterinary healthcare professionals often see insufficient added value [14], even though a greater awareness of the added value associated with collaboration would ultimately result in improved care [5, 15, 16].

Greater awareness of the added value brought about by collaboration on the part of healthcare professionals is consistent with the social desire for more intensive collaboration between human and veterinary healthcare [1, 8–10, 12]. These two groups of healthcare professionals speak the same 'language' and should therefore be able to understand each other well [17]. Despite the fact that, broadly speaking, both groups followed similar training programmes [18, 19] and perform similar clinical procedures, there is hardly any exchange of knowledge and experience [5]. In addition, a clear focus on common goals is lacking, and collaboration between human and veterinary healthcare professionals remains limited at present [5, 6, 20]. So far, collaboration has only taken place in a limited number of research areas and only occasionally during outbreaks of emerging diseases [1, 4]. Closer examinations have revealed that the limited scale of collaboration is due, among other things, to mutual prejudices [2] and psychological barriers between the parties concerned [5]. Such mutual judgements and prejudices may disrupt the development of collaboration, but research into these phenomena has so far remained very limited. The present study is aimed to help fill that gap.

Common ingroup identity theory

In order to gain a better understanding of what stimulates cooperation among healthcare professionals, we used the Common Ingroup Identity Model developed by Gaertner and Dovidio [17]. This theory provides insight into the relationship between individual perceptions and behaviours towards groups and lists possible causes which may influence these. According to the Common Ingroup Identity Model, sharing a common goal affects the degree of collaboration, but this relationship is also influenced by the perception of this degree and the means of categorization [17, 21]. The Common Ingroup Identity Model [17] focuses on the individual's perception with regard to the group. In essence, the model states that members who see themselves as belonging to a larger, common whole consciously classify themselves within that larger whole, as a result of which prejudices between groups or communities decrease.

According to Gaertner and Dovidio, collaboration is influenced by characteristics (in this study qualified as the common goal) which play a role in the individual perception of the situation: does the individual perceive the existence of a single overarching group, several groups or subgroups, or no group at all? If individuals feel that they belong to a group, in this case 'healthcare', this will lead to more positive thoughts, feelings and behaviours among the individuals in the groups concerned [17]. As explained above, when group members see themselves as part of a larger whole and when they classify themselves within this structure, prejudice between groups or communities is reduced. According to Kramer and Brewer [22], people within a group or an overarching whole are prepared to share communal resources and other supplies, but they will develop resistance if these have to be shared with others *outside* the group. Still, a change occurs if these outsiders can be placed within a perceived larger whole. The realization that there is in fact a larger whole means that the positive thoughts, feelings and behaviours (such as the sharing of resources and information) which would normally be reserved for the individual's own familiar group are extended to members of other communities who also belong to the larger overarching whole. Common endeavour and classifying thus go hand in hand, leading to feelings of 'us' rather than feelings of 'us versus them'. In other words, it depends on how an individual sees his group or subgroup within a larger whole [17].

Using the Common Ingroup Identity Model, we quantitatively assessed healthcare group interrelationships in order to gain insight into the contributions towards cooperation that can be made by means of a common goal for healthcare professionals formulated via their perception of group formation. In the past, the Common Ingroup Identity Model was researched primarily in experimental studies, with a main focus on perceived group formation [23]. A limitation of the model is that the duration of the effect of an intervention is unclear, as is the reduction of bias [24]. The current study will not only indicate whether the Common Ingroup Identity Model is useful for the respective groups of healthcare professionals, but it will also quantitatively assess the relationships between the common goal and collaboration in combination with associated mediating factors. In this way, the study will contribute to further theoretical development in terms of validation as well as to the quantitative usefulness of the Common Ingroup Identity Model. It will also examine whether the exchange of knowledge is an additional trigger for collaboration once healthcare professionals have become aware of the common goal.

Collaboration and common goal

In the social dilemma referred to earlier, where there is insufficient awareness of the possible advantages of collaboration, and in this case human and veterinary collaboration, crucial factors include the reasons why healthcare professionals place themselves in a particular category and identify with their 'own' professional group [2, 3, 5]. It is 'natural' for people to engage in social categorization: the brain is hard-wired to think in terms of categories, and categories form the basis for standard judgements and prejudices [25]. The advantages of social categorization are that individuals know where they stand and what is expected of them, and that a group or community contributes to a feeling of (social) well-being [17]. The same is true of human and veterinary healthcare professionals, although a certain distance is maintained between them [2, 5]. After all, what is qualified by the terms 'human' and 'animal' is placed in different categories. This is illustrated by the dichotomy between the two professional groups, established on the basis of typical activities, with 'human patient' being contrasted with 'animal patient', and hence on the basis of category-based thinking [2]. Still, mutual contact alone does not lead to productivity or better joint results; for good results, interdependence is necessary [26, 27]. If individuals perceive a common goal, in this case 'improving care through One Health', then according to the Common Ingroup Identity Theory this can be expected to lead to more positive thoughts, feelings and behaviours between individuals in the groups concerned [17], because there will then be more perceived interdependence between the two groups. According to the Common Ingroup Identity Theory, the awareness of a larger whole or a common ingroup, in this case a joint responsibility for improving care, will lead to the extension of positive thoughts, feelings and behaviours (such as the sharing of resources and information) that were traditionally reserved for the individual's own familiar group to members of other communities who also belong to the larger overarching whole.

In the case of common goals and interests, a clear interdependence can be seen: after all, the aim is to achieve a result which requires contributions from *both* groups. In their model, Gaertner and Dovidio [17] describe a common goal in terms of 'interdependence'. In this respect, collaboration between human and veterinary healthcare professionals is the result of addressing common goals and interests [2, 3, 6, 11, 16]. This is in line with the social interdependence theory which argues that interdependence results from a common goal [27–31]. Mutatis mutandis, this altruistic goal was recently incorporated in the One Health initiative (16). This means that One Health, as a common goal, can be expected to lead to greater collaboration. This brings us to our first hypothesis:

One Health as a common goal has a positive effect on collaboration between human and veterinary healthcare professionals.

The process of classifying concerns the individual's perception of the connection between – in this case – two groups of healthcare professionals: how an individual sees his group or subgroup within a larger whole and whether the individual perceives the existence of a single overarching group, multiple groups or subgroups, or no group at all [17]. As described earlier, One Health can affect how people see themselves as part of a larger, common whole and how they classify themselves within that larger whole. The Common Ingroup Identity theory distinguishes the following types of perception and reclassification: recategorization, decategorization and mutual differentiation [21]. These types are elaborated below.

Recategorization

Perceived commonality and perceived common goals (overlap between groups and a stronger feeling of 'us' rather than 'us and them', recategorization) result in greater collaboration [22, 32]. That being said, the feeling of 'us' is not by definition limited to a single group: a person can possess multiple identities because he or she can be a member of multiple groups [33]. This means that in addition to classifying themselves in the veterinarians' group, veterinarians could also classify themselves in the (overarching) group of healthcare providers [34]. We speak of recategorization when an overarching identity is perceived in which old groups are represented as a whole or in a new form, for example as a subgroup. Via the formation of a subgroup, collaboration between the two groups of healthcare professionals is further enhanced, for instance through awareness of a common goal. This brings us to our second hypothesis:

The positive relation between common goal and collaboration is mediated by the partial effect of recategorization.

Decategorization

According to Gaertner and Dovidio [17], a common goal causes perceptions to be reclassified into changed perceptions, thus leading to greater collaboration. It may be expected that if healthcare professionals become aware of a common goal, there will be room to recognize the overlap with the other group of healthcare professionals. This type of development is also known as decategorization. If a certain situation is perceived as a form of decategorization, the emotional group connections become less important, so that there will be room for individuals to recognize shared identities. In turn, this will lead individuals to have more extensive contacts with other individuals, as a result of which prejudices will decrease and positive attitudes towards people in a different group can be developed [17]. This brings us to our third hypothesis:

The positive relation between common goal and collaboration is mediated by the partial effect of decategorization.

Mutual differentiation

Brown and Wade [35] and Molleman, Broekhuis, Stoffels and Jaspers [36] conclude that if one wishes to stimulate collaboration, both groups must be able to retain their old identity. It is possible for the two groups to collaborate, but the researchers believe it is important that both groups continue to operate separately and that both fulfil a complementary role within the framework of their common goal. Such a structure, with interdependence and individual space for each group, will ultimately reduce prejudice and tension on either side [21, 37, 38]. This perceived commonality can then lead to greater collaboration [22, 32, 39].

A thorough understanding of interdependence and common endeavour has a psychological effect on interaction, interrelationships and collaboration: it leads to recognition, stimulation and interaction [27]. In the case of mutual differentiation as a social categorization perception, there is appreciation of the knowledge and expertise on the part of the other professional group. According to Gaertner and Dovidio [17], 'there is a win-win situation which produces positive feelings and stereotyping towards the other group, while the individual's own group can define it's own profile'. In the case of recategorization and mutual differentiation, it is important in both cases that the original identity is not abandoned when collaboration takes place. Both groups will then be able to retain some autonomy within a common whole and they will not stray too far into each other's territory [36].

Where the common goal (*in casu* One Health) is perceived as collaboration by mutual differentiation, a special focus lies on the importance of each of the groups with respect to their different qualities and expertise. Hewstone and Brown [40] state that collaboration should be focused on complementary knowledge and expertise. Collaboration will be triggered by paying attention to each other's knowledge and expertise, as a function of the clarity of a common goal. This brings us to our fourth hypothesis:

The positive relation between common goal and collaboration is mediated by the partial effect of mutual differentiation.

Knowledge sharing

Ives, Torrey and Gordon [41] argue that having a clear common interest leads to situations in which an exchange of knowledge can take place. In addition to what follows from the Common Ingroup Identity Model, it can be assumed that knowledge sharing leads to collaboration because individuals can use each other's expertise [42–44]. Knowledge sharing between teams and groups improves performance and effectiveness [45–47]. Added value can be achieved by having professionals from different backgrounds learning and working together, thanks to the possibilities offered in terms of exchanges, the integration of knowledge and innovation. Advantages are particularly associated with the sharing of implicit knowledge and new insights [42]. Collaboration is promoted by knowledge transfer through informal or small-scale processes and lateral, social contacts [48, 49]. Kramer and Brewer [22] showed that individuals were particularly inclined to share knowledge with others within their own group, but also that they can be more reticent with more distant contacts. In that case, and especially in the case of One Health, it is important to address perceived distance; when others are perceived as less distant, they will have fewer reservations to collaborate within the framework of One Health. Finally, Holmes [50] demonstrates a positive connection between (continuing) knowledge sharing and mutual ties, trust within a group and collaboration [22, 32, 51]. This brings us to our fifth hypothesis:

> *The positive relation between common goal and collaboration is mediated by the partial effect of knowledge sharing.*

Methods

Sample

Our study sample consisted of 368 respondents. By means of a digital newsletter from the professional organizations – the Royal Dutch Veterinary Association (KNMvD) and the Royal Dutch Medical Association (KNMG) – human and veterinary healthcare professionals were invited on a one-off basis to complete the questionnaire. The questionnaire was sent to 40,000 human and 5000 veterinary healthcare professionals. In addition to these professional associations, human and veterinary healthcare professionals were contacted via social media such as LinkedIn and Twitter.

A total of 595 healthcare professionals responded, 368 of whom completed the survey in full. Of the 368 respondents, 58 (16%) were human healthcare professionals; 310 (84%) were veterinary healthcare professionals. The low response rate demonstrated by the group of human healthcare professionals could be explained by their limited interest in the One Health topic [5]. An illustration of this can be found in the difference in attention paid to the topic in the professional body's journals. During the last five years, One Health was mentioned only nine times in the weekly Dutch journal of Human healthcare professionals; in contrast, every monthly issue of the veterinary journal elaborated on the topic. Of all our respondents, 57% were female. The average age of the respondents was 44, and respondents had been working in the profession for an average of approximately 16 years. 87% of respondents were still active in clinical practice and 10% were working outside clinical practice. Of the healthcare professionals, 289 respondents (79%) had completed their studies in Utrecht. 12% of respondents had studied abroad, and of these more than 90% had studied in Belgium. Of the 368 respondents, 283 (77%) were members of the professional association, over 75% regularly read a professional journal in their own field, and fewer than 25% regularly read a professional journal in another field. Of the 58 human healthcare professionals, 90% had a specialization listed in the Dutch healthcare professions register (BIG). In the veterinary sector, the 310 respondents included 179 domestic animal veterinarians, 27 equine veterinarians, 76 farm veterinarians and 6 special animal veterinarians. These general figures tally with the figures obtained from the professional associations; there are no indications of bias.

Measures

The variables were measured with a series of questions that had been compiled from various existing validated questionnaires. Many original items were adapted to the specific situation of human and veterinary healthcare professionals in order to ensure that the items were meaningful to them. The questionnaire took approximately 15 min to complete.

Apart from a number of open questions (related to age or the number of working years), all items were based on a Likert scale (1–7) and can be interpreted as continuous variables, thus following the fundamental Ordinary Least Square (OLS) principles. The seven-point scale was used to obtain greater dispersion and hence more nuance in the data [52]. Table 1 reports the general descriptives of the variables (mean, SD, alpha and correlations).

The dependent variable, *collaboration*, was based on Bock, Zmud, Kim and Lee [53] with a construct reliability score of 0.90, to which the one-item question on the perceived degree of overlap formulated by Schubert and Otten [54] was added (the OSIO – Overlap of Self Ingroup and Outgroup). An example of an item is 'I collaborate when the opportunity arises'.

Common goal was based on Fisman and Laupland [2] and Kahn [3] and has a construct reliability score of 0.89. Participants were asked the following:

Table 1 Construct descriptive statistics, these constructs are created based on the valid items of the PLS-SEM model

Construct	Theoretical range	Actual range	Mean	SD	Reliability
Collaboration	1–7	1.00–7.00	4.37	1.37	0.90
Common goal	1–7	1.00–7.00	5.33	1.04	0.89
Recategorization	1–7	1.00–7.00	4.04	1.01	0.85
Decategorization	1–7	1.00–7.00	4.40	1.07	0.91
Mutual differentiation	1–7	1.00–7.00	5.80	0.95	0.94
Knowledge sharing	1–7	2.75–7.00	5.56	0.78	0.82

"Thinking of possible collaboration between physicians and veterinarians, to what extent do you agree with the following statements?". An example of an item is 'I think more could be done to stimulate innovation in healthcare'.

Recategorization was measured with questions based on Edmondson [55] with a construct reliability of 0.85. An example of an item is 'In the collaboration between physicians and veterinarians in general, it is possible to raise problems and difficult subjects in the collaboration'.

Decategorization was measured with a combination of items based on the instruments developed by Doosje, Ellemers and Spears [56] and Shamir, Zakay, Breinin and Popper [57]. An example of an item is 'In the collaboration between physicians and veterinarians in general, it is considered important to make a lasting contribution to the collaboration'.

Mutual differentiation was measured with questions based on Berendsen, Benneker, Groenier, Schuling, Grol and Meyboom-de Jong [58] with a construct reliability of 0.94. An example of an item is 'In the collaboration between physicians and veterinarians in general, there is appreciation of the expertise of the other professional group and a readiness to pursue contact on it'.

Knowledge sharing was based on Connolly and Kellaway's study [59] with a construct reliability of 0.82. An example of an item is 'In the collaboration between physicians and veterinarians in general, I am prepared to share specific professional knowledge (expertise) with the other professional group'.

Analysis strategy

The study sample consisted of 368 respondents. This size is acceptable in view of the rule of thumb provided by Barclay, Higgins and Thompson [60], which suggests using ten times the maximum number of paths aiming at any construct in the outer model (this is not applicable as no formative constructs were used) and the inner model. All construct variables (Collaboration, Common Goal, Recategorization, Decategorization, Mutual Differentiation, and Knowledge Sharing) are reflective constructs.

For the outer model evaluation, internal consistency reliability and convergent validity were examined. The construct reliability scores ranged between 0.82 and 0.94, which was acceptable [61], and for the convergent validity the Average Variance Extracted (AVEs) of the constructs was also good [62]; this is included in Table 1. Secondly, indicator reliability was examined and all factor loadings were found to be higher than 0.6 and as such acceptable [63]. The construct and the factor loadings proved to be satisfactory for use in the analysis, although it can be said that the coefficients of the determinants are low – and that they are negligible in the case of Mutual Differentiation and Decategorization for collaboration. Finally, discriminant validity was checked, comparing the AVEs of the constructs with the inter-construct correlations [62]. Additionally, cross-loadings were checked. Evidence was found to exclude three items from Mutual Differentiation due to cross-factor loadings.

Partial Least Squares Path Modelling (PLS-SEM) was conducted with SmartPLS version 2.0 [64]. For the partial least square algorithm, the path weighting scheme was used, and the maximum number of iterations was set to 300. As stop criterion, 10^-5 was used. A uniform value of 1 was used as an initial value for each of the outer weights [65].

Results and discussion

Table 2 shows the correlations between de different variables. Reliability and convergent validity of the measurement model was also confirmed by computing standardized loadings for indicators (Table 2) and Bootstrap t-statistics for their significance [66], see Table 3. For this bootstrapping, 5000 subsamples were used with a bias-corrected bootstrap testing for a two-tailed significance of 95%. The coefficient of determination was found to be moderate for Collaboration (R^2 = 0.42). The effect size of Common Goal on Collaboration (f^2 = 0.12), Recategorization on Collaboration (f^2 = 0.03) and Knowledge Sharing on Collaboration (f^2 = 0.04) can be considered small [67]. The effect sizes of Decategorization on Collaboration (f^2 = 0.00) and Mutual Differentiation on Collaboration (f^2 = 0.00) were negligible.

To obtain the Q^2 values as an indicator of the model's predictive relevance, the blindfolding procedure was used, resulting in small predictive relevance for Collaboration

Table 2 Correlations between latent variables and square roots of average variance extracted, numbers shown in boldface denote the square root of the average variance extracted, correlations are significant at the 0.01 level (2-tailed)

	Construct	Mean	SD	1	2	3	4	5	6
1	Collaboration	4.37	1.37	**0.77**					
2	Common goal	5.33	1.04	0.58	**0.77**				
3	Recategorization	4.04	1.01	0.38	0.28	**0.86**			
4	Decategorization	4.40	1.07	0.41	0.36	0.63	**0.79**		
5	Mutual differentiation	5.80	0.95	0.30	0.36	0.15	0.29	**0.92**	
6	Knowledge sharing	5.56	0.78	0.51	0.61	0.24	0.40	0.34	**0.73**

(Q^2 = 0.24), Knowledge Sharing (Q^2 = 0.19), and Mutual Differentiation (Q^2 = 0.11). The effect size for the predictive relevance of Common Goal on Collaboration was very small (q^2 = 0.05), as was Knowledge Sharing on Collaboration (q^2 = 0.02). Finally, the procedures outlined by Preacher and Hayes [68] were followed to examine multiple mediation effects.

With the help of multiple mediation models, it is possible to observe not only the direct effect of Common Goal on Collaboration, but also the mediation effects. The mediation effects are a_1b_1 = .051 (through Recategorization), a_2b_2 = .037 (through Decategorization), a_3b_3 = .024 (through Mutual Differentiation), and a_4b_4 = .167 (through Knowledge Sharing).

Figure 1 was designed based on the calculated mediation effects. All paths show a significant relation. This makes the Common Ingroup Identity Model an effective model to provide a plausible explanation why human and veterinary healthcare professionals do or do not collaborate. Having a common goal, like One Health, leads to collaboration via Recategorization. This mediating relation is also present for Knowledge Sharing. However, for Decategorization and Mutual Differentiation, there is a significant relation with Common Goal and with Collaboration; Decategorization and Mutual Differentiation have a direct relation with Collaboration that is not a mediating relation.

The PLS analysis confirms that a common goal promotes collaboration. Hypothesis 1 is therefore accepted. Bootstrapping the indirect effects of Common Goal on Collaboration, we found that Recategorization (0,051) and Knowledge Sharing (0,167) are significant mediators, thus supporting hypotheses 2 and 5. The specific indirect effect through Knowledge Sharing is larger than through Recategorization (effect Recategorization is significantly smaller; see contrasts) [68].

Significant relations were found between Common Goal via Decategorization with Collaboration and for Mutual Differentiation with collaboration. No evidence was found to support hypotheses 2 (mediating effect of decategorization) and 3 (mediating effect of mutual differentiation). Nevertheless, the results indicate an intervening effect for Decategorization and Mutual Differentiation, resulting in a satisfactory explanation why human and veterinary healthcare professionals do or do not collaborate. All four elements (Recategorization, Decategorization, Mutual Differentiation and Knowledge Sharing) are relevant; Recategorization and Knowledge Sharing are mediating variables.

Common Goal proved to be an important factor for promoting collaboration between human and veterinary healthcare professionals. This relationship is partly explained by the mediating role of recategorizing and knowledge sharing, but also partly by the intervening

Table 3 Coefficients of determination and predictive relevance

	R^2 incl.	R^2 excl.	1-R^2 incl.	f^2
f^2 Common Goal - > Collaboration	0.42	0.35	0.58	0.12
f^2 Recategorization - > Collaboration	0.42	0.40	0.58	0.03
f^2 Decategorization - > Collaboration	0.42	0.42	0.58	0.00
f^2 Mutual Differentiation - > Collaboration	0.42	0.42	0.58	0.00
f^2 Knowledge Sharing - > Collaboration	0.42	0.40	0.58	0.04
	Q^2 incl.	Q^2 excl.	1-Q^2 incl.	q^2
q^2 Common Goal - > Collaboration	0.24	0.20	0.76	0.05
q^2 Recategorization - > Collaboration	0.24	0.23	0.76	0.01
q^2 Decategorization - > Collaboration	0.24	0.24	0.76	0.00
q^2 Mutual Differentiation - > Collaboration	0.24	0.24	0.76	0.00
q^2 Knowledge Sharing - > Collaboration	0.24	0.2296	0.76	0.02

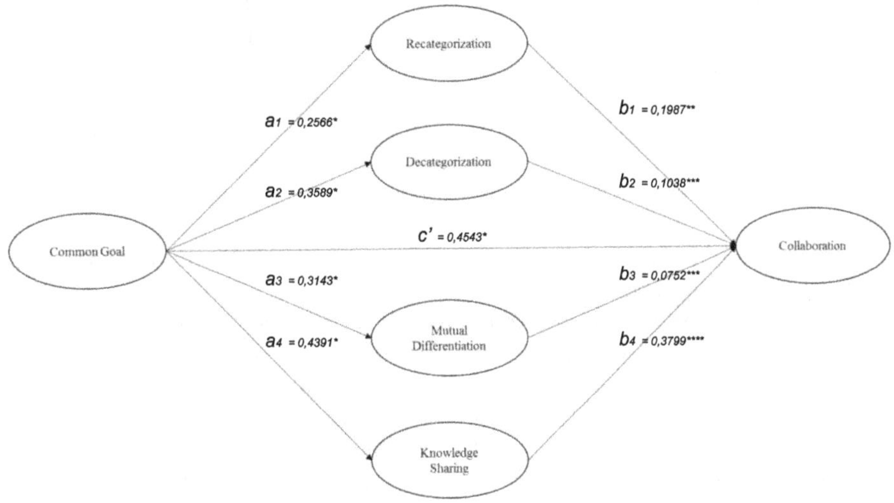

Fig. 1 Mediation effects, *p = ≤ .001; **p = ≤ .008; ***p = ≥ .05; ****p = ≤ .0003

effects of Decategorization and Mutual Differentiation. Having a common goal (*in casu* One Health) produces altered perceptions in the form of an overarching identity. Upon recognizing their interdependence, human and veterinary healthcare professionals will initiate collaboration [27]. Collaboration, if there is a common goal, must therefore be seen to a greater extent as interdependence, as described earlier by Mohr and Spekman [69], in which there is still scope to retain individual identity, as argued by Brown and Wade [35] and Molleman et al. [36]. In the case of recategorization, there is scope to retain individual identity since an overarching identity is created. Gaertner and Dovidio [17] showed that a common goal leads to a reduction of prejudice and resistance between groups (thus influencing the perception of the situation), which in turn has an influence on collaboration. The current findings point in the same direction.

This study shows that in addition to recategorization, knowledge sharing also has a mediating role with respect to the influence of a common goal (One Health) on cooperation. Findings indicate that One Health stimulates knowledge sharing and in this way enhances collaboration between human and veterinary healthcare professionals. It may therefore be concluded that knowledge sharing is a promoting factor for human and veterinary healthcare professionals to use each other's expertise [42–44]. The healthcare professionals have different backgrounds, but they improve their performance and make it more effective by learning from each other and by collaborating [45–47]. One Health is an important initiative to generate and promote knowledge sharing. This study has shown that knowledge sharing is in fact stimulated if the common goal of One Health is perceived as an invitation to work together on the basis of mutual interdependence. Seen in this way, continuous knowledge sharing will ultimately improve the ties and the forms of collaboration between the two groups of healthcare professionals [50].

This study has also shown that Decategorization has a significant effect in the relation between Common Goal and Collaboration, although this is not a mediating but an intervening effect. Our analyses show that this path, which has also been described by Gaertner and Dovidio [17], also applies to the human and veterinary healthcare professionals. Many healthcare professionals will be of the opinion that decategorization is not sufficiently concrete; they will therefore give it little importance, which might explain why we did not find a mediating effect.

This study has also revealed that Mutual Differentiation expresses a significant relation between Common Goal and Collaboration. However, as with Decategorization, there is no mediating effect between Collaboration and Common Goal for Mutual Differentiation. It may therefore be concluded that Mutual Differentiation helps to explain the collaboration between human and veterinary healthcare professionals. A possible explanation for the fact that no mediating effect was found for Mutual Differentiation may be limited insight in each other's sectors and expertise, and any untapped added value still to be discovered [2].

Practical implications

The current study's findings indicate that in order to achieve greater collaboration between human and veterinary healthcare professionals, it is first and foremost necessary to define a common goal. That being said, the concept of One Health is not yet sufficiently 'alive' in the heads of healthcare professionals. Most of these professionals will probably not have a clear idea of how to interpret it, particularly in their own practice. Having a clear common goal will likely help them overcome the social dilemma that healthcare professionals face. After all, these professionals will only be triggered to work together once the common goal is shaped and starts to come alive, as is also argued by Ives, Torrey and Gordon [41]. These researchers state that having a clear idea of the goal stimulates knowledge sharing. The social dilemma among healthcare professionals referred to earlier [14] is thus overcome, and the added value of interaction becomes clear to them. A common goal (as investigated in this study) only comes into existence as a result of this concreteness, and this will trigger the mechanisms required to create an overarching identity [21].

Furthermore, it is of importance for both groups of healthcare professionals to know each other and to realize that they have a shared responsibility, not only in terms of combatting infectious diseases, but also in terms of providing optimum care for patients. This insight is expected to facilitate cooperation between the groups of healthcare professionals [40]. The notion that there are differences between the two groups does not necessarily imply that there is no, or could not be any, collaboration between them [17]. On the other hand, a word of caution is needed here: we have to be careful not to facilitate or create too much interference concerning the other professionals' fields, because this could result in resistance [36].

Professional associations can play a facilitating role in creating a common goal, promoting recognition and fostering awareness with respect to common responsibilities. Knowledge sharing could be shaped, for example, by including articles from the other field in the professional journals of both professional groups. As respondents in the current study reported, fewer than 25% read a professional journal related to the other sector. The mutual inclusion of each other's articles could be a first step in creating a relatively simple form of knowledge transfer. In addition to the publication of articles in each other's professional journals, professional associations could offer joint interdisciplinary training programmes and refresher courses.

It has become increasingly clear that greater awareness of the added value of the common goal results in more extensive cooperation [21, 37, 38]. This awareness reveals not only what both groups of healthcare professionals have in common, but also that human and veterinary healthcare professionals have more in common than they themselves realize. This insight will lower the current psychological barriers between the two groups of healthcare professionals, resulting in more extensive collaboration between them [17]. This awareness among both groups of healthcare professionals could be further improved via the communications issued by their professional groups.

Limitations and future research

As the current study was a cross-sectional study, it has certain limitations concerning long-term effects or relations. In order to gain a deeper insight into possible causes and consequences, longitudinal research is needed. One Health is an interdisciplinary approach and less concrete for healthcare professionals. To stimulate collaboration on the basis of the arguments presented in the current study's introduction, additional and more detailed research is necessary: although One Health has been studied as an overarching concept, individual elements have been somewhat neglected. Beyond that, we recommend more qualitative research on this subject. This is needed to obtain greater insight not only into 'physicians' and veterinarians' thoughts and feelings, but also into the overlaps between the two groups. In addition, an international study is needed to compare the different worlds. For instance, to the best of our knowledge, in the Western world veterinarians generally are greater all-rounders than physicians, but in the developing countries we see that physicians are also all-rounders; one would expect that the psychological barrier will be lower between these health care professionals. We expect this to have an influence on their cooperation.

Conclusion

To the best of our knowledge, this study is the first research project in which the Common Ingroup Identity Model is quantitatively researched with the help of questionnaires. It is recommended that further research be conducted into this model with a view to using it in more quantitative analyses. Collaboration between healthcare professionals - the One Health approach - can be further investigated by focusing on other characteristics that influence the collaboration between the two groups. Possible options are stereotyping and social value orientation. The healthcare sector, and specifically the interaction between the human and veterinary fields, offers untapped potential, such as the development of treatments which could improve the healthcare as a whole.

Every study that analyzes the interaction between the two fields and addresses the healthcare professional's social dilemma will be of immense value to society and can possibly give indications how to improve the quality of life. This study has shown that the Common Ingroup Identity Model helps to explain why human and veterinary healthcare professionals do or do not collaborate. Stimulating the interdependency perception, which can be reached with a clear common goal like the One Health approach, could increase collaboration between these health care professionals.

Abbreviations
AVAs: Average variance extracted; BIG: Dutch healthcare professions register; CDCP: USA centres for disease control and prevention; GDP: Gross domestic product; KNMG: Royal Dutch Medical Association; KNMvD: Royal Dutch Veterinary Association; OLS: Ordinary least square; OSIO: Overlap of self ingroup and outgroup; PLS-SEM: Partial least squares path modelling; SARS: Severe acute respiratory syndrome; WHO: World Health Organization

Acknowledgements
We would like to thank the following people:
Prof. dr. L.J. Hellebrekers, for his support during the collection of data from veterinary healthcare professionals; Prof. emer. dr. L. Wigersma, for his support during the collection of data from human healthcare professionals; M.M. van Houten MSc MA, for revising the manuscript critically in terms of (intellectual) content and for textual corrections; L. Kuipers MA, for editing the English text.

Funding
Not applicable.

Authors' contributions
BE is the study's initiator who carried out the data acquisition and drafted the article. BE and JS contributed to the conception and design of the study, provided input on the interpretation of the data and revised the article critically for important intellectual content. MD performed the statistical analyses. RB contributed to the interpretation of data. All authors approved the final article.

Competing interests
The authors declare that they have no competing interests.

Consent for publication
Not applicable.

References
1. WHO/FAO/OIE. Report of the WHO/FAO/OIE joint consultation on emerging zoonotic diseases. 2004. http://apps.who.int/iris/bitstream/10665/68899/1/WHO_CDS_CPE_ZFK_2004.9.pdf. Accessed 5 Feb 2014.
2. Fisman DN, Laupland KB. The 'one health' paradigm: time for infectious diseases clinicians to take note? Can J Infect Dis med Microbiol. 2010;21(3):111–4.
3. Kahn LH. Confronting zoonoses, linking human and veterinary medicine. Emerg Infect Dis. 2006;12(4):556–61.
4. Krauss, H., Weber, A., Appel, M., Enders, B., Graevenitz, A., van, Isenberg, H.D., Schiefer, H.G., Slenczka, W. & Zahner, H. (2003). Zoonoses. Infectious diseases transmissible from animals to humans (3rd edition). Washington: ASM Press.
5. Natterson-Horowitz B, Bowers K. Zoobiquity. New York: Random House Inc.; 2012.
6. Zinsstag, J., Meisser, A., Schelling, E., Bonfoh, B. & Tanner, M. (2012). From "two medicines" to "one health" and beyond. Onderstepoort J vet res, 79(2), 492-497.
7. One health Initiative (n.d.a). *About the One Health Initiative.* http://www.onehealthinitiative.com/about.php. Accessed 13 Sept 2016.
8. United States General Accounting Office. West Nile Virus Outbreak — Lessons for Public Health Preparedness. 2000; http://www.gao.gov/new.items/he00180.pdf. Accessed 10 Feb 2014.
9. World Bank. People, pathogens and our planet - volume 1: towards a one health approach for controlling Zoonotic diseases. Washington D.C: The International Bank for Reconstruction and Development/World Bank; 2010.
10. World Bank (2011). Towards one health: interim lessons from the global program on avian and human pandemic influenza. Washington D.C.: The International Bank for Reconstruction and Development/World Bank.
11. Lee, J.W. & McKibbin, W.J. (2004). Estimating the global economic costs of SARS. S. Knobler, A. Mahmoud & S. Lemon, A. Mack, L. Sivitz & K. Oberholtzer (Eds.), Learning from SARS: preparing for the next disease outbreak: workshop summary. Washington (DC): National Academies Press (US).
12. Rijksinstituut voor Volksgezondheid en Milieu (2003). Is Dit Een Uitbraak? http://www.rivm.nl/Documenten_en_publicaties/Algemeen_Actueel/Uitgaven/Infectieziekten_Bulletin/Jaargang_22_2011/April_2011/Inhoud_april_2011/Is_dit_een_uitbraak. Accessed 20 Feb 2014.
13. Lange P, van Balliet DP, Parks CD, Van Vugt M. Social dilemmas: understanding human cooperation. New York: Oxford University Press; 2013.
14. Fleuren M, Wieferink K, Paulussen T. Determinants of innovation within health care organizations literature review and Delphi study. Int J Qual Health Care. 2004;16(2):107–23.
15. One health Sweden (n.d.a). *The One Health-perspective.* http://www.onehealth.se/ohs/node/21. Accessed 13 Sept 2016.
16. Lueddeke GR. Global population health and well-being in the 21st century. New York: Springer Publishing Company; 2016.
17. Gaertner SL, Dovidio JF. Reducing intergroup bias: the common Ingroup identity model. In: van Lange PAM, Kruglanski AW, Higgins ET, editors. Handbook of theories of social psychology. Thousand Oaks, CA: Sage; 2010. p. 439–57.
18. Universiteit Utrecht (n.d.b). *Onderwijs.* http://www.uu.nl/faculty/veterinarymedicine/NL/onderwijs/Pages/default.aspx. Accessed 20 Feb 2014.
19. Universiteit van Gent (n.d.a). *Onderwijs.* http://www.ugent.be/di/nl/onderwijs. Accessed 20 Feb 2014.
20. Kooistra, H. (2014, 11 september). "Primair hyperaldosteronisme (ziekte van Conn)". Speech for Zoobiquitycongres. Dierenpark Amersfoort.
21. Gaertner SL, Dovidio JF, Anastasio PA, Bachman BA, Rust MC. The common ingroup identity model: Recategorization and the reduction of intergroup bias. Eur rev soc Psychol. 1993;4(1):1–26.
22. Kramer RM, Brewer MB. Effects of group identity on resource utilization in a simulated commons dilemma. J Pers soc Psychol. 1984; 46(5):1044–57.
23. Vezzali L, Cadamuro A, Versari A, Giovannini D, Trifiletti E. Feeling like a group after a natural disaster: common ingroup identity and relations with outgroup victims among majority and minority young children. Br J soc Psychol. 2014;54(3):601–15.
24. Nier JL, Gaertner SL, Dovidio JF, Banker BS, Ward CM. Changing interracial evaluations, affective reactions, and behaviour: the effects of a common group identity. Group Process Intergroup Relat. 2001;4(4):299–316.
25. Allport GW. The nature of prejudice. Cambridge: Addison-Wesley; 1954.
26. Hwong N, Caswell A, Johnson DW, Johnson R. Effects of cooperative and individualistic learning on prospective elementary teachers' music achievement and attitudes. J soc Psychol. 1993;133(1):53–64.
27. Johnson RT, Johnson DW. An Educational Psychology success story: social interdependence theory and cooperative learning. Educ res. 2009; 38(5):366–7.
28. Lewin K. A dynamic theory of personality. New York: McGraw-Hill; 1935.
29. Lewin K. Resolving social conflicts. New York: Harper; 1948.
30. Deutsch M. A theory of cooperation and competition. Hum Relat. 1949; 2(2):129–52.
31. Deutsch M. Cooperation and trust: some theoretical notes. In: Jones MR, editor. Nebraska symposium on motivation. Lincoln: University of Nebraska Press; 1962. p. 275–319.
32. Park B, Rothbart M. Perception of out-group homogeneity and levels of social categorization: memory for the subordinate attributes of in-group and out-group members. J Pers soc Psychol. 1982;42(6):1051–68.
33. Turner JC, Hogg MA, Oakes PJ, Reicher SD, Wetherell MS. Rediscovering the social group. Oxford, England: Basil Blackwell; 1987.
34. Tajfel H. The achievement of group differentiation. In: Tajfel H, editor. Differentiation between social groups. Studies in the social psychology of intergroup relations. London: Academic Press; 1978. p. 77–98.
35. Brown RJ, Wade G. Superordinate goals and intergroup behaviour: the effect of role ambiguity and status on intergroup attitudes and task performance. Eur J soc Psychol. 1987;17(2):131–42.
36. Molleman E, Broekhuis M, Stoffels R, Jaspers F. How health care complexity leads to cooperation and affects the autonomy of health care professionals. Health Care Anal. 2008;16(4):329–41.
37. Banker BS, Gaertner SL. Achieving step-family harmony: an intergroup relations approach. J Fam Psychol. 1998;12(4):310–25.
38. Gaertner SL, Dovidio JF, Bachman BA. Revisiting the contact hypothesis: the induction of a common Ingroup identity. Int J Int Rel. 1996;20(3–4):271–90.

39. Wilder DA. Perceiving persons as a group: categorization and intergroup relations. In: Hamilton DL, editor. Cognitive processes in stereotyping and intergroup behaviour. Hillsdale: Erlbaum; 1981. p. 213–57.
40. Hewstone M, Brown R. Contact is not enough: an intergroup perspective on the "contact hypothesis.". In: Hewstone M, Brown R, editors. Contact and conflict in intergroup encounters. Oxford: Blackwell; 1986. p. 1–44.
41. Ives W, Torrey B, Gordon C. In: Morey D, Maybury MT, Thuraisingham BM, editors. Knowledge sharing is a human behavior. Knowledge management classic and contemporary work (pp 99–129). Massachusetts; 2000.
42. Bossche P, Van den Gijselaers WH, Segers M, Kirschner PA. Social and cognitive factors driving teamwork in collaborative learning environments Team learning beliefs and Behaviors. Small Group res. 2006;37(5):490–521.
43. Cummings JN. Work groups, Structural diversity, and knowledge sharing in a global Organization. Manag Sci. 2004;50(3):352–64.
44. Tsai W. Knowledge transfer in Intraorganizational networks: effects of network position and absorptive capacity on business unit innovation and performance. Acad Manag J. 2001;44(5):996–1004.
45. Farrell JB, Flood PC, MacCurtain SM, Hannigan A, Dawson J, West M. CEO Leadership, top Team trust and the combination and exchange of information. Ir J Manag. 2005;26(1):22–40.
46. Renzl B. Trust in management and knowledge sharing: the mediating effects of fear and knowledge documentation. Omega. 2008;36(2):206–20.
47. Srivastava, A; Bartol, K. M. & Locke, E. A. (2006). Empowering Leadership in management teams: effects on knowledge sharing, efficacy, and Team performance. Acad Manag J, 49(6), 1239–1251.
48. Bengtsson Sören Kock M. Cooperation and competition in relationships between competitors in business networks. J bus Ind Mark. 1999;14(3):178–94.
49. Tsai W. Social structure of "Coopetition" within a multiunit Organization: coordination, competition, and Intraorganizational knowledge sharing. Organ Sci. 2002;13(2):179–90.
50. Holmes JG. Trust and the appraisal process in close relationships. In: Jones WH, Perlman D, editors. Advances in personal relationships. London: Jessica Kingsley; 1991. p. 57–104.
51. Alavi M, Kayworth TR, Leidner DE. An empirical examination of the influence of organizational culture on knowledge management practices. J Manage Info Syst. 2005;22(3):191–224.
52. Dawes J. Do data characteristics change according to the number of scale points used. Int J Mark res. 2008;50(1):61–77.
53. Bock GW, Zmud RW, Kim YG, Lee JN. Behavioral intention formation knowledge sharing: examining roles of extrinsic motivators, social-psychological forces, and organizational climate. MIS q. 2005;29(1):87–111.
54. Schubert TW, Otten S. Overlap of self, Ingroup, and Outgroup: pictorial measures of self-categorization. Self Identity. 2002;1(4):353–76.
55. Edmondson A. Psychological safety and learning behavior in work teams. Adm Sci Q. 1999;44(2):350–83.
56. Doosje B, Ellemers N, Spears R. Perceived variability as a function of group status and identification. J exp soc Psychol. 1995;31(5):410–36.
57. Shamir B, Zakay E, Breinin E, Popper M. Correlates of charismatic leader behavior in military units: subordinates' attitudes, unit characteristics, superiors' appraisals of leader performance. Acad Manag J. 1998;41(4):387–409.
58. Berendsen AJ, Benneker WHGM, Groenier KH, Schuling J, Grol RPTM, Meyboom-de Jong B. DOC vragenlijst - een instrument om de waardering van huisartsen en specialisten over hun onderlinge samenwerking te meten. In: Berendsen AJ, editor. (Red.), *Samenwerking tussen huisarts en specialist. Wat vinden de patiënten en de dokters?* Houten: Bohn Stafleu Van Loghum; 2008. p. 57–70.
59. Connelly CE, Kelloway K. Predictors of employees' perceptions of knowledge sharing cultures. Leadersh org dev J. 2003;24(5):294–301.
60. Barclay D, Higgins C, Thompson R. The partial least squares (PLS) approach to causal modeling: personal computer adaptation and use as an illustration. Technol Stud. 1995;2(2):285–309.
61. Nunnally JC, Bernstein IH. The assessment of reliability. Psychometric Theory. 1994;3(1):248–92.
62. Fornell C, Larcker D. Evaluating Structural Equation models with unobservable variables and measurement error. J Mark res. 1981;18(1):39–50.
63. Hair JF, Hult GTM, Ringle CM, Sarstedt M. A primer on partial least squares Structural Equation Modeling (PLS-SEM). Thousand Oaks: Sage; 2014.
64. Ringle C, Wende S, Will A. SmartPLS. 2005:2.0. http://www.smartpls.de. Accessed 1 Mar 2015.
65. Henseler J. On the convergence of the partial least squares path modeling algorithm. Comput Stat. 2010;25(1):107–20.
66. Anderson JC, Gerbing DW. Structural Equation Modeling in practice: a review and recommended two-step approach. Psychol Bull. 1988;103(3): 411–23.
67. Cohen J. Statistical power analysis for the Behavioral sciences. 1st ed. Hillsdale: Lawrence Erlbaum Associates; 1969.
68. Preacher KJ, Hayes AF. Asymptotic and resampling strategies for assessing and comparing indirect effects in multiple mediator models. Behav res Methods. 2008;40(3):879–91.
69. Mohr J, Spekman R. Characteristics of partnership success: partnerschip attributes, communication behaviour, and conflict resolution techniques. Strateg Manag J. 1994;15(2):135–52.

13

Normal patellofemoral kinematic patterns during daily activities in dogs

Erica J. Moore[†], Stanley E. Kim[*†], Scott A. Banks, Antonio Pozzi, Jason D. Coggeshall and Stephen C. Jones

Abstract

Background: Patellar abnormalities are a common cause of pain and lameness in dogs; however, in vivo the relative motion between the femur and patella in dogs is not well described. The objective of this study was to define normal in vivo sagittal plane patellofemoral kinematics in three axes of motion using non-invasive methods. We hypothesized patellofemoral alignment in the sagittal plane would tightly correlate with the femorotibial flexion angle. Six healthy dogs without orthopedic disease underwent computed tomography (CT) of their hind limbs to create 3-D models of the patella and femur. Normal stifle joint motion was captured via flat-panel imaging while each dog performed a series of routine activities, including sitting, walking, and trotting. The 3-D models of the patella and femur were digitally superimposed over the radiographic images with shape-matching software and the precise movement of the patella relative to the femur was calculated.

Results: As the femorotibial joint flexed, the patellofemoral joint also flexed and the patella moved caudally and distally within the femoral trochlea during each activity. Patellar flexion and distal translation during walk and sit were linearly coupled with the femorotibial flexion angle. Offset was evident while trotting, where patella poses were significantly different between early and late swing phase ($p \leq 0.003$). Patellar flexion ranged from 51 to 6° while trotting. The largest flexion angle (92°) occurred during sit. The patella traversed the entire proximodistal length of the femoral trochlea during these daily activities.

Conclusions: Using single-plane flat-panel imaging, we demonstrated normal in vivo patellofemoral kinematics is tightly coupled with femorotibial kinematics; however, trot kinematic patterns did not follow the path defined by walking and stand-to-sit motions. Our normal data can be used in future studies to help define patellofemoral joint kinematics in dogs with stifle abnormalities.

Keywords: Gait analysis, Dog, Kinematic, Patellofemoral

Background

The stifle is a complex synovial joint consisting of the femorotibial and patellofemoral joints. Stifle motion occurs in three planes resulting directly from the intricate anatomical relationship between the distal femur, proximal tibia and fibula, patella, pelvic limb musculature, and the stifle joint capsule and its associated ligaments [1]. Patellofemoral abnormalities are common in dogs [2]. Patellar luxation is a highly prevalent disorder affecting the stifles of dogs and alters stifle mechanics [2]. Cranial cruciate ligament insufficiency is also common in dogs and has been shown to disrupt normal patellofemoral joint motion [3, 4].

Abnormal motion or kinematics of joints can lead to cartilage degradation, inflammation, pain, lameness, and progressive osteoarthritis [1]. The traditional method utilized for analyzing canine stifle kinematics involves attaching reflective markers to the overlying skin of tissue landmarks with movement captured by digital cameras [5–8]. These studies, while non-invasive, do not provide precise data regarding movement of the underlying bones; instead these studies only yield general information on the angles and velocities of femorotibial flexion-extension movement. Imprecise placement of the reflective markers and skin motion can introduce variability in femorotibial kinematic data during gait analysis [8]. Other methods for evaluating stifle kinematics

* Correspondence: stankim@ufl.edu
[†]Equal contributors
Comparative Orthopaedics Biomechanics Laboratory, College of Veterinary Medicine, University of Florida, PO Box 1001262015 SW 16th Ave, Gainesville, FL 32610-0126, USA

include radiography and goniometry; however, these methods are not able to track the position of the patella during motion in dogs in vivo [9, 10].

Patellar kinematics is well described in humans and is typically referenced in relation to the femoral trochlea; of which tilt, rotation, flexion, and shift are of particular importance [11, 12]. Despite the high prevalence of patellofemoral problems in dogs, a similar description of normal patellar motion in this species has not been well described. Research evaluating the patellar kinematics following cranial cruciate ligament transection using a 2-D digital technique in a cadaveric model found patellar flexion angle was altered, suggesting abnormal patellofemoral biomechanics may play a role in the development of patellofemoral osteoarthritis in dogs with cranial cruciate insufficiency [3]. Cadaveric studies, however, have several limitations and cannot fully simulate complex in vivo stifle biomechanics.

Joint kinematics can be quantified in a precise manner in-vivo by using fluoroscopic or flat-panel methods, where the region of interest is imaged while the subject performs tasks such as walking. In-vivo femorotibial kinematics in normal and cranial-cruciate ligament deficient stifles of dogs have been characterized using continuous horizontal-beam imaging [13–15]. To the investigators' knowledge, in vivo dynamic patellofemoral kinematics has not been studied in dogs. The objective of this study was to define the normal in vivo sagittal plane patellofemoral kinematics in dogs during daily activities using horizontal-beam flat-panel imaging. We hypothesized patellofemoral alignment in the sagittal plane (patellar flexion-extension angle, craniocaudal translation, and proximodistal translation) would tightly correlate with the femorotibial flexion angle. We also hypothesized patellar movement would be restricted to the length of the femoral trochlea.

Methods

Six healthy Labrador Retrievers (four males, two females) were studied. All procedures were approved by the University of Florida Institution's Animal Care and Use Committee. Dogs underwent complete physical and orthopedic examinations prior to data collection. The mean age was 4 years (range 1–7 years) and mean weight was 28 kg (range 26–32 kg). These dogs were confirmed via computed tomographic (CT) analysis to be free of pelvic limb orthopedic abnormalities.

Data collection

Computed tomography analyses[1] were conducted to obtain stationary images of both hind limbs from the coxofemoral to the tarsocrural joint. Transverse images were obtained with a slice thickness of 0.5 mm.

Horizontal-beam lateral projection flat-panel images[2] of stifles were acquired while each dog walked at a velocity of 1.1 m/s (2.5 mph) and trotted at a velocity of 2 m/s (4.5 mph) on a treadmill for three separate trials with three to five strides per trial, and while the dog underwent a stand-to-sit motion for two separate trials. Images were acquired using a pulse width of 1 ms at 30 frames per second and an image area of 400 × 300 mm, producing a pixel size of 0.39 mm × 0.39 mm and image resolution of 1,024 × 1,024 pixels. Radiographic configurations supplied a 72 kV beam with a 50 mA beam current.

Three-dimensional model creation and coordinate assignation

Three-dimensional models of the patella and femur were constructed from the CT analyses of the subjects using the Digital Imaging and Communication in Medicine (DICOM) images and an open source 3-D-segmentation program.[3] The bone models were imported into reverse-engineering software[4] and coordinate systems were assigned based on local anatomical landmarks of the patella and femur [13, 16]. Femoral coordinates were applied such that the mediolateral axis (x-axis) passed through the center of the lateral and medial femoral condyles with the femoral origin located at the midpoint between the condyles (Fig. 1). The proximodistal axis (y-axis) passed proximally along the femoral shaft, perpendicular to the mediolateral axis in the plane common to the center of both femoral condyles and the femoral head. Patellar coordinates were applied such that the mediolateral axis (x-axis) passed through the most medial and lateral points on the circumference of the bone with the patellar origin defined as the midpoint of the axis. The proximodistal axis (y-axis) was defined as a line that passed through the most proximal and distal aspects of the patella, perpendicular to the mediolateral axis. The craniocaudal axes (z-axis) for the femur and patella were created from the cross product of the mediolateral and proximodistal axes, thus creating a Cartesian coordinate system.

Three-dimensional to Two-dimensional shape-matching

The 3-D bone models of the patella and femur and the single-plane flat-panel images were imported into open-source shape-matching software[5] (JointTrack). The 3-D models were digitally superimposed over the lateral flat-panel images with JointTrack and the model's projected silhouettes were manipulated via translation and rotation such that the anatomic contours of the models precisely overlapped the corresponding contours of the 2-D flat-panel images (Fig. 2). The patella was positioned centrally within the trochlea groove, such that the center of the patella's articulating surface remained as congruent

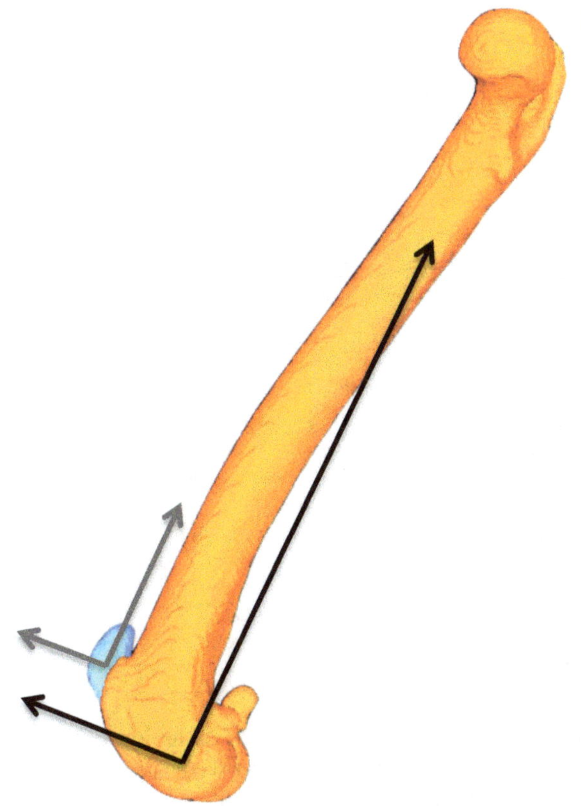

Fig. 1 Femur and patellar coordinate systems. Patellar coordinates are indicated in gray; femoral coordinates indicated in black

as possible with the trochlear groove in the axial plane. This process was performed by one individual (EM) and was repeated for each frame of the various activities and cycles performed. The orientation of the shape-matched bone models was used to calculate the relative alignment between the patella and femur for patellar flexion-extension angle (degrees), proximodistal translation (mm), and mediolateral translation (mm) using the custom-written Matlab[6] program. The custom Matlab program transformed the data into clinically relevant patellofemoral poses in six degrees of freedom [17]. The program was utilized such that the degrees of freedom were reported as patella relative to femur. Kinematic poses were normalized and interpolated to allow for comparative analysis of each cycle shape-matched. The kinematic properties were described in relation to femorotibial flexion angle, which have been reported for this exact data set in a separate study [15].

Statistical analysis

A statistical package[7] was used for all analyses. Differences between single points during the gait cycle at equivalent flexion angles (offset) were determined by a paired *t*-test. A Pearson's correlation coefficient was performed on the interpolated patellofemoral and femorotibial data to determine the extent of a linear relationship. The data was considered as strongly correlated if the $r > 0.8$ and weakly correlated in $r < 0.3$. For all statistical analyses performed, $p < 0.05$ was considered statistically significant.

Results

As the femorotibial joint flexed, the patella also flexed (Fig. 3) and translated caudally (Fig. 4) and distally (Fig. 5) within the femoral trochlea for each activity. Patellar flexion, caudal translation, and distal translation during sit were linearly correlated with femorotibial flexion angle (Figs. 3, 4 and 5). All three measured degrees of freedom were correlated during walk and sit, however no correlation was found for these parameters during trot (Table 1). Offset, defined as significant differences in patellofemoral alignment at identical femorotibial flexion angles, was evident during trot, where the patella poses differed in early and late swing phase in each of the three measured degrees of freedom (Fig. 6; flexion-extension, $p = 0.002$; craniocaudal, $p = 0.003$; proximodistal, $p = 0.002$). Patellar flexion ranged from a mean of 51 to 6° during trot, and the largest patellar flexion angle of 92° was evident during sit (Table 1). Patellar flexion during the swing phase of walk ranged from 10° to a maximum of 33°, while a range of 7 to 13° was observed during stance (Table 2). During trot, patellar flexion angles ranged from 13 to 51° during swing

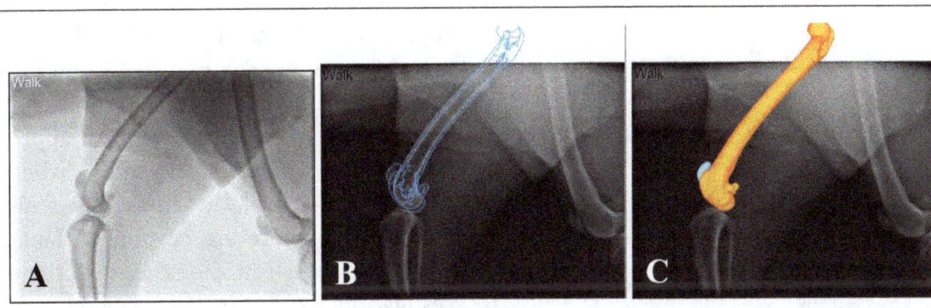

Fig. 2 Shape-matching process. **a** Flat-panel radiographic image imported into JointTrack. **b** Contoured silhouettes based on the 3-D models of the femur and patella utilized for shape-matching over the radiographic image. **c** Shape-matched 3-D projections of the femur and patella

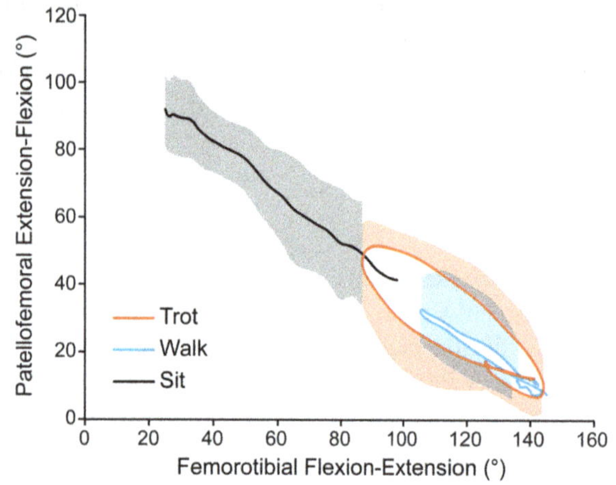

Fig. 3 Patellofemoral flexion-extension over the course of femorotibial flexion-extension. Each color represents a daily activity of dogs and the flexion-extension patellofemoral kinematic properties are compared over the course of femorotibial flexion-extension. For the x-axis, higher values indicate greater femorotibial extension. For the y-axis, higher values indicate greater patellofemoral flexion, where the patellar long axis is less parallel to the femoral long axis

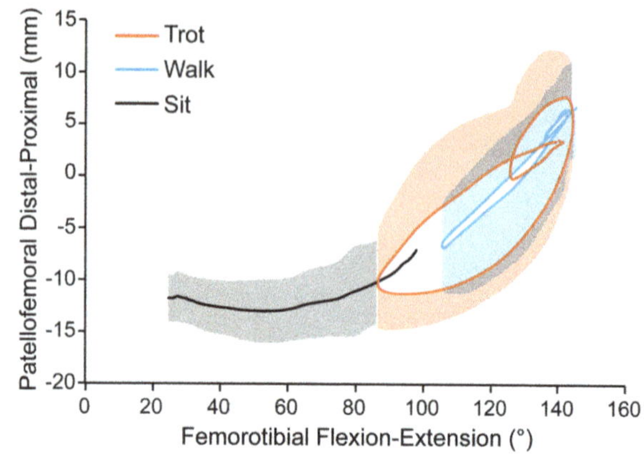

Fig. 5 Patellofemoral proximodistal translation over the course of femorotibial flexion-extension. Each color represents a daily activity of dogs and the proximodistal patellofemoral kinematic properties are compared over the course of femorotibial flexion-extension. Proximodistal translation measurements of the patella relative to the femur in mm. For the x-axis, higher values indicate greater femorotibial extension. For the y-axis, higher values indicate greater proximal translation of the patella, where the patellar origin is displaced more proximally to the femoral origin

and from 7 to 17° during stance (Table 2). The patella also traversed the length of the femoral trochlea during these daily activities, with nearly the entire patella positioned distal to the trochlear groove in deep flexion during sit (Fig. 7). The patella was confined within the proximal aspect of the trochlear groove during extension of all activities (Fig. 7).

Discussion

Using single-plane flat-panel imaging, we demonstrated non-invasively that normal in vivo patellofemoral kinematics are tightly coupled with femorotibial kinematics. When the daily activities were assessed collectively, we observed patellar flexion angle increased and the patella translated distally as the femorotibial joint flexed. The highest demand activity, trotting, produced kinematic patterns that did not follow the same pathways seen during walking and stand-to-sit motions. Although a portion of the patella was positioned distal to the trochlear groove during deep flexion while sitting, the base of the patella always remained positioned within the femoral trochlea during the activities analyzed in these dogs.

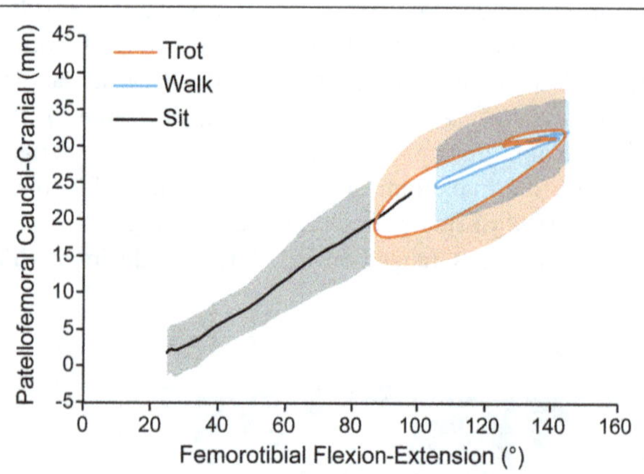

Fig. 4 Patellofemoral craniocaudal translation over the course of femorotibial flexion-extension. Each color represents a daily activity of dogs and the craniocaudal patellofemoral kinematic properties are compared over the course of femorotibial flexion-extension. Craniocaudal translation measurements of the patella relative to the femur in mm. For the x-axis, higher values indicate greater femorotibial extension. For the y-axis, higher values indicate greater cranial translation of the patella, where the patellar origin is displaced more cranially to the femoral origin

Our results are similar to the findings from a canine cadaveric investigation, in which passive patellofemoral joint motion was described over a smaller range of femorotibial motion [3]. Both studies demonstrated that all three kinematic parameters were linearly related to the femorotibial flexion angle. Our results, however, differ slightly with respect to the magnitude of observed change; for example, changes in femorotibial flexion angle from 90 to 150° induced proximodistal patella translation of approximately 13 mm in the cadaver study versus approximately 18 mm in our in vivo study [3]. The change in patellar flexion of approximately 25° was reported in the cadaver study, whereas we found a change of 44° over the equivalent femorotibial range of motion [3]. There are several explanations for the discrepancies between the studies. Most obviously, our investigation was an in vivo dynamic analysis, accounting for all the complex forces acting on the patella in vivo. Anatomic differences between breeds may have been a

Table 1 Average maximum, minimum, and range of motion kinematics during all three activities

	Flexion angle	Proximal translation	Cranial translation
Trot			
Maximum	51° (5)	7.8 mm (4.1)	32.4 mm (5.5)
Minimum	6° (4)	−11.3 mm (3.2)	17.6 mm (3.8)
Range of Motion	45° (6)	19.1 mm (4.1)	14.8 mm (2.7)
r	0.064	−0.029	0.008
p	0.006	0.224	0.732
Walk			
Maximum	33° (11)	6.8 mm (3.6)	32.1 mm (4.6)
Minimum	7° (4)	−6.8 mm (4.1)	24.4 mm (5.4)
Range of Motion	26° (9)	13.6 mm (2.6)	7.7 mm (3.4)
r	−0.86	0.858	0.672
p	0	0	<0.001
Sit			
Maximum	92° (12)	−13.0 mm (2.9)	23.7 mm (7.4)
Minimum	41° (19)	−7 mm (5.4)	1.7 mm (3.4)
Range of Motion	51° (20)	6.0 mm (5.1)	22.0 mm (7.5)
r	−0.951	0.346	0.893
p	0	<0.001	0

Pearson correlation coefficient (r) and p values listed in relation to femorotibial flexion angle
Data in parentheses indicate ± 1 standard deviation

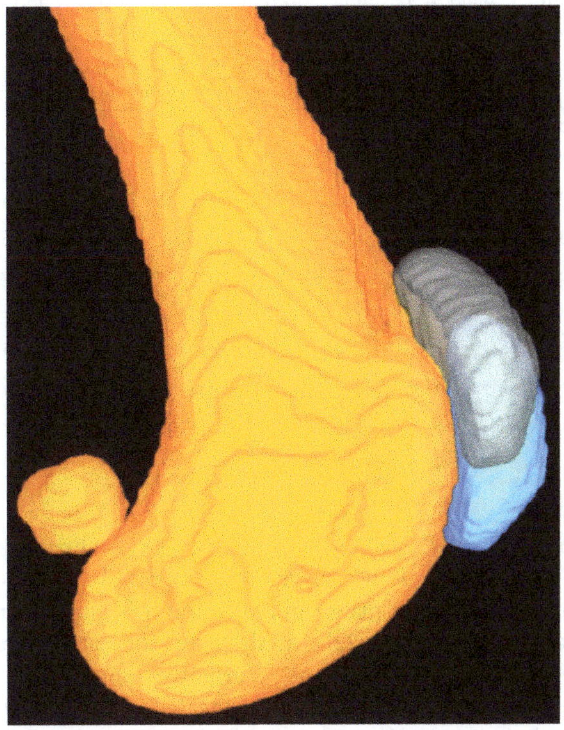

Fig. 6 Representative image of off-set of patellofemoral poses during trot. The same femorotibial flexion angle is represented by the *orange* femur. The solid *blue* patella is the patellar orientation when entering swing phase and the *white* patella is the patellar orientation when exiting swing phase

factor, as our study used Labrador Retrievers while the cadaver study used mix-breed dogs. Equally importantly, variations in coordinate assignation and reference points have been shown to dramatically affect patellar tracking patterns in humans, even within the same individual [12]. To the author's knowledge, this is only the second report characterizing patellar kinematics in dogs. Standardized coordinate systems and reference points for future studies would allow more meaningful comparison between investigations.

The most significant finding of the study was that the relationship between patellar poses and femorotibial flexion angle varied according to the phase of the gait cycle during trotting; the patella was positioned more proximal, more cranial, and more flexed in early swing phase when compared to late swing phase at the identical femorotibial flexion angle (Fig. 6). This offset likely contributed to the lack of a statistical linear correlation with the femorotibial flexion angle. The cause of this offset upon entering and exiting swing during trotting remains to be clarified. Potential causes include the varying magnitude at which the pelvic limb musculature, particularly the quadriceps muscle group, are contracting and acting on the patella, as well as the secondary motions of the tibia such as internal-external rotation and craniocaudal tibial translation. While an increased force of quadriceps contraction did not have significant effect on patellar movement in a human cadaveric study, an in vivo MRI study demonstrated the resting patellar position in the trochlea groove could be altered by muscular contraction during either open- or closed-chain exercises [18, 19]. Surface electromyographic studies in dogs have demonstrated widely varying patterns of vastus lateralis contraction according to differing activities, which could alter patellofemoral poses during different phases of the gait cycle as observed in our study [20]. Electromyographic studies performed concurrently with radiographic kinematic analyses might improve our understanding of how muscular contraction alters patellar kinematics in dogs.

The single-plane flat-panel imaging and shape-matching methodology utilized in this study was previously validated for femorotibial kinematics in dogs [15, 21]. The precision of this methodology for this joint was determined to be within 1.28 mm and 1.58° with an intraobserver variability of less than 0.52 mm and 0.91° for translation and rotations, respectively [21]. These values reported for the femorotibial joint are unlikely to be directly applicable for the patellofemoral joint due to differences in bone geometry. Studies performed in

Table 2 Average maximum and minimum during swing and stance phase during walking and trotting activities

	Flexion angle	Proximal translation	Cranial translation
Trot			
Swing Maximum	51°	3.1 mm	31 mm
Swing Minimum	13°	−11.6 mm	17.6 mm
Stance Maximum	17°	7.8 mm	32.4 mm
Stance Minimum	7°	−0.2 mm	30.2 mm
Walk			
Swing Maximum	33°	6.1 mm	31.4 mm
Swing Minimum	10°	−6.8 mm	24.4 mm
Stance Maximum	13°	6.8 mm	32.1 mm
Stance Minimum	7°	3.6 mm	31.5 mm

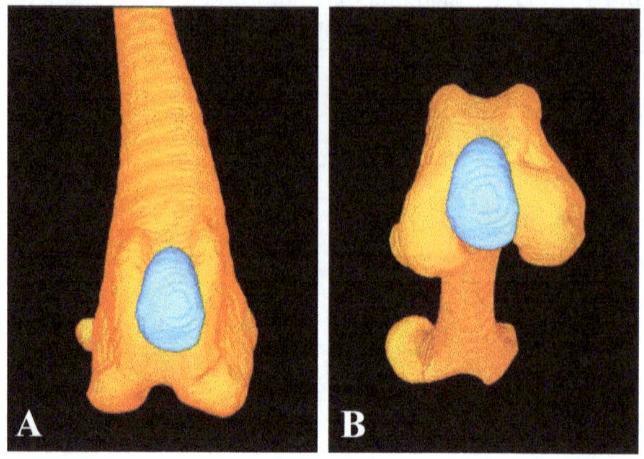

Fig. 7 Free-view of the femur and patella during stand-to-sit motion. **a** Mean position of the femur and patella in extension at the beginning of sit. The *gray line* designates the proximal aspect of the femoral trochlea. **b** Position of the femur and patella in the flexion phase of sit with the patella appearing far distal in the femoral trochlea

humans using similar methodology to evaluate the patellofemoral joint kinematics reported accuracy within 0.6° for in-plane rotations and 1.5 mm for in-plane translations [22]. Analysis in this study was confined to sagittal plane translations and rotation due to the uniplanar nature of the technique and the patellofemoral joint anatomy. Although studies have not been performed to specifically validate the accuracy of our methodology for determining patellofemoral joint kinematics in dogs, a pilot series assessing repeatability of 3-D to 2-D image registration for this joint appeared to consistent with the results observed in other studies [23, 24].

The 3-D patella model was approximated to remain central within the trochlear groove such that the center of the patella's articulating surface remained as congruent as possible with the trochlear groove in the axial plane. We utilized the 3-D geometry of the trochlear groove to define medial-lateral translation as well as patellar tilt. The kinematic parameters in the sagittal plane may have been different if the assumptions were not made. Studies in humans have shown the axial plane topography of the trochlear groove could be used to predict axial plane patellar kinematics, supporting our methodology [25]. However, coronal plane rotation, conventionally known as patellar rotation, was not readily predictable by trochlear anatomy in humans [25]. Bi-plane radiographic analysis would be required to gain a more thorough intricate understanding of canine patellofemoral joint motion in vivo.

Our data should be useful as a baseline of normal patellofemoral kinematics in dogs, against which comparisons can be made in future studies. The main goal of this study was to characterize normal patellofemoral motion in order to define the change in kinematics caused by cranial cruciate ligament rupture in a future study by our group. Because the most profound femorotibial kinematic abnormalities with cranial cruciate ligament rupture occur in the sagittal plane, it is logical to expect that the patellofemoral kinematics we reported, including patellar flexion, proximodistal translation, and craniocaudal translation, may be disrupted by the condition. Indeed, cadaveric studies have found the cranial cruciate ligament rupture can alter patella alignment and patellofemoral contact mechanics [4]. Patellofemoral mechanics are also of particular interest with the surgical treatment of cranial cruciate ligament rupture as stifle extensor mechanism abnormalities frequently occur following various procedures used to address the disease [26]. Our results are likely less applicable to patellar luxation, where the major abnormalities in motion are in the coronal plane.

Conclusions

The study used CT based models and single-plane flat-panel imaging to quantify patellofemoral motion during commonly performed daily activity in dogs. There was significant linear correlation between femorotibial flexion angle and each of the three degrees of freedom in the sagittal plane during sit and walk. The patella utilizes the full length of the trochlear groove during daily activity. Trotting induced offset, where patellar poses differed according to the phase of the gait cycle, despite identical femorotibial flexion angles. By defining normal in vivo kinematic patterns non-invasively, new knowledge of the normal canine stifle has been generated which may lead to the improvement and development of new surgical correction methods for stifle abnormalities.

Endnotes

[1]Toshiba Aquilon 8, Toshiba American Medical Systems Inc, Tustin, CA.

[2]Toshiba Infinix-I flat panel C-arm fluoroscope, Toshiba American Medical Systems Inc, Tustin, CA.

[3]ITK-SNAP, Paul A. Yushkevich et al., http://www.itksnap.org.

[4]Geomagic Studio, Geomagic Inc., Research Triangle Park, NC.

[5]JointTrack, University of Florida, FL, http://sourceforge.net/projects/jointtrack/.

[6]Matlab, MathWorks, Natick, MA.

[7g] SigmaPlot 12, Systat Software, Inc. San Jose, CA.

Abbreviations

CT: Computed tomography; DICOM: Digital imaging and communication in medicine

Acknowledgements

The authors thank Mr Tim Vojt for assisting with producing the graph figures.

Funding

This study was funded by grants for the Merial Veterinary Student Scholars Program and Departmental Funds at the University of Florida College of Veterinary Medicine.

Authors' contributions

EJM shape-matched the 3-D bone models of the femur and patella onto the flat-panel images, analyzed the data, and drafted the manuscript. SEK participated in the design of the study, assisted in data analysis, and helped draft the manuscript. JC created the 3-D bone models and trained EJM in shape-matching. SCJ provided the shape-matched data for femorotibial kinematics. SAB, DDL and AP participated in the design of the study, as well as drafting of the manuscript. All authors read and approved the final manuscript.

Competing interests

The authors declare that they have no competing interests.

Consent for publication

Not applicable.

References

1. Carpenter DH, Cooper RC. Mini review of canine stifle joint anatomy. Anat Histol Embryol. 2000;29:321–9.
2. Johnson JA, Austin C, Breur GJ. Incidence of canine appendicular musculoskeletal disorders in 16 veterinary teaching hospitals from 980 through 1989. Vet Comp Orthopaed. 1994;7:56–69.
3. Pozzi A, Dunbar NJ, Kim SE. Effect of tibial plateau leveling osteotomy on patellofemoral alignment: a study using canine cadavers. Vet J. 2013;198:98–102.
4. Guerrero TG, Pozzi A, Dunbar N, Kipfer N, Haessig M, Horodyski MB, et al. Effect of tibial tuberosity advancement on the contact mechanics and the alignment of the patellofemoral and femorotibial joints. Vet Surg. 2011;40:839–48.
5. Durant AM, Millis DL, Headrick JF. Kinematics of stair ascent in healthy dogs. Vet Comp Orthopaed. 2011;2:99–105.
6. Holler PJ, Brazda V, Dal-Bianco B, Lewy E, Mueller MC, Peham C, et al. Kinematic motion analysis of the joints of the forelimbs and hind limbs of dogs during walking exercise regimens. Am J Vet Res. 2010;71:734 40.
7. Agostinho FS, Rahal SC, Miqueleto NSML, Verdugo MR, Inamassu LR, El-Warrak AO. Kinematic analysis of Labrador retrievers and rottweilers trotting on a treadmill. Vet Comp Orthopaed. 2011;3:185–91.
8. Torres BT, Whitlock D, Reynolds LR, Fu YC, Navik JA, Speas AL, et al. The effect of marker location variability on noninvasive canine stifle kinematics. Vet Surg. 2011;40:715–9.
9. Thomas TM, Marcellin-Little DJ, Roe SC, Lascelles BDX, Brosey BP. Comparison of measurements obtained by use of an electrogoniometer and a universal plastic goniometer for the assessment of joint motion in dogs. Am J Vet Res. 2006;67:1974–9.
10. Torres BT, Punke JP, Fu YC, Navik JA, Speas AL, Sornborger A, et al. Comparison of canine stifle kinematic data collected with three different targeting models. Vet Surg. 2010;39:504–12.
11. Katchburian MV, Bull AMJ, Shih YF, Heatley FW, Amis AA. Measurement of patellar tracking: assessment and analysis of the literature. Clin Orthop Relat R. 2003;412:241–59.
12. Bull AMJ, Katchburian MV, Shih YF, Amis AA. Standardisation of the description of patellofemoral motion and comparison between different techniques. Knee Surg Sport Tr A. 2002;10:184–93.
13. Tashman S, Anderst W. In vivo measurement of dynamic joint motion using high speed biplane radiography and CT: application to canine ACL deficiency. J Biomech Eng. 2003;125:238–45.
14. Rey J, Fischer MS, Böttcher P. Sagittal joint instability in the cranial cruciate ligament insufficient canine stifle. Caudal slippage of the femur and not cranial tibial subluxation. Tierarztl Prax Ausg K Kleintiere Heimtiere. 2014;42:151–6.
15. Kim SE, Jones SC, Lewis DD, Banks SA, Conrad BP, Tremolada G, et al. In-vivo three-dimensional stifle kinematics during daily activities in dogs. J Orthop Res. 2015;33:1603–10.
16. Goh JCH, Lee PYC, Bose K. A cadaver study of the function of the oblique part of vastus medialis. J Bone Joint Surg. 1995;77:225–31.
17. Grood ES, Suntay WJ. A joint coordinate system for clinical description of three-dimenstional motions. Application to the knee. J Biomech Eng. 1983;105:136–44.
18. Nagamine R, Otani T, White SE, McCarthy DS, Whiteside LA. Patellar tracking measurement in the normal knee. J Orthop Res. 1995;13:115–22.
19. Felicio LR, Saad MC, Liporaci RF, Baffa Ado P, dos Santos AC, Bevilaqua-Grossi D. Evaluating patellar kinematics through magnetic resonance imaging during open- and closed-kinetic-chain exercises. J Sport Rehabil. 2010;19:1–11.
20. Breitfuss K, Franz M, Peham C, Bockstahler B. Surface electromyography of the vastus lateralis, biceps femoris, and gluteus medius muscle in sound dogs during walking and specific physiotherapeutic exercises. Vet Surg. 2014. doi:10.1111/j.1532-950X.2014.12302.x.
21. Jones SC, Kim SE, Banks SA, Conrad BP, Abbasi AZ, Tremolada G, et al. Accuracy of noninvasive, single-plane fluoroscopic analysis for measurement of three-dimensional femorotibial joint poses in dogs. Am J Vet Res. 2014;75:477–85.
22. Akbarshahi M, Schache AG, Fernandez JW, Baker R, Banks S, Pandy MG. Non-invasive assessment of soft-tissue artifact and its effect on knee joint kinematics during functional activity. J Biomech. 2010;43:1292–301.
23. Fregly BJ, Rahman HA, Banks SA. Theoretical accuracy of model-based shape matching for measuring natural knee kinematics with single-plane fluoroscopy. J Biomech Eng. 2005;127:692–9.
24. Mahfouz MR, Hoff WA, Komistek RD, Dennis DA. A robust method for registration of three-dimensional knee implant models to two-dimensional fluoroscopy images. IEEE Trans Med Imaging. 2003;22:1561–74.
25. Varadarajan KM, Freiberg AA, Gill TJ, Rubash HE, Li G. Relationship between three-dimensional geometry of the trochlear groove and in vivo patellar tracking during weight-bearing knee flexion. J Biomech Eng. 2010. doi:10.1115/1.4001360.
26. Mattern KL, Berry CR, Peck JN, De Han JJ. Radiographic and ultrasonographic evaluation of the patellar ligament following tibial plateau leveling osteotomy. Vet Radiol Ultrasoun. 2006;2:185–91.

14

Phenotypic and genetic characterization of *Piscirickettsia salmonis* from Chilean and Canadian salmonids

Alexander Otterlei[1], Øyvind J. Brevik[2], Daniel Jensen[1], Henrik Duesund[2], Ingunn Sommerset[3], Petter Frost[3], Julio Mendoza[4], Peter McKenzie[5], Are Nylund[1] and Patricia Apablaza[2*]

Abstract

Background: The study presents the phenotypic and genetic characterization of selected *P. salmonis* isolates from Atlantic salmon and rainbow trout suffering from SRS (salmonid rickettsial septicemia) in Chile and in Canada. The phenotypic characterization of the *P. salmonis* isolates were based on growth on different agar media (including a newly developed medium), different growth temperatures, antibiotics susceptibility and biochemical tests.

Results: This is the first study differentiating Chilean *P. salmonis* isolates into two separate genetic groups. Genotyping, based on 16S rRNA-ITS and concatenated housekeeping genes grouped the selected isolates into two clades, constituted by the Chilean strains, while the Canadian isolates form a branch in the phylogenetic tree. The latter consisted of two isolates that were different in both genetic and phenotypic characteristics. The phylogenies and the MLST do not reflect the origin of the isolates with respect to host species. The isolates included were heterogeneous in phenotypic tests.

Conclusions: The genotyping methods developed in this study provided a tool for separation of *P. salmonis* isolates into distinct clades. The SRS outbreaks in Chile are caused by minimum two different genetic groups of *P. salmonis*. This heterogeneity should be considered in future development of vaccines against this bacterium in Chile. Two different strains of *P. salmonis*, in regards to genetic and phenotypic characteristics, can occur in the same contemporary outbreak of SRS.

Keywords: *P. salmonis*, Phenotyping, Genotyping, 16S rDNA-ITS, Housekeeping genes, Phylogeny, MLST

Background

The Chilean aquaculture industry has constantly faced problems with *Piscirickettsia salmonis*, which causes salmonid rickettsial septicemia (SRS) [1]. This disease causes high mortalities in several salmonids species Atlantic salmon (*Salmo salar*), Rainbow trout (*Onchorhyncus mykiss*), Coho salmon (*Onchorhyncus kisutch*), and was responsible for 90 % of the total use of antibiotics in Chile in 2014 [2]. *P. salmonis* has been detected in several countries including Norway, Canada, Scotland, Ireland and Chile [3, 4], but opposed to the situation in Chile, SRS is considered manageable in these countries.

* Correspondence: Patricia.Apablaza@cermaq.com
[2]Cermaq Group AS, Dronning Eufemias gate 16, P.O. Box 144 SentrumN-0102 Oslo, Norway
Full list of author information is available at the end of the article

The present knowledge on *P. salmonis* is restricted in several aspects such as characterization (phenotypical and genetic), geographical distribution, host specificity, presence of natural reservoirs and transmission routes. Although several vaccines are available [5–7] none of them are able to induce complete protection against SRS. This lack of protection suggests that more basic knowledge is needed about the biology of *P. salmonis*.

P. salmonis is a Gram-negative, predominantly coccoid, aerobic, non-encapsulated, and highly fastidious bacterium of approx. 0.5–1.5 μm diameter [3]. The pathogen was first described as an obligatory intracellular bacterium and has traditionally been cultured on Chinook salmon embryos cells (CHSE-214) and others fish cell lines [8]. In 2008 it was shown that *P. salmonis* could be grown on artificial cell-free media [9–11].

However, work at our laboratory has shown that not all isolates growth well at these media, hence, we developed a new improved medium for isolation and culturing of *P. salmonis* strains.

This study present new basic knowledge of *P. salmonis* isolated from sub-acute, acute and chronic outbreaks of SRS. These isolates are compared to the type strain, LF-89. The new knowledge presented could form a better basis for development of efficient strategies for control and treatment of SRS, and possibly a new basis for future development of vaccines against *P. salmonis.*

Methods

Collection of *P. salmonis*

The isolates of *P. salmonis* were obtained in 2011 and 2012 from Atlantic salmon and Rainbow trout suspected or diagnosed with SRS. The Chilean isolates, were obtained from a pool of homogenized fish tissues (kidney, spleen, liver, brain). The Canadian isolates were collected from the same site during a single outbreak of SRS, and from kidney. All the isolates were sent to the Fish Diseases Research Group at the University of Bergen where they were sub-cultured on CHAB agar [10] and stored at −80 °C for later characterization. An overview of all the isolates included in the study is presented in the Table 1. The geographical origins of the isolates are presented in Fig. 1. The *P. salmonis* type isolate (LF-89) was also included in the study.

This study followed the recommendations of the Norwegian Animal Welfare Act (01.01.2010) and the work was done under the regulations given by the Norwegian Food Safety Authority. The bacterial samples were obtained from the fish after they has been anaesthetized by a blow to the head and killed by instantly decapitation. This procedure complies with the Norwegian fish welfare regulations.

New growth medium

To improve the growth of *P. salmonis* on solid media, a new optimized SRS blood agar (SRS-BA) was developed. The composition of this agar was 40 g of TSA (BD, Difco); 20 g of Red Sea Salt (RSS) (Red Sea, USA); 50 ml of defibrinated sheep blood (DSB) (Oxoid Limited, UK); 1 g of L-cysteine (Sigma-Aldrich); 5 g of D-glucose

Table 1 Data for all the selected *P. salmonis* isolates included in the study

Isolate code	Country	County (Region)	Sampling date	Mortality (%)	Host	Sample tissue	Clinical condition
LF-89	Chile	Puerto Montt (X)	1989	na	Coho salmon	kidney	na
Ch2-As-I	Chile	Chiloé Sur (X)	08.08.2012	7,8	Atlantic salmon	k-l-sp-b	acute
Ch3-Rt-L	Chile	Calbuco (X)	03.10.2012	6,7	Rainbow trout	lession	sub-acute
Ch4-Rt-L	Chile	Calbuco (X)	05.10.2012	6,7	Rainbow trout	lession	sub-acute
Ch5-As-I	Chile	Chiloé Centro (X)	18.07.2012	5,1	Atlantic salmon	k-l-b	sub-acute
Ch6-Rt-L	Chile	Calbuco (X)	10.08.2012	13,2	Rainbow trout	lession	sub-acute
Ch7-As-L	Chile	Aysén (XI)	na	na	Atlantic salmon	muscle	chronic
Ch8-Rt-K	Chile	Chiloé Centro (X)	17.06.2011	1,9	Rainbow trout	kidney	sub-acute
Ch9-As-na	Chile	Chiloé Centro (X)	27.03.2012	2,4	Atlantic salmon	na	sub-acute
Ch10-As-I	Chile	Chiloé Sur (X)	24.07.2012	21,5	Atlantic salmon	k-l-sp-b	acute
Ch11-As-I	Chile	Chiloé Centro (X)	04.05.2012	2,2	Atlantic salmon	k-l-b	sub-acute
Ch12-As-I	Chile	Chiloé Centro (X)	07.05.2012	14,8	Atlantic salmon	k-l-b	acute
Ch13-As-I	Chile	Chiloé Centro (X)	18.04.2012	3,6	Atlantic salmon	k-l-sp-b	chronic
Ch14-As-I	Chile	Chiloé Centro (X)	13.01.2012	14,8	Atlantic salmon	k-sp	acute
Ch15-As-I	Chile	Chiloé Centro (X)	23.08.2012	5,4	Atlantic salmon	k-l-b-sp	sub-acute
Ch16-As-I	Chile	Chiloé Centro (X)	June 2012	14,8	Atlantic salmon	k-l-b	acute
Ch17-As-I	Chile	Chiloé Centro (X)	23.05.2012	14,8	Atlantic salmon	k-l-b	acute
Ch18-As-I	Chile	Chiloé Centro (X)	22.06.2012	3,6	Atlantic salmon	k-l-b-sp	chronic
Ca19-As-I	Canada	British Columbia	11.12.2012	<0,03	Atlantic salmon	kidney	chronic
Ca20-As-I	Canada	British Columbia	11.12.2012	<0,03	Atlantic salmon	kidney	chronic

Codes indicates the country of isolation, Chile (Ch), Canada (Ca); number of isolate (1–20); fish species, Atlantic salmon (As), Rainbow trout (Rt), Coho salmon (Cs); and tissue, kidney (K), liver (l), spleen (sp) and brain (b). The samples were obtained from a pool of internal organs. The codes are: I from internal lesions, L from external lesions, and K from kidney. Sub-acute and acute clinical conditions frequently present hemorrhages in the brain, splenomegaly and extensive congestion particularly in the swimbladder. In chronic conditions typical findings are whitish nodules in the liver which becomes brownish and finally progress as granuloma. Mostly in Atlantic salmon and rainbow trout, the dermis present speckle erosions which progress to pustules and finally caverns. It has also seen splenomegaly and hepatomegaly; pericarditis with fibrin deposits in Atlantic salmon and rainbow trout. In Coho salmon the fibrin deposits are located mostly internally in the abdomen. Mortality percentage is described as percentage of dead fish due to SRS, from necropsy findings, in one production cycle. In most of the farms antimicrobials were used for treatment. Na: information not available

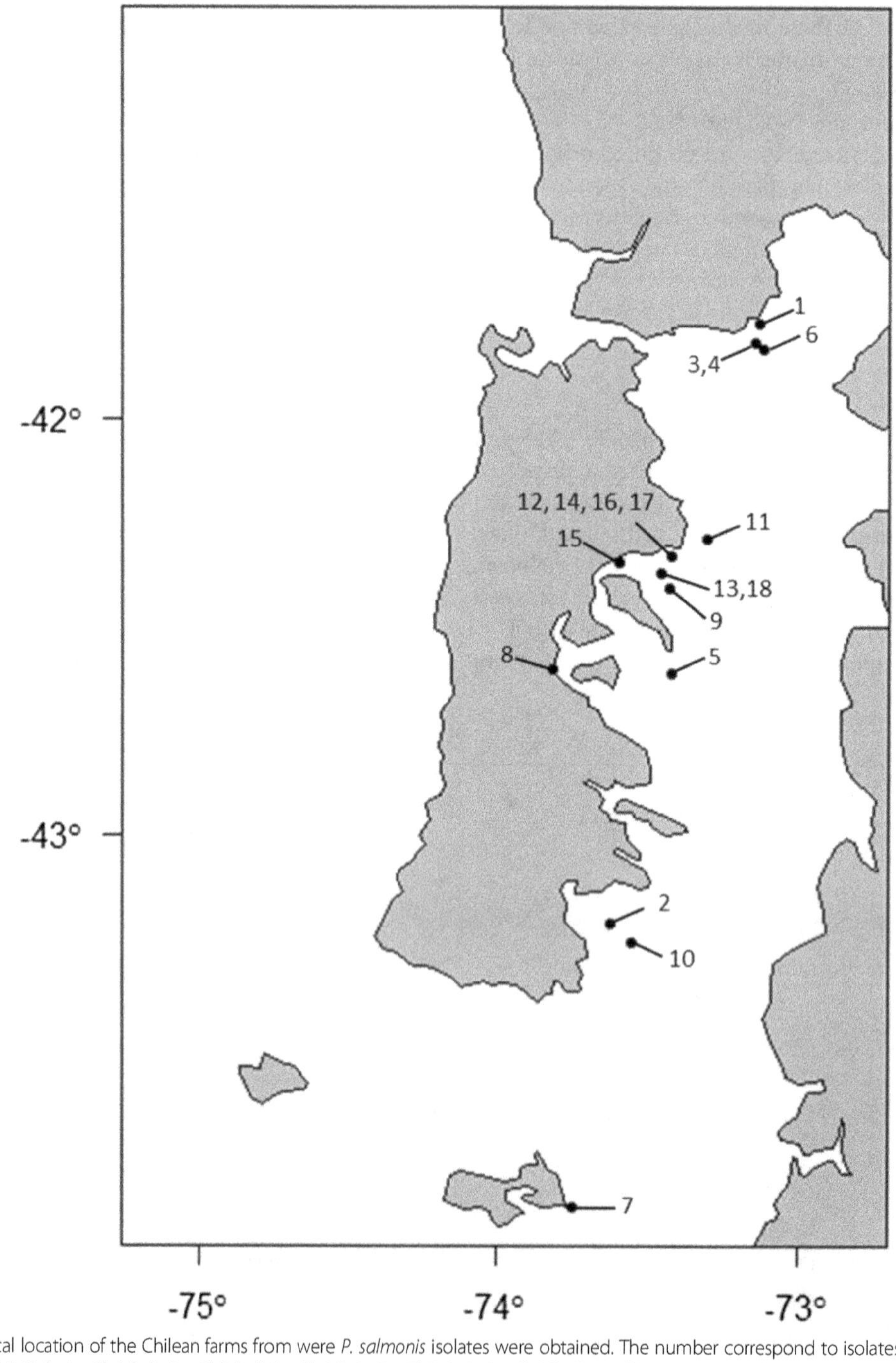

Fig. 1 Geographical location of the Chilean farms from were *P. salmonis* isolates were obtained. The number correspond to isolates: 1 = LF-89, 2 = Ch2-As-I, 3 = Ch3-Rt-L, 4 = Ch4-Rt-L, 5 = Ch5-As-I, 6 = Ch6-Rt-L, 7 = Ch7-As-L, 8 = Ch8-Rt-K, 9 = Ch9-As-na, 10 = Ch10-As-I, 11 = Ch11-As-I, 12 = Ch12-As-I, 13 = Ch13-As-I, 14 = Ch14-As-I, 15 = Ch15-As-I, 16 = Ch16-As-I, 17 = Ch17-As-I, and 18 = Ch18-As-I

(Sigma-Aldrich); 50 ml of fetal bovine serum (FBS) (Thermo Scientific Hyclone, USA); 0.2 mM ferric nitrate (Sigma-Aldrich) and reverse osmosis water (RO) to a final volume of 1000 ml. RSS was chosen to simulate natural sea water composition. RO water, TSA and RSS were autoclaved at 121 °C for 15 min. DSB was added after cooling from autoclaving. Subsequently, the agar was cooled down to 50 °C and L-cysteine, D-glucose, FBS and ferric nitrate were added. The pH was adjusted to 6.8 ± 0.2.

Phenotypic characterization

Colonies > 1 mm were used for morphological characterization and bacteria from these colonies were

Gram-stained for the description of cell morphology and other phenotypic characteristics.

Testing of different growth media was performed using two colonies from each isolate streaked on the following media: SRS-BA, Austral-TSHem [11], CHAB [10], CHAB with 0.2 mM Fe, blood agar (BA), BA with 2 % NaCl, marine agar (MA) and tryptone-yeast extract-salts with glucose agar (FLPA) [12] and incubated at 19 ° C for 14 days. The temperature range for bacterial growth measured as number of colonies and colony size was tested using three colonies streaked out on SRS-BA and incubated at 8, 11, 16, 19, 22, and 25 °C. The growth was recorded at days 3, 7, 10 and 14 in both tests.

Test of the susceptibility to antimicrobial drugs was performed by the agar diffusion method using tablets as described by Justesen et al. [13], with some modifications. 19 °C was used for incubation, as this is within the common optimum temperature range of all isolates. The inhibition zone was measured after 10 days of incubation, to ensure sufficient growth. The antimicrobial sensitivity was tested for all the isolates against: streptomycin (10 μg); oxytetracycline (30 μg); penicillin (1 unit); ceftazidime (30 μg); ampicillin (2 μg); and florfenicol (30 μg). The inhibition zone was measured, in millimeters, from the tablet border towards to all the extension of the inhibition area.

Indole and oxidase tests were performed with BBL™ DrySlide™ (BD BBL™, U.S.A) kits. The cefinase test using BBL™ Cefinase™ Paper Disc (BD BBL™, U.S.A) was used to determine the production of β-lactamases. Catalase was detected by adding a drop of hydrogen peroxide 3 % (Sigma-Aldrich, Germany) to a microscope slide before transferring a small amount of bacteria onto the H_2O_2 solution. The API ZYM galleries (BioMérieux, U.S.A) for the detection of bacterial enzymes were used according to the manufacturer's protocol, except that the incubation temperature was set at 19 °C and the incubation time at 24 h. A 6.0 McFarland standard, as recommended by BioMérieux, was made in advance for turbidity comparison. H_2S production was done using hydrogen Sulfide Test Strips (Sigma-Aldrich, Switzerland). All the phenotypical and biochemical tests were performed in triplicate, with the exception of the antimicrobial susceptibility analysis, which was done in duplicate.

Genetic characterization

The DNA extraction from pure cultures of all *P. salmonis* was performed with an E.Z.N.A Tissue DNA kit. The quality of DNA was tested using NanoDrop (Saveen Werner, Life Science) before storing at −20 °C.

PCR, purification and visualization of products by gel electrophoresis, and sequencing were performed as described by Apablaza et al. [14]. Sequencing of the 20 isolates was performed using specific primers for 16S rDNA and ITS, and for the housekeeping genes, HK (dnaK, groEL, tbpB, mltB, ospA, radA, airA, bax, tnpA, elfP). The primers are presented in Table 2. The Vector NTI® v9.0 Software package (Invitrogen) was used for sequence assembling and alignment. Manual adjustments and verification of reading frames for the protein coding genes were conducted in GeneDoc (Karl Nicholas ©2000). The evolutionary analysis and calculation of the best fit model for the 16S rDNA-ITS dataset (2191 base pairs) was conducted in MEGA6 [15]. The maximum likelihood method using the Hasegawa-Kishino-Yano [16] model with discrete Gamma distribution was applied.

The software KAKUSAN4 was used for construction of concatenated sequences of the 10 HK genes (8969 base pairs), calculation of substitution rate, and the best fit model for the individual loci and codon positions [17]. The data were exported into an MrBays-block (V. 3.2.2 x86) for analysis. The phylogenetic analysis was performed with Proportional Codon, Proportional model and a mcmc of 40 000 000 generations. The phylogram was constructed using TreeAnotator and viewed in FigTree [18]. A statistics report of percentage identity (PID) and average nucleotide identity (ANI) was made in GeneDoc (Karl Nicholas ©2000).

The multi locus sequence typing (MLST) method was applied as described by Apablaza et al. [14]. Briefly, the different allele types (AT) within the 10 HK were used to create the sequence types (ST). Based on the different STs, a data matrix from the 18 isolates of *P. salmonis* was exported as a nexus file into PAUP 4.0. A dendrogram was constructed using neighbor-joining (NJ) distance method.

All the nucleotide sequences were deposited in the GenBank database. Accession numbers are presented in Additional file 1: Table S1.

Results

Phenotypic characterization

The colonies grown on SRS-BA were slightly convex, grey-white, shiny, and centrally opaque with translucent, slightly undulating margins. At the microscopic level, the cells were Gram-negative, coccoid shaped, measuring from 0.4 to 1.8 μm in diameter. No distinctive colony or cell morphology differences were observed among the isolates.

The results of the growth at the different media are presented in Table 3. The minority of the isolates were classified as 'fastidious' (LF-89, Ch5-As-I, Ch6-Rt-L, and Ca20-As-K) while the rest of the isolates were defined as 'less fastidious'. Five of the isolates (Ch3-Rt-L, Ch4-Rt-L, Ch5-As-I, Ch6-Rt-L and Ca20-As-I) grew on SRS-BA only. No growth was recorded on MA and FLPA media.

Table 2 Primers used for PCR analysis in the present study

Target gene	Primer	Direction	Sequence (5´–3´)	Reference
16 s rDNA	Eug B27F	Fwd	AGAGTTTGATCMTGGCTCAG	[25]
	Eug A1518R	Rev	AAGGAGGTGATCCANCCRCA	[25]
ITS	SRS-ITS/F	Fwd	GTACACACCGCCCGTCACAC	Present study
	SRS-ITS/R	Rev	CCTCACGGTACTAGTTCACTATCGG	Present study
dnaK	SRS-dnaK/F2	Fwd	CCGTGTCGTGTGGCGCTAAAA	Present study
	SRS-dnaK/R2	Rev	TTGAGATTGAGCCTGCTCCGC	Present study
	SRS-dnaK3/F1	Fwd	CCGCGTGTGATTGAGAGTGC	Present study
	SRS-dnaK3/R1	Rev	CGTCATCACCCCACCCATGG	Present study
groEL	SRS-groEL/F1	Fwd	CTTCGGTACCGGTTCCCGTC	Present study
	SRS-groEL/R1	Rev	TCTTGCAGTTTCTCGCGGTCG	Present study
	SRS-groEL/F2	Fwd	GTGAAGCTCTGGCAACACTCGTC	Present study
	SRS-groEL/R2	Rev	AGGAAGCTCTGCAACCATCGC	Present study
tbpB	SRS-tbpB/F1	Fwd	AACTGGGCAGGCGTCACTGTT	Present study
	SRS-tbpB/R1	Rev	CGGCGCGTCTCTAATGTTCG	Present study
	SRS-tbpB2/F2	Fwd	CCAAGCTGGATCACCGCCAT	Present study
	SRS-tbpB2/R2	Rev	AAAGATAGGCCCAGCCACGC	Present study
mltB	SRS-mltB/F	Fwd	ACCACTCACGCGGCATCTAA	Present study
	SRS-mltB/R	Rev	ACTCAAATCATACACCGCCATTGCA	Present study
ospA	SRS-ospA/F	Fwd	AGCCGTCAAGAAGTCGGAGCT	Present study
	SRS-ospA/R	Rev	TGCCAACGACCATCCGCTTG	Present study
radA	SRS-radA/F1	Fwd	ATCAGTCGCCAGCCTGTTGG	Present study
	SRS-radA/FR1	Rev	GTCCTCGTTGCACTGGACGA	Present study
airA	SRS-air/F1	Fwd	GGGTGCGTCCGGGGATTATG	Present study
	SRS-rairA/R1	Rev	TAAGGTGCACGCAGTGGCAT	Present study
bax	SRS-bax/F1	Fwd	TCAAGGGATCTGGGAAGTGCT	Present study
	SRS-bax/R1	Rev	ACCACTGCCTATCTTGCTCAACA	Present study
tnpA	SRS-tnpA/F1	Fwd	ACCTGTTAAGTTCTCGGCCATT	Present study
	SRS-tnpA/R1	Rev	AGCCTTCACAAATGTCAACAAGTGA	Present study
elfP	SRS-elfP/F	Fwd	GCCACKGCTAATTCAGCAA	Present study
	SRS-elfP/R	Rev	STGGAATGGTCAGCCACYT	Present study

The isolate Ch15-G2-As-I produced the highest number of colonies in SRS-BA. Ch14-As-I induced α- (dark green/brown discoloration around colonies) and β-hemolysis (medium translucence under the colonies) on BA with 2 % NaCl. This isolate grew on all the tested media, with exception of MA and FLPA (Fig. 2).

The maximum temperature range for the isolates growth was from 8 to 25 °C on SRS-BA (data not shown). Ch2-As-1, Ch7-As-L, Ch8-Rt-K, Ch12-As-I, Ch18-As-I, and Ca19-As-K had the ability to grow at 25 °C, while the type strain LF-89 did not grow at this temperature. After three days of incubation all isolates showed growth at 16, 19 and 22 °C. The optimum temperature for maximum growth was in the range 19–22 °C for the less fastidious isolates (including Ca19-As-K), and 16 to 19 °C for the remaining strains, including Ca20-As-K (Table 4).

The study of the antibiotic sensitivity of the isolates with respect to different antibiotics shows large variation in the inhibition zones. The strain Ch3-Rt-L seems to be resistant to the most of the antibiotics tested (Table 5). All isolates were sensitives to oxytetracycline, while florfenicol yielded the largest inhibition zones with the exception of above mentioned strain. Ch10-As-I had the largest inhibition zones in all antibiotics with the exception of penicillin.

Indole and oxidase tests were negative for all of the isolates, while catalase and cefinase tests were positive.

Table 3 Summary of growth of *P. salmonis* isolates on different culture media

Isolate	SRS-BA	CHAB	CHAB w/Fe	Austral-TSHem	BA	BA w/2 % NaCl
Ch11-As-I	+++	+++	+++	++	++	+++
Ch7-As-L	+++	+++	+++	++	++	++
Ch14-As-I	+++	++	++	++	++	+++
Ch9-As-na	+++	+++	+++	++	+	+
Ch13-As-I	+++	++	++	++	++	+++
Ch17-As-I	++	++	+	+	++	++
Ch2-As-I	+++	++	++	+	++	++
Ch12-As-I	+++	++	++	+	+	++
Ch15-As-I	+++	+	+	W	+	+
Ch10-As-I	++	++	++	+	+	++
Ch8-Rt-K	+++	+	+	+	+	+
Ch18-As-I	+++	+	+	+	-	+
Ca19-As-I	+++	++	++	-	+	+
Ch16-As-I	++	+	+	-	+	++
LF-89	+++	++	++	-	+	+

Symbols: (−), no growth; (+), scant growth; (++), moderate growth; (+++), vigorous growth; and (w), weak growth. Isolates Ch3-Rt-L, Ch4-Rt-L, Ch5-As-I, Ch6-Rt-L, and Ca20-As-I were grew only in SRS-BA

In the APY ZYM galleries, the results which differentiate the isolates are shown in Table 6. The tests were negative for all the isolates in the remaining enzymes included in the gallery. The Canadian isolate Ca19-As-I and the Chilean Ch8-Rt-K were the only ones positive for the enzyme esterase lipase and esterase, respectively. In addition, the isolate Ch14-As-I gave a positive reaction for β-galactosidase and α-glucosidase while the rest of the isolates were negative.

Genetic characterization

Phylogenetic analysis of the 18 partial (2198 bp) sequences of the 16S rDNA-ITS genes identified two clades (G1 and G2) as shown in the Fig. 3. The Canadian isolates are distinct and belong to the same branch in the phylogenetic tree. The analysis of the genetic relationships of the concatenated HKs is presented in Fig. 4. After several PCR attempts it was not possible to obtain all the expected PCR products for the isolates Ch13-As-I and Ch9-As-na, therefore they were not includes in the genetic analysis.

Comparison of 10 housekeeping sequences from the isolates, included in the MLST scheme, revealed 438 variable nucleotide positions across 11176 nucleotides (nts) (Table 7). The highest percentage of variable nucleotide positions (5.6 %) was seen in the tnpA locus and the lowest (2.4 %) in mltB. The putative amino acid sequence showed variation in 7.2 positions of a total of 2985 amino acids. The highest percentage of variable amino acid positions (4.4 %) was seen in the airA and bax loci; and the lowest (0.0 %) in elfP. In the analysis of the genetic relationships of *P. salmonis*

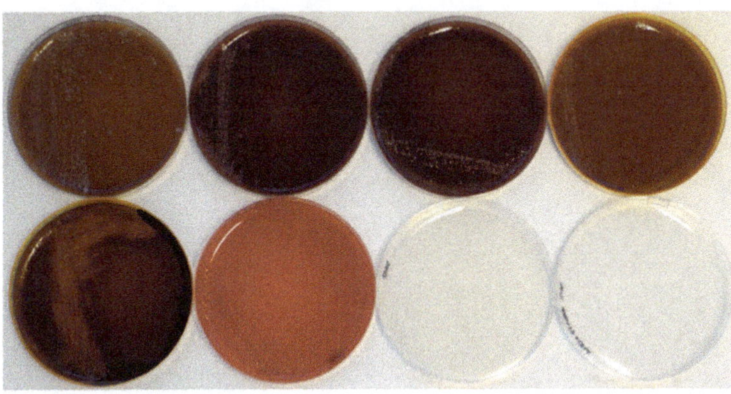

Fig. 2 Isolate Ch14-As-I cultured in eight different growth media: from upper left to the right, SRS-BA, CHAB, CHAB supplemented with ferric nitrate; Austral-TSHem; BA w/2 % NaCl, BA, MA, and FLPA

Table 4 Optimum growth temperature for the *P. salmonis* isolates

Isolate	Optimum growing temp (°C)
LF-89	16–19
Ch2-As-I	16–19
Ch3-Rt-L	16–19
Ch4-Rt-L	16–19
Ch5-As-I	16–19
Ch6-Rt-L	16–19
Ca20-As-K	16–19
Ch7-As-L	19–22
Ch8-Rt-K	19–22
Ch9-As-na	19–22
Ch10-As-I	19–22
Ch11-As-I	19–22
Ch12-As-I	19–22
Ch13-As-I	19–22
Ch14-As-I	19–22
Ch15-As-I	19–22
Ch16-As-I	19–22
Ch17-As-I	19–22
Ch18-As-I	19–22
Ca19-As-K	19–22

isolates, based in the analysis of concatenated HK, it were found two clades with similar grouping shown by the phylogenetic analysis of 16S rDNA-ITS genes. However, a better separation was seen in the clades G1 and G2 (Fig. 4).

The MLST analyses (Fig. 5) resulted in 12 STs based on the different ATs. The Chilean isolates presented 10 STs and the Canadian, two. The MLST analysis reflects the 16S rDNA-ITS phylogeny, arranging the isolates in three groups (Fig. 5).

Discussion

The present study shows the 18 Chilean *P. salmonis* isolates as two genetically distinct groups, a separation supported by all three genotyping methods. Clade G1, containing isolates from Puerto Montt area and two isolates from Chiloe; and clade G2, including isolates retrieved from sites along the East coast of Chiloé Island and Melinka Island (Fig. 1). The present study, which does not included European isolates, clearly shows that the 18 Chilean isolates are genetically distinct from the two Canadian isolates of *P. salmonis* (Figs. 3, 4 and 5). Previous studies have shown genetic variations among Chilean isolates of *P. salmonis* and that Chilean strains are more genetically related to each other than to European and Canadian isolates [19–21]. However, these phylogenetic studies

Table 5 Antibiotic inhibition zones (mm) of the *P. salmonis* isolates

Isolate	Streptomycin	Oxytetracycline	Penicilin	Ceftazidime	Ampicilin	Florfenicol
LF-89	5	23	12	15,5	19,5	24
Ch2-As-I	0,5	0,5	1,5	10	3	14,5
Ch3-Rt-L	3,5	8,5	0,5	0,5	2,5	4
Ch4-Rt-L	2	18	6,5	17,5	14	19
Ch5-As-I	1	17	12	16,5	12,5	19,5
Ch6-Rt-L	0	16,5	13	15,5	13	18
Ch7-As-L	0	10	10	13,5	10,5	14,5
Ch8-Rt-K	1	21	2	13,5	13,5	24,5
Ch9-As-na	2	25	7	16	9,5	24
Ch10-As-I	32,5	27,5	1,5	18,5	22	23,5
Ch11-As-I	1	21	4	5	7,5	19
Ch12-As-I	0,5	17	9,5	12,5	1,5	22
Ch13-As-I	0,5	22	2,5	10	10	25
Ch14-As-I	0	22	9,5	11,5	11,5	24,5
Ch15-As-I	1	20	6	12	9	20,5
Ch16-As-I	0	3,5	6,5	12,5	8	17,5
Ch17-As-I	0,5	24,5	5,5	11	14,5	23
Ch18-As-I	2,5	20	0	10	1,5	15,5
Ca19-As-I	2	17	21,5	22	25	24,5
Ca20-As-I	2,5	24	13	13,5	15	27,5

Table 6 *P. salmonis* differential enzymatic reactions in API ZYM galleries

Isolate	AP	E	EL	LA	VA	CA	AP	NP
LF-89	W	W	W	+	+	W	+	+
Ch2-As-I	W	W	W	+	+	–	W	W
Ch3-Rt-L	W	W	W	+	+	–	W	+
Ch4-Rt-L	W	W	W	+	+	–	W	+
Ch5-As-I	W	W	W	+	+	–	W	W
Ch6-Rt-L	W	W	W	+	+	W	+	+
Ch7-As-L	+	W	W	+	W	W	+	W
Ch8-Rt-K	+	+	W	W	W	–	+	W
Ch9-As-na	+	W	W	+	+	–	+	W
Ch10-As-I	+	W	W	+	+	+	+	+
Ch11-As-I	+	W	W	+	+	–	+	W
Ch12-As-I	+	W	W	+	+	–	+	+
Ch13-As-I	+	W	W	W	W	+	+	W
Ch14-As-I	+	W	W	+	+	–	+	+
Ch15-As-I	+	W	W	+	+	–	+	+
Ch16-As-I	+	W	W	+	+	–	+	W
Ch17-As-I	+	W	W	+	+	–	+	+
Ch18-As-I	+	W	W	+	+	–	+	+
Ca19-As-K	+	W	+	+	+	–	+	+
Ca20-As–K	+	W	W	+	+	–	+	+

W: weak reaction; +: positive reaction; –: negative reaction

have only consisted of five or less Chilean isolates [19, 20], and were therefore not able to have sufficient resolution to separate them in phylogenetic clades.

All three genetic methods used in this study are suitable for separation of *P. salmonis* isolates, and we present the first MLST typing system for *P. salmonis*. However, more isolates from a wider geographical area are needed for mapping of geographical distribution, reservoirs, possible transmission routes, host specificity, and variation in tissue tropism. Other methods, like variable number of tandem repeats (VNTR), giving a better separation of the isolates, are needed for studies of virulence.

The isolates studied were separated in two groups under the optimum growing temperature tests which correlate to a large extent with the results of genotyping. An optimal cultivation temperature at 16–19 °C was seen for isolates includes in clade G1 isolates confirming the findings of Fryer et al. [22]. Whereas, the less fastidious isolates, included in clade G2, had an optimal temperature between at 19–22 °C, which correlates with data presented by Mikalsen et al. [10].

The Canadian isolates differed both in genetic and phenotypic characteristics, as both were isolated from

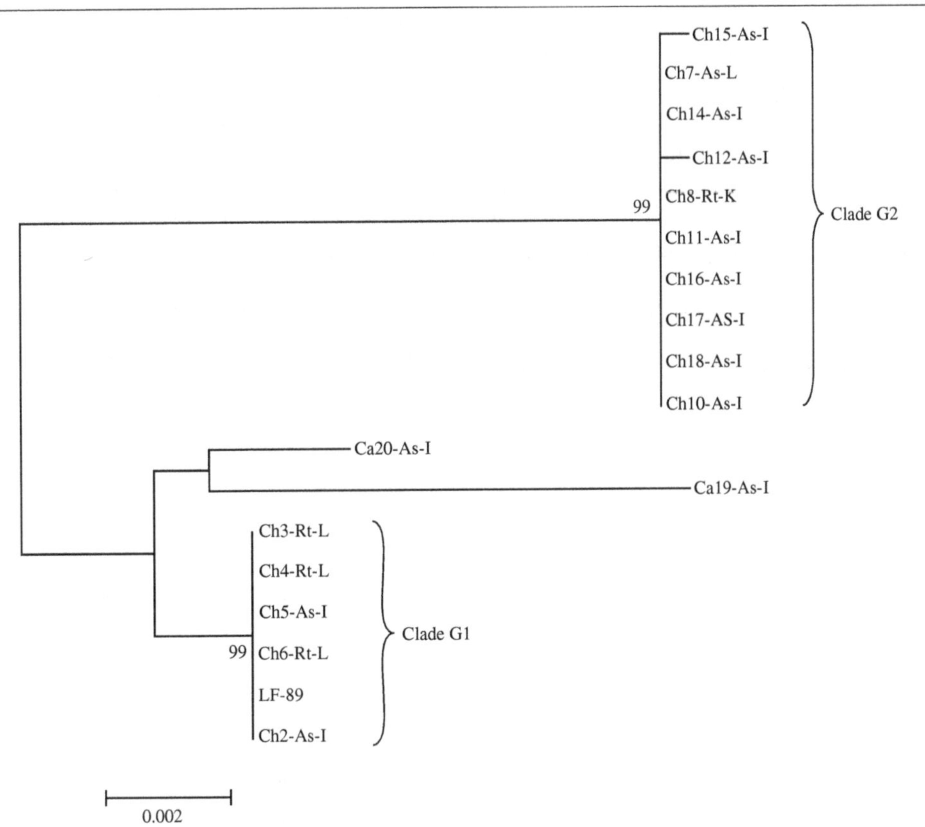

Fig. 3 The phylogenetic relationships of the 18 isolates of *P. salmonis*, based in the analysis of 2198nt within 16S rDNA-ITS genes. The phylogenetic tree was obtained by Mega 6.05 software. The codes for all the isolates are explained in the Table 1

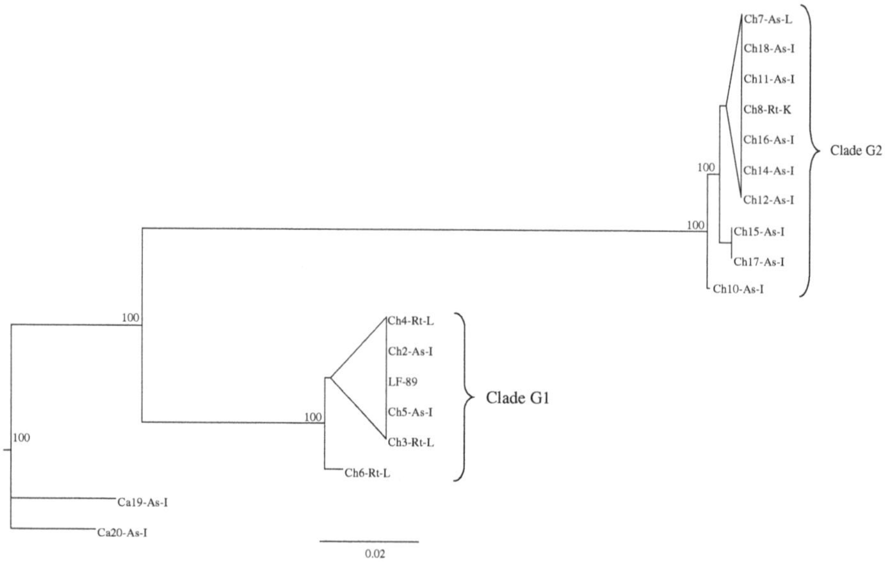

Fig. 4 The genetic relationships of the 18 isolates of *P. salmonis*, based in the analysis of concatenated HK. The phylogenetic three was obtained by the mrBayes software. The codes for all the isolates are explained in the Table 1

the same site during a contemporary outbreak SRS, showing that two different strains of *P. salmonis* can occur during a single outbreak of SRS.

Comparison of the different culture media clearly shows that SRS-BA is the best medium for culturing all the isolates included. Ch14-As-I had the fastest growth and was the only isolate positive for β-galactosidase and α-glucosidase in the API ZYM test. The presences of α-glucosidase and β-galactosidase have also been described to vary for strains of the related intracellular bacterium *Francisella philomiragia* subsp. *philomiragia* [23]. β-galactosidase and α-glucosidase participate in metabolic pathways in Gram negative bacteria [24] and might influence the bacterial growth.

Conclusions

This is the first study showing that there are two genetic groups of *P. salmonis* present in Chile, and that more than one strain of *P. salmonis* can occur under a contemporary outbreak of SRS. The two Canadian isolates were genetically separate when compared to the 18 Chilean isolates, although belong to the same branch. Other isolates should be

Table 7 Overview of the number of variable nucleotide and putative aminoacids positions in the alignment of 16S rDNA, ITS and the ten housekeeping genes of *P. salmonis* included

Gene	N	No. Nucleotides	Variable positions	%	No. Amino acids	Variable positions	%
16S	18	1433	14	1,0	-	-	-
ITS	18	765	34	4,4	-	-	-
dnaK	18	1684	66	3,9	560	3	0,5
groEL	18	1454	73	5,0	484	10	2,1
tbpB	18	1879	95	5,1	626	26	4,2
mltB	18	843	20	2,4	280	5	1,8
ospA	18	364	14	3,8	121	3	2,5
radA	18	906	37	4,1	301	5	1,7
airA	18	407	21	5,2	135	6	4,4
bax	18	612	18	2,9	203	9	4,4
tnpA	18	356	20	5,6	118	5	4,2
elfP	18	473	26	5,5	157	0	0,0
MLST	216	11176	438	4,1	2985	7,2	2,6

Symbols: N: number of *P. salmonis* sequences

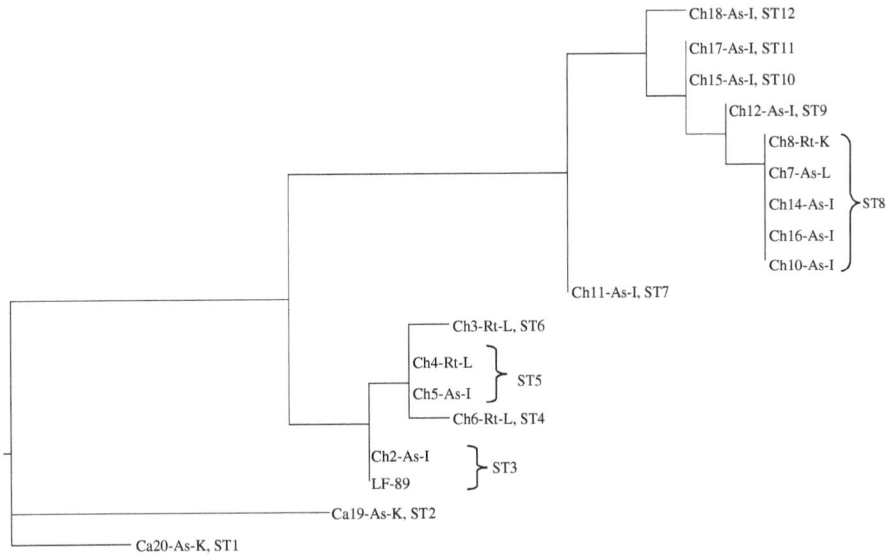

Fig. 5 Dendrogram showing the sequence type relations in the multilocus sequence typing scheme (MLST) of the 18 isolates of *P. salmonis*. The MLST analysis was constructed using 11176nt from the HK dnaK, groEL, trpB, mltB, ospA, radA,alr, bax, tnpA, and elfP. The analysis was performed using the distance method in PAUP 4.0. The codes for all the isolates are explained in the Table 1

included in further genotyping studies on Canadian strains of *P. salmonis*. The genotyping methods used are suitable for separation of the isolates; however, other molecular tools are most likely needed for separating isolates with different virulence. The phenotypic tests showed variation among the isolates, with the temperature test giving the best separation. In future studies the SRS-BA should be the preferred agar for isolation and culturing of *P. salmonis*. Studies of geographical distribution and host specificity will have to include more isolates from different fish hosts in all areas with production of salmonids and presence of *P. salmonis*.

The MLST and the sequences alignments for 16S rRNA-ITS and the concatenated housekeeping genes are made available at the TreeBASE data base (http://purl.org/phylo/treebase/phylows/study/TB2:S18993).

Abbreviations
ANI: average nucleotide identity; DSB: defibrinated sheep blood; HK: housekeeping genes; ITS: internal transcriber space; MA: marine agar; MLST: multi locus of sequence typing; RO: reverse osmosis water; RSS: red sea salt; SRS: salmonid rickettsial septicemia; SRS-BA: salmonid rickettsial septicemia-blood agar; TSA: tryptic soy agar; VNTR: variable number of tandem repeats.

Competing interests
The authors declare that they have no competing interests.

Authors' contributions
AO was the main responsible for the experimental work and data analysis, ØJB identified the HK genes, contributed to the genetic data analysis and writings, DJ performed experimental work, HD coordinated the project, contributed to the experimental design and writings, IS and PF contribute to the experimental design and writings, JM coordinated the project and gave the critical review of the different drafts, PMK contributed with the writing of the manuscript, AN contributed with different parts of the project design and reviewed all the drafts and PA coordinated the laboratory work and was the main responsible for the writing of the manuscript. All authors read and approved the final manuscript.

Acknowledgements
Thanks to the field veterinarians Luis Almonacid, Carlos Bertin and Karin Ruiz (Cermaq Chile), and Kathleen Frisch (Cermaq Canada), for providing detailed description of the clinical findings of SRS in the different host species. This work was financed by a collaboration project between Cermaq Chile, Cermaq Group AS, Norway, and the University of Bergen.

Author details
[1]Fish Diseases Research Group, Department of Biology, University of Bergen, P.O. 7803N-5020 Bergen, Norway. [2]Cermaq Group AS, Dronning Eufemias gate 16, P.O. Box 144 SentrumN-0102 Oslo, Norway. [3]MSD Animal Health, Thormølensgt. 55, 5008 Bergen, Norway. [4]Cermaq Chile, Diego Portales 2000, piso 10, Puerto Montt, Chile. [5]Cermaq Canada, 203 - 919 Island Highway, Campbell River, BC V9W 2C2, Canada.

References
1. Portnoy DS, Hollenbeck CM, Vidal RR, Gold JR. A comparison of neutral and immune genetic variation in Atlantic salmon, *Salmo salar* L. in Chilean aquaculture facilities. PLoS ONE. 2014;9(6):e99358.
2. Sernapesca. Report of the use of antimicrobials in the national salmoniculture. National Service of Fisheries, Subdivision of Aquaculture, Animal Health Unit. Chile; 2015. (In Spanish).
3. Fryer JL, Hedrick RP. *Piscirickettsia salmonis*: a Gram-negative intracellular bacterial pathogen of fish. J Fish Dis. 2003;26(5):251–62.
4. Rozas M, Enríquez R. Piscirickettsiosis and *Piscirickettsia salmonis* in fish: a review. J Fish Dis. 2014;37(3):163–88.
5. Kuzyk MA, Burian J, Machander D, Dolhaine D, Cameron S, Thornton JC, Kay WW. An efficacious recombinant subunit vaccine against the salmonid rickettsial pathogen *Piscirickettsia salmonis*. Vaccine. 2001;19(17–19):2337–44.
6. Wilhelm V, Huaracan B, Martínez R, Rosemblatt M, Burzio LO, Valenzuela PDT. Cloning and expression of the coding regions of the heat shock roteins HSP10 and HSP16 from *Piscirickettsia salmonis*. Biol Res. 2003;36(3–4): 421_8.

7. Tobar JA, Jeréz S, Caruffo M, Bravo C, Contreras F, Bucarey SA, Harel M. Oral vaccination of Atlantic salmon (*Salmo salar*) against salmonid rickettsial septicaemia. Vaccine. 2011;29(12):2336–40.
8. Fryer JL, Lannan CN, Giovannoni SJ, Wood ND. *Piscirickettsia salmonis* gen. nov., sp. nov., the causative agent of an epizootic disease in salmonid fishes. Int J System Bacteriol. 1992;42(1):120–6.
9. Mauel MJ, Ware C, Smith PA. Culture of *Piscirickettsia salmonis* on enriched blood agar. J Vet Diag Inv. 2008;20(2):213–4.
10. Mikalsen J, Skjaervik O, Wiik-Nielsen J, Wasmuth MA, Colquhoun DJ. Agar culture of *Piscirickettsia salmonis*, a serious pathogen of farmed salmonid and marine fish. Fems Microbiol Letters. 2008;278(1):43–7.
11. Yañez AJ, Silva H, Valenzuela K, Pontigo JP, Godoy M, Troncoso J, Romero A, Figueroa J, Cárcamo JG, Avendaño-Herrera R. Two novel blood-free solid media for the culture of the salmonid pathogen *Piscirickettsia salmonis*. J Fish Dis. 2013;36(6):587–91.
12. Cepeda C, García-Márquez S, Santos Y. Improved growth of *Flavobacterium psychrophilum* using a new culture medium. Aquaculture. 2004;238(1–4):75–82.
13. Justesen US, Acar Z, Olsson K, Jensen TG, Kerrn MB, Skov RL, Gahrn-Hansen B. Comparison of Rosco Neo-Sensitabs with Oxoid paper disks in EUCAST disk diffusion antimicrobial susceptibility testing on Mueller-Hinton agar. Eur J Clin Microbiol Infect Dis. 2013;32(5):621–5.
14. Apablaza P, Loland AD, Brevik OJ, Ilardi P, Battaglia J, Nylund A. Genetic variation among *Flavobacterium psychrophilum* isolates from wild and farmed salmonids in Norway and Chile. J Appl Microbiol. 2013;114(4):934–46.
15. Tamura K, Stecher G, Peterson D, Filipski A, Kumar S. MEGA6: Molecular evolutionary genetics analysis version 6.0. Mol Biol Evol. 2013;30:2725–9.
16. Hasegawa M, Kishino H, Yano T. Dating the human-ape split by a molecular clock of mitochondrial DNA. J Mol Evol. 1985;22:160–74.
17. Tanabe AS. Kakusan4 and Aminosan. two programs for comparing nonpartitioned, proportional and separate models for combined molecular phylogenetic analyses of multilocus sequence data. Mol Ecol Res. 2011;11(5): 914–21.
18. Drummond AJ, Suchard MA, Xie D, Rambaut A. Bayesian phylogenetics with BEAUti and the BEAST 1.7. Mol Biol Evol. 2012;29(8):1969–73.
19. Reid HI, Griffen AA, Birkbeck TH. Isolates of *Piscirickettsia salmonis* from Scotland and Ireland show evidence of clonal diversity. Appl Env Microbiol. 2004;70(7):4393–7.
20. Mauel MJ, Giovannoni SJ, Fryer JL. Phylogenetic analysis of *Piscirickettsia salmonis* by 16S, internal transcribed spacer (ITS) and 23S ribosomal DNA sequencing. Dis Aquatic Org. 1999;35(2):115–23.
21. Heath S, Pak S, Marshall S, Prager EM, Orrego C. Monitoring *Piscirickettsia salmonis* by denaturant gel electrophoresis and competitive PCR. Dis Aquatic Org. 2000;41(1):19–29.
22. Fryer JL, Lannan CN, Garces LH, Larenas JJ, Smith PA. Isolation of a rickettsiales-like organism from diseased coho salmon (*Oncorhynchus kisutch*) in Chile. Fish Pathol. 1990;25(2):107–14.
23. Ottem KF, Nylund A, Karlsbakk E, Friis-Moller A, Kamaishi T. Elevation of *Francisella philomiragia* subsp *noatunensis* Mikalsen et al. (2007) to *Francisella noatunensis* comb. nov. [syn. *Francisella piscicida* Ottem et al. (2008) syn. nov.] and characterization of *Francisella noatunensis* subsp. *orientalis* subsp. nov., two important fish pathogens. J Applied Microbiol. 2009;106(4):1231–43.
24. Juers DH, Heightman TD, Vasella A, McCarter JD, Mackenzie L, Withers SG, Matthews BW. A structural view of the action of *Escherichia coli* (lacZ) beta-galactosidase. Biochemistry. 2001;40(49):14781–94.
25. Giovannoni SJ, Rappe MS, Vergin KL, Adair NL. 16S rRNA genes reveal stratified open ocean bacterioplankton populations related to the Green Non-Sulfur bacteria. Proc Natl Acad Sci U S A. 1996;93(15):7979–84.

15

Evaluation of biomarker canine-prostate specific arginine esterase (CPSE) for the diagnosis of benign prostatic hyperplasia

Dora Pinheiro[1], João Machado[2], Carlos Viegas[3,4], Cláudia Baptista[5], Estela Bastos[6], Joana Magalhães[7], Maria A. Pires[3,8], Luís Cardoso[2,3] and Ana Martins-Bessa[2,3*]

Abstract

Background: Benign prostatic hyperplasia (BPH) is the most common canine prostatic disorder. Although most or even all intact male dogs may develop BPH by 5–8 years of age, many show no clinical signs. Taking into account the non-specific character of clinical and ultrasonographic findings, a new diagnostic approach has recently been proposed based on the augmentation of blood canine prostate-specific arginine esterase (CPSE) in hyperplasic dogs. The aim of the present study was to verify CPSE levels in negative controls and hyperplasic dogs, considering cytological findings as the reference method and taking into account the fact that controls were middle-aged intact dogs (median of 5.0 years), contrarily to previous studies carried out with very young control dogs.

Results: Significant differences of median CPSE levels were found between controls and hyperplasic dogs (29.1 versus 160.7 ng/mL, respectively); and significant positive correlations were found between median CPSE levels and age or prostatic volume ($r = 0.549$ and 0.448, respectively; $p < 0.001$). Sensitivity, specificity, positive and negative likelihood ratios put into evidence the good performance of the test. The agreement between methods was found to be very high, notably between CPSE levels and cytological results (Cohen's kappa coefficients above 0.8).

Conclusions: Considering the results all together, measurement of CPSE is confirmed as a useful and accurate method and should be considered as an alternative or complementary tool to conventional methods for the diagnosis of BPH in middle-aged dogs.

Keywords: Prostate, Benign prostate hyperplasia, BPH, Canine prostate-specific arginine esterase, CPSE, Biomarker

Background

Diseases of the prostate are common in middle-aged to older intact dogs. The canine prostate can be affected by benign prostatic hyperplasia (BPH), squamous metaplasia, cysts, inflammation and neoplasia. BPH, the most common prostatic disorder, is a spontaneous disease of intact male dogs that begins as glandular hyperplasia as early as 2 years of age [1]. Dihydrotestosterone is accepted as a key hormone in the pathogenesis of the disease, stimulating enlargement of the prostate by enhancing growth of both the stromal and glandular components [2]. Oestrogens, in particular the ratio of 17β-oestradiol/testosterone, are also involved in the development of BPH, as is potentially prolactin [3] and also other mitogenic growth factors [4, 5].

When present, clinical signs of BPH include serosanguinous urethral discharge not associated with urination [6], hemospermia and hematuria, tenesmus, poor semen quality and infertility, and prostatomegaly [7], as well as constipation and dysuria [3]. The diagnosis of BPH is usually based on history, physical and/or andrologic exam and abdominal ultrasonography; and seldom on cytology by fine needle-aspiration (FNA). Palpation usually reveals a symmetrically enlarged and non-painful prostate. The presence of prostatomegaly confirmed by ultrasonography (with a heterogeneous or hyperechoic parenchyma with or without fluid-filled cysts) is frequently

* Correspondence: abessa@utad.pt
[2]Veterinary Teaching Hospital, UTAD, Vila Real, Portugal
[3]Department of Veterinary Sciences, School of Agrarian and Veterinary Sciences, UTAD, Vila Real, Portugal
Full list of author information is available at the end of the article

sufficient to reach a conclusive diagnosis of BPH [7]. However, BPH can be difficult to differentiate from other prostatic diseases, including squamous metaplasia, prostatitis, prostatic cysts and abscesses, and prostatic neoplasia, due to the similarity of clinical and ultrasonographic findings. Under these circumstances, other methods should be used, i.e., cytology or biopsy, and more recently the seric quantification of canine prostate-specific arginine esterase (CPSE) [8].

CPSE, a serine protease similar to the human prostate-specific antigen ("PSA"), is the most important specific androgen-dependent protein of prostatic secretion in dog and a remarkable marker of androgenic stimulation [9, 10]. Serum CPSE concentrations, as determined by immunoprecipitation, were found to be significantly elevated in dogs with BPH compared to normal dogs [11]. CPSE determination by enzyme-linked immunosorbent assay (ELISA) is currently an interesting method for BPH diagnosis, especially indicated to early detect dogs with a subclinical pathological condition, and opens new perspectives to the follow-up of medical treatment [8]. However, there is scarce information on CPSE levels in middle-aged healthy dogs. In such animals, the determination of CPSE concentration is a feasible procedure that can be of high importance for early BPH diagnosis.

The aims of the present study were: a) to compare CPSE levels in dogs with BPH (study group) and without BPH (control group); and b) to compare clinical, ultrasonographic and CPSE performances in the diagnosis of BPH, considering the cytological marks as the reference method for this study.

Methods

Clinical, ultrasonographic and cytological evaluations

All the dogs ($n = 60$) were evaluated only after an informed consent obtained from their owners. Each dog underwent clinical examination including a thorough history, physical and digital rectal examination (DRE) of the prostate, ultrasonography and cytological evaluation. Clinical manifestations compatible with BPH or cystic prostatic hyperplasia (CPH) comprised constipation, ribbon-like stools, hemorrhagic urethral discharge and/or intermittent hematuria, weight loss, rear limbs pain and abnormal DRE, such as palpable prostatomegaly and painful or abnormal prostate such as nodularity, indurations or asymmetry [12]. Prostatitis was suspected when clinical signs were more severe than BPH, as caudal abdominal or pelvic pain, and a diffuse to asymmetrical enlargement and/or prostatic pain was noted at DRE [13].

Additional procedures carried out comprised prostatic ultrasonography, prostatic massage or prostatic FNA for cytological evaluation (Figs. 1 and 2). Transabdominal ultrasonography of the prostate was performed with a Philips HD3 Ultrasound system (Philips Healthcare, USA), using a sectorial 3.0-7.0 MHz and linear 5.0-9.0 MHz transducers. The ultrasonographic examination enabled the evaluation of the prostate size, namely length (L) and height in the longitudinal plan (HL), and height (HT) and width (W) in the transverse one, plus shape, position, internal echogenicity and margins. The values for L, HL/HT and W were the average of three consecutive measurements. Prostatic volume (PV) was determined by the formula PV (cm^3) = $0.487 \times L \times W \times (HL \times HT/2) + 6.38$; and the expected volume (EV) was determined by the formula EV (cm^3) = $8.48 + [0.238 \times$ body weight (kg)$]$ [14]. All variations of the normal ultrasonographic aspect were recorded (i.e., asymmetric

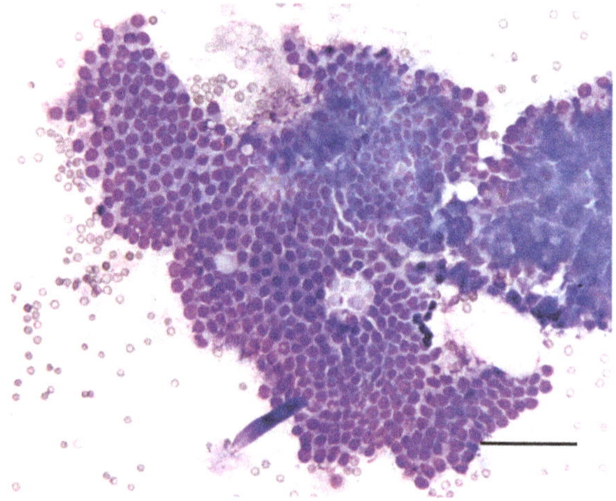

Fig. 1 Fine needle-aspirate from a prostate with benign hyperplasia (group A dog). Cells are arranged in clusters and show a uniform morphology with round nucleus and basophilic cytoplasm (Diff-quick staining; bar = 500 μm)

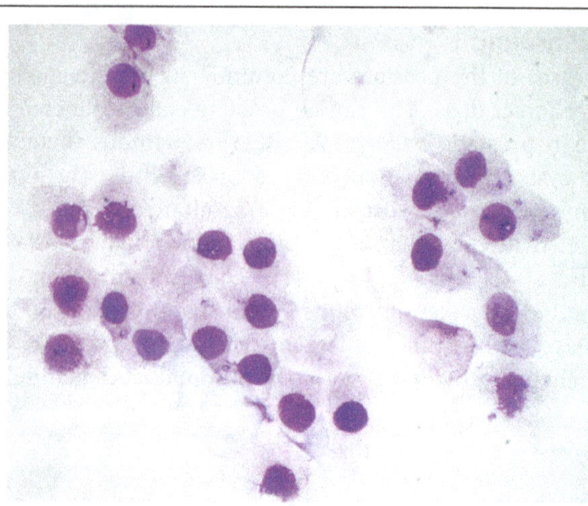

Fig. 2 Fine needle-aspirate from a normal prostate (group C dog). Cells are arranged in small clusters with a uniform morphology, showing round nucleus and clear cytoplasm (Diff-quick staining; ×600 magnification)

shape, size, and aspect of focal or multifocal variations of echogenicity; size and echogenicity of retention cysts or areas of cavitation; and irregular margins). Abnormal records of ultrasonography included BPH-suggestive, cystic prostatic hyperplasia (CPH)-suggestive and prostatitis-suggestive ultrasonograms. Ultrasonographic findings were subdivided into simple BPH, CPH and prostatitis. Findings compatible with BPH included symmetrical prostatic enlargement and diffusely hyperechoic parenchyma, whereas CPH showed hyperechoic parenchyma background with cavitary lesions of varying architecture and distal acoustic enhancement. Prostatitis was suspected when ultrasonographic findings were more pronounced than BPH, being the prostate variably hyperechoic with a more complex contour [13].

For cytology, samples were collected by ultrasound-guided transabdominal FNA, as previously described [6] or by prostatic massage, namely when ultrasonography suggested prostatitis [15]. The cells were then smeared on a slide, air-dried, stained with Diff-Quick and mounted with Entellan™ (Merck Millipore, USA). The presence of uniform sheets or clusters of prostatic cells with middle anysokaryosis and increased size with round and small nucleus, with a basophilic, moderate cytoplasm are the cytological criteria to determine the presence of BPH [16]. These clusters could be in a high quantity but their cells appeared as normal epithelial prostatic ones. The cytology of prostatitis is determined by the presence of a large number of neutrophils associated with a variable numbers of macrophages (more common in chronic prostatitis). Bacteria could be present, both freely or intracytoplasmatically (i.e., inside neutrophils and macrophages). Finally, squamous metaplasia is determined by the presence of prostatic cells with squamous epithelial characteristics such as large and clear to basophilic cytoplasm with small dense nucleus [16].

Groups of animals

Based on cytological results, two groups of adult intact male dogs were formed, i.e., a study group (A; Table 1; Additional file 1) and a control group (C; Table 2; Additional file 2).

Group A included eight mongrels and 21 other dogs from 13 defined breeds, i.e., Labrador Retriever ($n = 4$), Boxer ($n = 3$), Estrela Mountain Dog ($n = 3$), Golden Retriever ($n = 2$), Beagle ($n = 1$), Brittany ($n = 1$), Chow-Chow ($n = 1$), Cocker Spaniel ($n = 1$), Dalmatian ($n = 1$), Pekingese ($n = 1$), Portuguese Sheepdog ($n = 1$), Rottweiler ($n = 1$) and Siberian Husky ($n = 1$). Weight ranged from 8 to 59 kg, with a median of 30.0 kg (interquartile range [IQR]: 23.0-35.2). Age ranged from 5 to 15 years, with a median of 9.0 years (IQR: 7–11.5).

Group C included eight mongrels and 23 other dogs from 15 defined breeds, i.e., Beagle ($n = 5$), Brittany ($n =$ 2), German Shepherd ($n = 2$), Golden Retriever ($n = 2$), Cocker Spaniel ($n = 1$), Drever ($n = 1$), Estrela Mountain Dog ($n = 1$), French Bulldog ($n = 1$), German Spitz Klein ($n = 1$), German Spitz Mittel ($n = 1$), Labrador Retriever ($n = 1$), Miniature Pinscher ($n = 1$), Portuguese Pointer ($n = 1$), Portuguese Water Dog ($n = 1$), St. Bernard ($n =$ 1) and Transmontano Mastiff ($n = 1$). Weight ranged from 4 to 70 kg, with a median of 19.0 kg (IQR: 13.0-33.0). Age ranged from 1 to 12 years, with a median of 5.0 years (IQR: 2.0-7.0).

Table 1 Records from clinical examination, ultrasonography and cytology in 29 dogs (group A) diagnosed with benign prostatic hyperplasia (BPH) by cytological examination of prostatic aspirates

Clinical examination		Ultrasonography-suggested condition		Cytology (BPH+)	Dogs (n)
Physical signs	DRE	BPH	CPH	Prostatitis	
Absent	Normal	No	No	Yes	1
	Abnormal	No	Yes	No	2
				Yes	1
		Yes	No	No	3
Present	Normal	No	Yes	No	3
				Yes	2
		Yes	No	No	1
	Abnormal	Yes	No	No	5
		No	Yes	No	7
				Yes	4

CPH cystic prostatic hyperplasia, *DRE* digital rectal examination

Canine prostate-specific arginine esterase (CPSE)

Blood was collected from all the dogs, left to clot for 4 h at room temperature and the collected serum kept frozen at −25 °C until use. In order to measure plasma CPSE concentrations, an enzyme-linked immunosorbent assay (ELISA) was used strictly following the manufacturer's instructions (Odelis® CPSE, Virbac, France). Briefly, dilutions of the ELISA stock solution were done to obtain the different calibrator solutions (20, 10, 5.0, 2.5 and 0.0 ng/ml) and to define the standard curve. All the plasma samples were diluted at 1:10 and incubated at 37 °C for 1 h before being assayed. The horseradish peroxidase conjugate were placed into each well after washing cycle and incubated again at 37 °C for 1 h. After another washing cycle, tetramethylbenzidine was added for 10 min and the reaction then stopped. The optical density ("OD") of each sample was read at 450 nm and CPSE plasma concentrations calculated based on the standard curve plotted with calibrator concentrations. A CPSE value of 61 ng/ml was set as the cut-off for BPH (i.e., values equal to or greater that the cut-off were regarded as positive), according to the manufacturer's instructions.

Table 2 Records from clinical examination, ultrasonography and cytology in 31 dogs (group C) without benign prostatic hyperplasia (BPH) as determined by cytological examination of prostatic aspirates

Clinical examination		Ultrasonography-suggested condition			Cytology (BPH⁻)		Dogs (n)
Physical signs	DRE	BPH	CPH	Prostatitis	Prostatitis	Metaplasia	
Absent	Normal	No	No	No	No	No	23
					Yes	No	2
	Abnormal	No	Yes	No	Yes	No	1
Present	Normal	No	No	No	No	No	1
				Yes	Yes	No	1
	Abnormal	No	Yes	No	No	Yes	1
					Yes	Yes	1
		Yes	No	No	Yes	No	1

CPH cystic prostatic hyperplasia, *DRE* digital rectal examination

Data analysis

The agreement beyond chance between binomial results (i.e., positive or negative) of CPSE and those of the clinical, ultrasonographic and cytological evaluations for BPH was measured with Cohen's kappa coefficient (k). Sensitivity (true positive [TP]/TP + false negative), specificity (true negative [TN]/TN + false positive), positive likelihood ratio (sensitivity/1 − specificity) and negative likelihood ratio (1 − sensitivity/specificity) were calculated for CPSE binomial results taking cytology as the reference method. Exact binomial 95% confidence intervals (CI) were established for proportions. Differences in the CPSE levels between groups A and C were assessed by means of the Mann-Whitney U test. The association between CPSE levels and other quantitative variables (i.e., age, PV and EV) was measured by Spearman's rank correlation coefficient r [17]. Analyses were performed with SPSS 21.0 software for Windows, with a p value < 0.05 as statistically significant.

Results

CPSE levels between groups

The levels of CPSE (Fig. 3) were significantly different ($p < 0.001$) between group A (median: 160.7 ng/ml; IQR: 80.8–220.5) and group C (median: 29.1 ng/ml; IQR: 19.3–45.5). Significant ($p < 0.001$) correlations were found between age and CPSE level ($r = 0.549$) and CPSE and PV ($r = 0.448$); but not between CPSE and EV ($r = 0.193$; $p = 0.139$).

Clinical, ultrasonographic and cytological records

In Group A (study group), all 29 dogs evidenced BPH confirmed by cytology; moreover, eight (of these) dogs showed prostatitis concomitant with BPH (proved by the presence of a large number of neutrophils and associated macrophages, and variable amounts of uniform clusters of prostatic cells with middle anysokaryosis and increased size, round and small nucleus, with a clear or moderately basophilic cytoplasm, a characteristic of prostatitis with BPH). In Group C (control group; 31 dogs without BPH proved by cytology), six dogs had prostatitis and two other had squamous metaplasia (presence of large epithelial prostatic cells with a clear to basophilic cytoplasm, and a small dense nucleus similar to that of keratinocytes).

Comparison between CPSE levels, clinical, ultrasonographic and cytological evaluations

The k values from comparisons between binomial CPSE levels and clinic evaluation, ultrasonography and cytology were 0.83, 0.83 and 0.87, respectively (Table 3). A k value above 0.80 represents an almost perfect agreement beyond chance.

Three out of the 31 dogs of group C had a positive CPSE result. Two of those three dogs had prostatitis and CPSE values of 174.0 and 183.0 ng/ml; the other animal

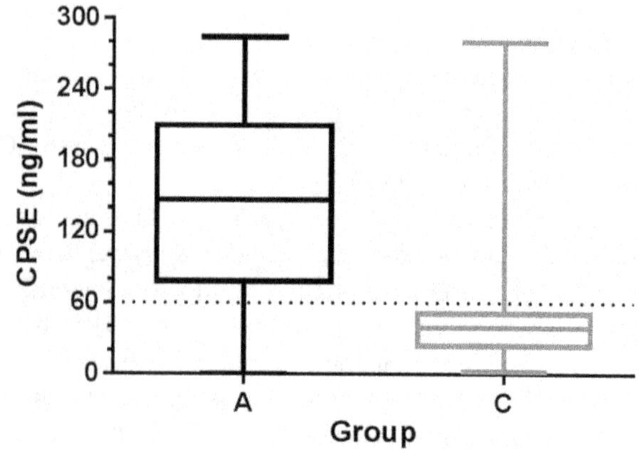

Fig. 3 Canine prostate-specific arginine esterase (CPSE) levels in 29 dogs (group A) with benign prostatic hyperplasia (BPH), as diagnosed by cytology; and in 31 dogs (group C) without BPH ($p < 0.001$). The *dotted line* represents the cut-off value for CPSE (i.e., values ≥ 61 ng/ml were regarded as a positive result)

Table 3 Comparison between the binomial results of canine prostate-specific arginine esterase (CPSE; a value ≥ 61 ng/ml was regarded as positive) and those of clinical evaluation, ultrasonography and cytology for the diagnosis of benign prostatic hyperplasia (BPH) in dogs

CPSE[a, b, c]	Clinical evaluation[a]		Ultrasonography[b]		Cytology[c]	
	+ve	−ve	+ve	−ve	+ve	−ve
+ve	30	1	29	2	28	3
−ve	4	25	3	26	1	28
Total	34	26	32	28	29	31

[a]: $k = 0.83$; [b]: $k = 0.83$; [c]: $k = 0.87$; +ve: positive; −ve: negative

had squamous metaplasia and a CPSE value of 147.0 ng/ml.

One dog of group A had a CPSE level of 45.2 ng/ml. Sensitivity of the CPSE binomial results (positive or negative) was 96.6% (95% CI: 82.2–99.4), specificity 90.3% (95% CI: 74.2–97.9), positive likelihood ratio 10.0 (95% CI: 3.4–29.3) and negative likelihood ratio 0.04 (95% CI: 0.01–0.26). A positive likelihood ratio of 10.0 reveals a moderate to large and often conclusive increase in the likelihood of BPH if the CPSE result is positive. On the other side, a negative likelihood ratio of 0.04 stands for a large and often conclusive decrease in the likelihood of BPH if the CPSE result is negative.

Discussion

Prostatic diseases are frequent age-related conditions in intact dogs. The importance of applying a systematic diagnostic protocol that allows an accurate identification of prostatic disorders should be emphasized, as this provides the chance of an early control of the disorder without development of chronic disease, which is hard to manage and causes deterioration of fertility [18].

Several diagnostic methods can be used to evaluate the prostate, from physical examination (i.e., DRE) to ultrasonography, assessment of ejaculate's third fraction, prostatic massage, prostatic FNA and biopsy [19]. Data obtained from clinical examination are important as starting points for further evaluation of the prostate. Nevertheless, clinical signs of prostatic disease can be transitory and unspecific, precluding a desirably early and conclusive diagnosis. Assessment of the ejaculate's third fraction could have been an adequate criterion to evaluate prostatic disease. However, taking into account that males included in the study were not breed dogs, semen collection was not attempted. Prostatic ultrasonography is an excellent method in the evaluation of the position, size, contours, and parenchymal echogenicity, as well as in the evaluation of the prostatic urethra. Jointly, clinical evaluation of the prostate and ultrasonography could allow a presumptive diagnosis of the prostatic condition in a reasonable number of cases, but sensitivity would not be optimal (i.e., the ability of detecting all the positive cases). Other methods should then be carried out, such as the prostatic massage and/or the invasive FNA and biopsy [15]. Ultrasound-guided transabdominal FNA was used in this study as the preferred method to obtain prostatic tissue and fluid, and then as the gold standard to which the other methods were compared, considering the very high agreement between FNA and histopathological diagnosis [20] and also the availability of this technique. Besides, the thin monolayer obtained with cytological smears often allows better assessment of individual cytomorphology, as well as improved detection of etiologic agents [21]. Prostatic biopsy is only considered in cases where less invasive diagnostic tests do not render a conclusive diagnosis [6, 19].

Under the above-mentioned circumstances, when it comes to obtain an accurate diagnosis prior to initiating a treatment, several tests can be carried out, taking always into account the benefits, costs and risks of each procedure. Also considering the fact that there is still room for improvement, novel molecular tools have been proposed to early detect prostatic diseases such as the CPSE ELISA kit, which allows determination of CPSE levels in an expeditious manner. In the present study, CPSE levels were determined after the formation of two defined groups, i.e., a study and a control, in which animals were cytologically confirmed as having BPH or not having-BPH, respectively. CPSE serum values were significantly higher in BPH than in non-BPH dogs, which indicate an increased production and secretion of this marker by prostatic epithelial cells in animals with BPH, and further confirm the diagnostic value of the test. Furthermore, seven dogs in group A (BPH positive) had at least one clinical sign but no changes at DRE, while seven other showed no clinical signs. Considering that these dogs were older than 5 years old, the present study highlights the importance of systematic CPSE quantification in middle-aged dogs even when apparently healthy. An early BPH diagnosis in these dogs is always desirable considering the impact of the disorder in fertility [22]. CPSE determination is furthermore useful when ultrasonography is not available or for diagnosis in large and obese dogs in which DRE could be impossible, and also of great utility in the follow-up of BPH medical treatment. CPSE determination does not preclude the attainment of other complementary tests used to exclude the coexistence of other prostatic diseases, such as prostatitis, squamous metaplasia or neoplasia, which are especially recommended when clinical examination and/or ultrasonography are suggestive of disorders other than BPH.

CPSE levels were moderately correlated with prostatic volume (PV), which could be explained by the elevated secretion of CPSE in enlarged hyperplasic prostates. There was no correlation between CPSE and the expected volume (EV) of the prostate, as the latter adjusts prostate size to the weight of dogs. Another important finding is the fact that, although there were significant differences between median weights of the dogs in the two groups, no statistically significant correlation was detected between weight and CPSE levels, a fact which indicates reliability of the test for large breeds.

In group A (study), seven out of 29 dogs with BPH – i.e., with high CPSE values – also presented prostatitis. The association of various prostatic disorders is not uncommon; in fact, diseased prostate glands are commonly affected by multiple and even co-existing pathological conditions [18]. CPH could predispose prostate to inflammation by providing a favorable medium for bacterial growth or by interference with normal defense mechanisms [4]. The hypothesis that inflammation emerges as the major contributor for the development of BPH has been suggested in men [23]. On the other hand, in group C (control), six out of 31 dogs presented prostatitis, with two of them showing CPSE increased values, which could indicate the need of following up these animals. Previous studies have found no difference between serum concentrations of CPSE in dogs with BPH and in those with bacterial prostatitis and carcinoma, which was attributed to the existence of concurrent BPH [11]. However, the method for CPSE determination was different from the current one. In the present study, this could be excluded considering that cytological analysis ruled out BPH in group C. The remaining dogs of group C with prostatitis showed low CPSE values, like the dogs without BPH in the same group. Further studies with large numbers of dogs should contribute to clarify these findings.

Conclusions

Results of the present study revealed a very high agreement (i.e., almost perfect) between CPSE test and other diagnostic tools for BPH diagnosis. Previous studies have suggested cytological evaluation as one of the methods with higher accuracy in the diagnosis of prostatic diseases [20], which was also observed in the present study, with the highest agreement found between the CPSE test and cytological diagnosis. The CPSE test can very accurately differentiate between dogs with and without BPH and may be considered as an alternative or complementary tool to conventional methods for BPH diagnosis. Finally, its systematic use can increase the likelihood of early diagnosing BPH in apparently healthy middle-aged dogs.

Additional files

Additional file 1: ("Group A_Hyperplasic dogs"): signalment, clinical diagnosis, ultrasonographic features, cytological diagnosis, prostatic dimensions and CPSE levels in 29 dogs with BPH as determined by cytology.

Additional file 2: ("Group C_Control Dogs"): signalment, clinical diagnosis, ultrasonographic features, cytological diagnosis, prostatic dimensions and CPSE levels in 31 dogs without evidence of BPH by cytology.

Abbreviations

BPH: Benign prostatic hyperplasia; CI: Confidence interval; CPH: Cystic prostatic hyperplasia; CPSE: Canine prostate-specific arginine esterase; ELISA: Enzyme-linked immunosorbent assay; EV: Expected volume; FNA: Fine needle-aspiration; IQR: Interquartile range; PV: Prostatic volume; RDE: Rectal digital examination

Acknowledgements

The authors would like to gratefully acknowledge Virbac (Portugal and France), for providing Odelis®-CPSE ELISA kit, and also to the Veterinary Teaching Hospital (Hospital Veterinário), UTAD, Vila Real, Portugal, and Hospital Referência Veterinária Montenegro, Porto, Portugal, for providing clinical cases. Prof. Augusto Matos (ICBAS, U. Porto, Portugal), is acknowledged for his help with case sampling.

Funding

The Portuguese Foundation for Science and Technology (FCT) sponsored this work under the Project PEst-OE/AGR/UI0772/2011.

Authors' contributions

Study design: DP and AM-B; clinical evaluation and sample collection: DP, JM, CV, CB and AM-B; laboratory work: JM, EB and MAP; data analysis: LC; writing of the manuscript: DP, LC and AM-B. All the authors revised and approved the final version of the manuscript.

Competing interests

The authors declare that they have no competing interests.

Consent for publication

Not applicable.

Author details

[1]University of Trás-os-Montes e Alto-Douro (UTAD), Vila Real, Portugal. [2]Veterinary Teaching Hospital, UTAD, Vila Real, Portugal. [3]Department of Veterinary Sciences, School of Agrarian and Veterinary Sciences, UTAD, Vila Real, Portugal. [4]Centre for the Research and Technology of Agro-Environmental and Biological Sciences (CITAB), UTAD, Vila Real, Portugal. [5]Department of Veterinary Clinics, UPVet, Instituto de Ciências Biomédicas Abel Salazar, Universidade do Porto, Oporto, Portugal. [6]Department of Genetics and Biotechnology, School of Life and Environment Sciences, UTAD, Vila Real, Portugal. [7]UCIBIO, REQUIMTE, Department of Chemical Sciences, Faculdade de Farmácia, Universidade do Porto, Oporto, Portugal. [8]Animal and Veterinary Research Centre (CECAV), UTAD, Vila Real, Portugal.

References

1. Berry SJ, Strandberg JD, Saunders WJ, Coffey DS. Development of canine benign prostatic hyperplasia with age. Prostate. 1986;9:363–73.
2. Johnston SD, Root MVK, Olson PNS. Disorders of the canine prostate. In: Johnston SD, Root Kustritz MV, Olson PNS, editors. Canine and Feline Theriogenology. Philadelphia: WB Saunders; 2001. p. 337–55.
3. Wolf K, Kayacelebi H, Urhausen C, Piechotta M, Mischk R, Kramer S, Einspanier A, Oei CHY, Gunzel-Apel A. Testicular steroids, prolactin, relaxin

and prostate gland markers in peripheral blood and seminal plasma of normal dogs and dogs with prostatic hyperplasia. Reprod Dom Anim. 2012; 47 Suppl 6:243–6.

4. Parry NMA. The canine prostate gland: Part 1. Non-inflammatory diseases. UK Vet. 2007;12:1–5.
5. Krakowski L, Wachockaa A, Brodzkia P, Wronaa Z, Piecha T, Wawrona W, Chałabis-Mazurek A. Sperm quality and selected biochemical parameters of seminal fluid in dogs with benign prostatic hyperplasia. Animal Reprod Sci. 2015;160:120–5.
6. Kustritz MVR. Collection of tissue and culture samples from the canine reproductive tract. Theriogenology. 2006;66:567–74.
7. Romagnoli S, 2007. The canine prostate: what it does and why does it grow so much. Proceedings of the Southern European Veterinary Conference, Barcelona, Spain, October 2007. SEVC and AVEPA (eds), 3 pp.
8. Lévy X, Nizanski W, von Heimendahl A, Mimouni P. Diagnosis of common prostatic conditions in dogs: an update. Reprod Dom Anim. 2014;49 Suppl 2:50–7.
9. Chapdelaine P, Dubé Y, Frenette G, Tremblay RR. Identification of arginine esterase as the major androgen dependent protein secreted by dog prostate and preliminary molecular characterization in seminal plasma. J Androl. 1984;5:206–10.
10. Frenette G, Dubé JY, Lacoste D, Tremblay RR. Radioimmunoassay in blood plasma of arginine esterase: the major secretory product of dog prostate. Prostate. 1987;10:145–52.
11. Bell FW, Klausner JS, Hayden DW, Lund EM, Liebenstein BB, Feeney DA, Johnston SD, Shivers JL, Ewing CM, Isaacs WB. Evaluation of serum and seminal plasma markers in the diagnosis of canine prostatic disorders. J Vet Intern Med. 1995;9:149–53.
12. Mukaratirwa S, Chitura T. Canine subclinical prostatic disease: histological prevalence and validity of digital rectal examination as a screening test. Tysdskr S Af vet Ver. 2007;78:66–8.
13. Parry NMA. Inflammatory diseases of the canine prostate gland. UK Vet. 2006;11:1–4.
14. Atalan G, Holt PE, Barr FJ, Brown PJ. Ultrasonographic estimation of prostatic size in canine cadavers. Res Vet Sci. 1999;67:7–15.
15. Williams J, Niles J. Prostatic disease in the dog. In Practice. 1999;21:558–75.
16. Solano-Gallego L. Reproductive system. In: Raskin RE, Meyer DJ, editors. Canine and feline cytology. A color atlas and interpretation guide. 2nd ed. Philadephia: Elsevier-Saunders; 2010. p. 274–308.
17. Petrie A, Watson P. Statistics for animals and veterinary science. 3rd ed. Oxford: Wiley-Blackwell; 2013.
18. Paclikova K, Kohout P, Vlasin M. Diagnostic possibilities in the management of canine prostatic disorders. Vet Med Czech. 2006;51:1–13.
19. Smith J. Canine prostatic disease: a review of anatomy, pathology, diagnosis, and treatment. Theriogenology. 2008;70:375–83.
20. Powe JR, Canfield PJ, Martin PA. Evaluation of the cytologic diagnosis of canine prostatic disorders. Vet Clin Pathol. 2004;33:150–4.
21. Kraft M, Brown M, LeRoy E. Cytology of the canine prostate. Irish Vet J. 2008;61:320–4.
22. Fontbone A. Infertility in male dogs: recent advances. Rev Bras Reprod Anim. 2011;35:266–73.
23. Alcaraz A, Hammerer P, Tubaro A, Schroder FH, Castro R. Is there evidence of a relationship between benign prostatic hyperplasia and prostate cancer? Findings of a literature review. Eur Urol. 2009;55:864–75.

16

Epidemiology, presentation and population genetics of patent ductus arteriosus (PDA) in the Dutch Stabyhoun dog

Marjolein L. den Toom[1*], Agnes E. Meiling[1], Rachel E. Thomas[2], Peter A. J. Leegwater[1] and Henri C. M. Heuven[1,3]

Abstract

Background: Patent ductus arteriosus (PDA) is one of the most common congenital heart defects in dogs and is considered to be a complex, polygenic threshold trait for which a female sex predisposition has been described. Histological studies in dogs suggest that smooth muscle hypoplasia and asymmetry of the ductus tissue is the major cause of PDA. The Stabyhoun population is small and a predisposition for PDA has been suggested. The aims of this study were to describe the incidence, presentation from a clinical and histopathological perspective, and the population genetics of PDA in the Dutch Stabyhoun population.

Results: Forty-six cases were identified between 2000 and 2013. Between 2009 and 2012 the birth incidence of PDA in the Stabyhoun breed was 1.05 %. We estimated this to be 7–13 times higher than expected in the general dog population. Twelve of the 46 cases were part of a litter in which more than one sibling was affected. There was no sex predilection in our case cohort. Dogs diagnosed in adulthood showed severe cardiomegaly. The mean inbreeding coefficient of the reference population of Stabyhoun dogs was 31.4 % and the actual and effective numbers of founders were 14 and 6.5, respectively. The heritability of PDA was 0.51 (±0.09) for the reference population and 0.41 (±0.10) for the phenotyped population. Histopathology of sections of the PDA from two dogs showed findings similar to those described in other breeds although the smooth muscle of the ductus adjacent to the pulmonary artery appeared more hypoplastic than that in the ductus adjacent to the aorta.

Conclusions: The Stabyhoun breed shows a strong predisposition for PDA. Apart from the absence of a higher incidence in females, no other significant features distinguish PDA in Stabyhouns from the condition in other dog breeds. Heritability and the mean inbreeding coefficient are both very high making the Dutch Stabyhoun breed particularly suited to the study of inherited risk factors for PDA.

Keywords: Canine, Genetics, Heritability, Patent ductus arteriosus, PDA, Prevalence, Sex predisposition

Background

Patent ductus arteriosus (PDA) is a condition in which the ductus arteriosus (DA), also known as the *ductus Botalli*, fails to close after birth. During foetal growth the DA carries blood from the pulmonary artery to the aorta, to bypass the fluid-filled, not yet functioning lungs. In dogs, the DA closes within the first week of life [1] by contraction of the DA muscle, enabling normal blood flow through the lungs and aorta. Before birth prostaglandin E_2 (PGE2) from the placenta maintains the patency of the DA by relaxing the DA muscle [2]. When the lungs open, oxygen tension rises in the blood, inducing closure of the DA through the endothelin signalling pathway [2]. In cases of PDA, however, the DA fails to close, causing a shunt through which blood flows in a pattern that deviates from the normal route of the circulatory system. The direction of the abnormal blood flow is determined by the left and right heart pressures ("left to right", i.e. systemic to pulmonary or "right to left", i.e. pulmonary to systemic). At birth, all shunts are "left to right", due to the higher pressures in the left heart. However, over time a complication known as pulmonary hypertension can develop. If the pulmonary

* Correspondence: M.L.denToom@uu.nl
[1]Department of Clinical Sciences of Companion Animals, Faculty of Veterinary Medicine, Utrecht University, Yalelaan 108, 3508, TD, Utrecht, The Netherlands
Full list of author information is available at the end of the article

hypertension is severe enough, the direction of blood flow through the shunt can reverse into a "right to left" shunt. This "reversal" occurs in approximately 5 % of dogs with PDA [3]. Blood flowing from the aorta into the pulmonary artery (left to right shunt) typically causes a continuous heart murmur, increased pulmonary vascularity, left atrial and left ventricular enlargement and dilation of the aortic arch. If untreated, most dogs develop left heart failure within the first year of life [4, 5]. In dogs with reversed PDA, the murmur disappears and dogs will show cyanosis, secondary polycythemia and hyperviscosity. This can lead to exercise intolerance, intermittent hind limb weakness and seizures [6, 7]. Some breeds of dog appear to have a strong predisposition for this defect [8] and inheritance has been clearly demonstrated in the Miniature Poodle [9]. Different modes of inheritance for PDA have been proposed [8, 9], but it is currently accepted that hereditary PDA in the dog is not a simple Mendelian trait. A study demonstrated that the defect has a graded phenotypic expression and that more severely affected parents had more severely affected progeny [9]. A high proportion of the offspring of test matings had a fully patent ductus arteriosus, while a smaller proportion had a blind diverticulum of the ductus arteriosus which communicated with the aorta, but not with the pulmonary artery. This is considered to be a *forme fruste* of PDA, representing incomplete closure. Based on these findings, it was concluded that PDA resembles a quasi-continuous or threshold trait with a high degree of heritability and with the likelihood of defective closure of the ductus arteriosus being increased with the proportion of the genome received from dogs with PDA [9]. The population of Stabyhoun dogs, a Dutch hunting breed, is small (approximately 5500 animals worldwide) and seems to be predisposed to PDA. In a retrospective study, evaluating PDA in a referral population, the number of presented PDA positive Stabyhoun dogs was approximately 15 times higher than expected [10].

PDA is the second most common type of congenital heart disease in man with an estimated incidence of approximately two to eight cases per 10,000 births in full-term infants whilst it accounts for the majority of all cases of congenital heart disease in preterm infants [11, 12]. Two retrospective twin studies have suggested a familial component to PDA in preterm infants [13, 14]. Familial clustering of PDA has also been reported in full-term infants [15]. In human patients causative mutations have been found in a gene encoding smooth muscle myosin heavy chain *(MYH11)* [16] and a gene encoding transcription factor AP-2 beta *(TFAP2B)* [17, 18], found in neural crest derived cells. However, many human cases with a suspected genetic background remain unsolved [19]. In dogs, a relationship between prematurity and PDA has not been described. Histological studies of PDA's in dogs suggest that abnormal tissue architecture (mainly smooth muscle hypoplasia and asymmetry) is the major cause of PDA [20]. As PDA is one of the most common congenital heart defects in dogs and recent studies suggest a more important role for genetic factors in the occurrence of PDA in human infants, research into the etiology and inherited risk factors in dogs and humans has gained more interest. We propose that the Stabyhoun dog is a good model for further research. The aims of this study were to describe the incidence, presentation from a clinical and histopathological perspective, and the population genetics of PDA in the Dutch Stabyhoun dog population.

Methods

Animals and incidence

Records from the database of the the Dutch Kennel Club (Raad van Beheer) and the Utrecht University Companion Animal Clinic for the period 2000 to 2013 were evaluated. Forty-six cases of PDA were identified and included in this study and the recorded data were reviewed retrospectively. This included, when available, age at diagnosis, gender, number of affected siblings, direction of blood flow in the shunt, and presence of cardiomegaly.

The birth incidence for the three years from 2009 to 2012 was calculated from the number of known PDA positive cases and the total number of dogs born in this period.

To be able to include dogs in an "unaffected phenotyped" population, dogs were examined by a resident or board certified diplomate in veterinary cardiology on a yearly breeders day of one of the Dutch Stabyhoun breeding clubs (Nederlandse Vereniging voor Stabij-en Wetterhounen (N.V.S.W.). A dog was included in the unaffected phenotyped population if the dog was asymptomatic and did not show any abnormalities on cardiovascular examination.

Histopathology

Histology of the PDA was performed in two puppies by one of the authors (RT) under supervision of a board certified pathologist. Results were compared to the described histological presentation in other breeds [20]. Samples were trimmed to obtain a transverse section that includes a transverse to diagonal section of the ductus with the adjacent aorta and pulmonary artery attached to the PDA. Tissues were fixed in 10 % neutral buffered formalin, embedded in paraffin according to standard procedures and cut into 4 μm tissue sections. Sections were stained with hematoxylin and eosin and picosirius red with alcian blue to visualize type I collagen and glycosaminoglycan (GAG)-rich intercellular matrix. Immunohistochemistry for smooth muscle actin (α-SMA) was performed on subsequent sections. Briefly, mouse anti-smooth muscle actin antibody[1] as the primary antibody and dog anti-mouse/biotin[2] as the secondary antibody were used according to manufacturers' instructions to demonstrate the presence of smooth muscle.

Population genetics

Pedigree data from the Dutch Kennel Club (Raad van Beheer) were retrieved for the period 1940 to 2013. For each dog the database records contained: registration number, registration number of both parents, date of birth, and sex. In the pedigree analysis, Stabyhoun dogs born from 2000 to 2013 were used as a reference population (in this study referred to as "REFPOP"). PDA positive dogs are referred to as "POSDOGS". Pedigree files were analyzed with the Pedig package [21] and the following programs of this package were used: verification of the pedigree was successfully performed with *verif_ped*, checking for individuals present in their own pedigree; *Prob_orig* was used to determine both the actual number of founders and the effective number of founders by use of the classical approach [22]; *Meuw* was used to calculate the inbreeding coefficient for all individuals with the algorithm of Meuwissen and Luo [23]. To find common ancestors of all PDA positive dogs *anc_comm* was used. The percentage of contribution to each individual by the common ancestors was compared to the contribution of those individuals to the reference population. The total numbers of males and females were compared with the numbers of sires and dams used for breeding. Also, the maximum number of offspring per individual was assessed for both sires and dams.

Statistical analysis

Heritability and variance components (σ^2) were calculated using ASReml software [24]. Because of the proposed complex polygenic threshold trait [9], the following logistic model was applied to estimate the genetic and environmental variance, which were used to calculate heritability: $y = \mu + \text{animal} + e$ where μ is the overall mean. Animal is a random effect. Normal distributions are assumed for the random effects: animal ~ N $(0, A\sigma_a^2)$, where A contains the additive genetic relationship between animals. The residual variance (σ_e^2) was fixed at 3.289 in order to scale the animal effects. The heritability was calculated using the formula: $h^2 = \sigma_a^2/(\sigma_a^2 + \sigma_e^2)$ where σ_a^2 is the additive genetic variation and $\sigma_a^2 + \sigma_e^2$ is the phenotypic variation. Variance components (including relationship matrices) and heritability were estimated in two datasets. Once over the entire REFPOP, assuming all individuals that did not have a known PDA were healthy, and once over the phenotyped population: the population of Stabyhoun dogs that were confirmed to be either PDA positive ($n = 46$) or PDA negative, based on clinical examination by a resident or board certified diplomate in veterinary cardiology ($n = 213$). For significance testing the software PASW Statistics 18 was used.

Results & discussion

Incidence

Between 2000 and 2013, 46 cases of PDA were identified in this study population. Twenty-nine cases were born between 2009 and 2012 and in total over the same period, 2749 pups were born and registered. Based on this, the minimal birth incidence in the Stabyhoun breed was 1.05 % during this period. In a large retrospective study performed in a university clinic, the prevalence rate for all combined cardiovascular malformations in dogs, was 0.68 % [8]. In reality we expect this number to be lower, as animals referred to a university clinic are usually not representative of the general population. The percentage of PDAs amongst these congenital cardiac defects is estimated to be between 11 and 28 % [7, 8, 25, 26]. Therefore, we estimated the incidence of PDA to be lower than 0.08–0.14 % in the overall dog population and our results show the incidence in the Stabyhoun dog is approximately 7.5–13 times higher. Furthermore, the actual birth incidence may be even higher, as it is possible that not all cases are reported. For example, as PDA can cause death at a very young age [8] necropsy is often not performed in these dogs. In addition, when PDA is diagnosed, cases are not always reported to the breeders associations and/or Dutch Kennel Club.

Clinical presentation

Of the 46 PDA positive dogs, 12 dogs were part of a litter in which more than one dog was known to be affected. We recorded three litters with two affected siblings and two litters with three affected siblings. Mean age at diagnosis was 316 days with a range of 39–2865 days. Most dogs were diagnosed as young pups, but four dogs were diagnosed as adults (14, 21, 52 and 96 months old). These four dogs were still asymptomatic but showed cardiomegaly at the time of diagnosis. Only one dog, aged approximately six months at presentation, was diagnosed with a "reversed" PDA. Twenty-three dogs were male and twenty-three dogs were female. Apart from the absence of a higher incidence in females, no other significant features distinguish PDA in Stabyhouns from the condition in other dog breeds. In both canine and human studies a clear predisposition for females has been reported [8, 10, 26, 27]. The reason for this female predisposition is unclear. Surprisingly, no sex predilection was seen in this case cohort. The reason for the absence of a female predisposition in the Stabyhoun breed is unclear as the number of animals should be sufficient to show a significant difference if present. This could be an important distinguishing feature of PDA in this breed and further studies are necessary to further investigate this phenomenon.

Histopathology

The ductus arteriosus in both puppies was approximately 0.5 cm in length with a lumen of 0.5–1 cm. The tissues of both puppies have similar histological characteristics. The wall of the pulmonary artery is composed of little collagen and consists predominantly of smooth muscle and GAG-rich extracellular matrix. The type I collagen in the aortic wall is regularly, circumferentially distributed between smooth muscle cells. In general the type I collagen in the wall of the PDA appears to be less densely organized than that in the walls of the aorta and pulmonary artery. In the wall of the PDA adjacent to the aorta the collagen fibers are arranged concentrically and separated by evenly distributed GAG-rich extracellular matrix (Fig. 1a). In the wall of the PDA adjacent to the pulmonary artery the collagen is irregularly arranged with short crisscrossing bundles separated by irregular deposits of GAG-rich extracellular matrix (Fig. 1b). Similar to the collagen bundles, the smooth muscle cells are also more haphazardly organized and appear less dense in the side of the PDA adjacent to the pulmonary artery (Fig. 1c and d). The histological results from these dogs show some agreement with the results described by Buchanan et al. [20], however there are also some differences which may reflect the differences in the technique used for histological assessment: Whereas Buchanan made a quantitative analysis over the whole length of the PDA our images are from a small number of sections. In the cases presented here, the structure of the wall of the PDA in both puppies is asymmetric in terms of the organization of the distribution of collagen and smooth muscle fibers with regards to one another and the GAG-rich component of the extracellular matrix. However, as only a single site was analyzed, it is possible that these differences reflect differences in depth and angle of sectioning. Future studies could analyze the wall structure of non-persistent ductus arteriosus in age-matched Stabyhoun control dogs.

Population genetics

Pedigree structure

The entire evaluated Stabyhoun pedigree consisted of 14,955 dogs, bred between 1940 and 2013. In the reference population (REFPOP) from 2000 to 2013, 7008 dogs were born. The number of males did not differ significantly from the number of females in both the entire

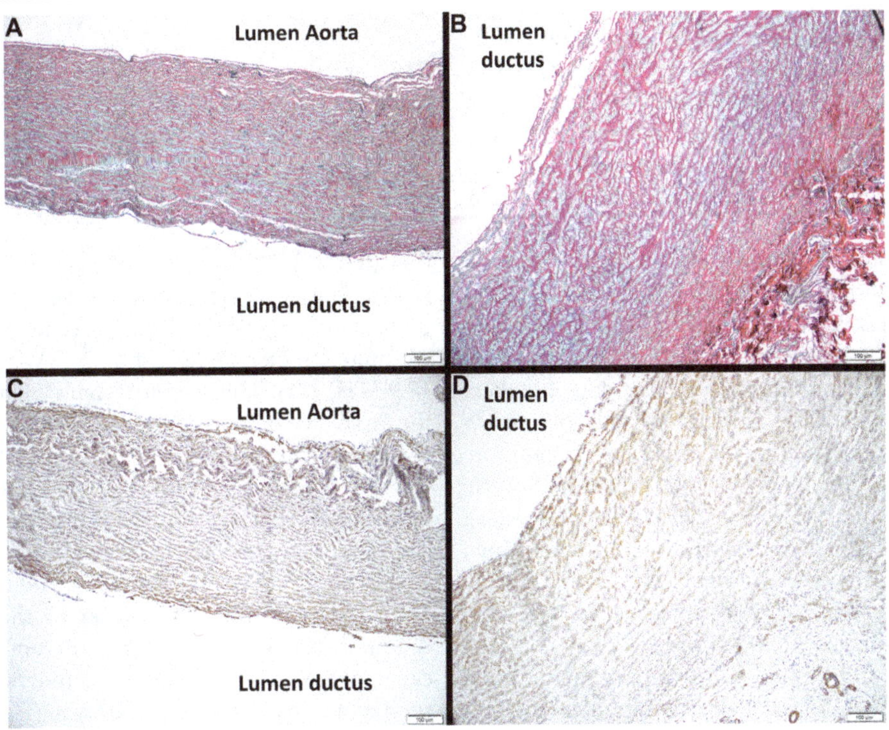

Fig. 1 Histopathology of PDA in Stabyhoun dogs. **a** Picosirius red with Alcian blue: Wall of the persistent ductus arteriosus adjacent to the aorta showing approximately evenly distributed collagen and GAG-rich extracellular matrix. ×100. **b** Picosirius red and Alcian blue: Wall of the PDA adjacent to the pulmonary artery; the collagen is irregularly arranged with short crisscrossing bundles separated by irregular deposits of GAG-rich extracellular matrix. ×100. **c** Smooth muscle actin: Wall of the persistent ductus arteriosus adjacent to the aorta with immunohistochemical staining of smooth muscle actin highlighting the concentric and relatively even distribution of smooth muscle cells. ×100. **d** Smooth muscle actin: Wall of the persistent ductus arteriosus adjacent to the pulmonary artery; bundles of smooth muscle cells are short and irregularly distributed. ×100

($p = 0.139$) and reference populations ($p = 0.173$). Additionally, equal numbers of males and females were affected with PDA (POSDOGS; 23 males and 23 females). The number of founders in the studbook for the entire population is 38. The actual number of founders for the reference population was 14. In other words, all individuals born between 2000 and 2013 descended from a total of 14 individuals. The effective number of founders was lower, only 6.5. This indicates that in an idealized population, were all matings are at random, only 6.5 founders would give the same level of inbreeding. The percentage of females that are mothers was 22.2 % in the REFPOP, whereas the percentage of males that are fathers was only 11.8 %. Over the entire population the percentage of females that are mothers was 15.1 %, which is lower than 22.2 %, indicating that more females were used for breeding in the current population compared to before 2000. The same is true for males, where only 6.8 % fathered at least one litter, over the entire population, compared to 11.8 % in the REFPOP. The maximum number of offspring per sire was 392 for the entire population and 127 for the REFPOP. Per dam the maximum number of offspring was 78 for the entire population and 52 for the REFPOP.

Table 1 Genealogical parameters for PDA positive cases, reference population and total of the Stabyhoun population

	POSDOGS	REFPOP	Total
N	46	7008	14,955
F mean	0.315	0.314	0.268
F max	0.360	0.389	0.466
Proportion $F > 0.1$	1.0	1.0	0.951
Founders	–	14	38
Effective # founders	–	6.5	–
# males	23	3424	7387
# sires	–	403	503
% of males that sire	–	11.8	6.8
Max. offspring per sire		127	392
# females	23	3541	7568
# dams	–	787	1139
% of females that sire	–	22.2	15.1
Max offspring per dam		52	78

POSDOGS: PDA positive cases, registered at databases of the Dutch Kennel Club and/or the Utrecht University Companion Animal Clinic between 2000 and 2013. *REFPOP*: the total reference population of Stabyhoun dogs born from 2000 to 2013 and registered in database of the Dutch Kennel Club. *N:* number of individuals, *F mean:* mean inbreeding coefficient, *F max:* maximal inbreeding coefficient, proportion $F > 0.1$: the proportion of dogs in the population with an inbreeding coefficient higher than 0.1

Inbreeding coefficients

There was no significant difference in inbreeding coefficient (F) between the REFPOP and the POSDOGS. The mean inbreeding coefficient of the REFPOP was 31.4 % and the mean inbreeding coefficient of the POSDOGS was 31.5 %. Results of the pedigree structure analysis and inbreeding coefficients are summarized in Table 1. Both inbreeding coefficients are higher than the inbreeding coefficient of a brother-sister or parent-offspring mating, which give the highest level of inbreeding in a single generation (25 %). This is notably higher when compared to other dog breeds [28–30]. However, for most of the breeds in these studies not all known ancestry data is taken into account. In this study we analysed approximately 12 generations of Stabyhoun dogs, since the recognition of the breed in 1942. In other studies, records were mainly reviewed from the 1970 – 1990's and they generally assumed that all individuals present at that time were nonrelated. However, in three scent-hound breeds from the alpine region, pedigrees since founding in the 1930s were investigated. In these breeds, after correcting for pedigree completeness, inbreeding coefficients of 6.4, 9.1 and 13.6 % for Bavarian mountain hound (BMH), Hanoverian hound (HH) and Tyrolean hound (TH), respectively, were demonstrated [31]. The BMH has a similar population size to the Stabyhoun, whereas HH and TH have significantly smaller populations. As population size is a strong predictor for inbreeding coefficients, it could be expected that the Stabyhoun and BMH would have similar inbreeding coefficients, but the Stabyhoun population shows a higher level of inbreeding. This can be explained by the low number of founders for the Stabyhoun population. Although the Stabyhoun studbook contains 38 potential founders, only 14 of these founders are actual ancestors of the current day population (the REFPOP) and the effective number of founders is 6.5. The scent-hound breeds had actual numbers of founders of 353 (BMH), 226 (HH) and 98 (TH) and effective numbers of founders of 43.7 (BMH), 41.6 (HH) and 18.9 (TH) [31]. This is considerably higher and facilitates the avoidance of inbreeding. A French study examining all members of nine different dog breeds that were registered between 1975 and 2001 reported founder numbers of 13 (Barbet) to 1158 (Epagneul Breton) and corresponding effective founder numbers of 6.9–70.7 [28]. The effective number of founders of the Stabyhoun is below this range, whereas the actual number of founders is within the range. Breeding practices that cause uneven contribution of founders to the REFPOP, such as the use of popular sires, may underlie this discrepancy. In the Stabyhoun breed there are indications of the use of popular sires, as only 11.8 % of males father at least one litter. In addition, within the entire population one particular sire fathered 392 offspring. For the current day population the maximum number of offspring for one sire is 127, approximately corresponding to

18 litters for a single male. The maximum number of offspring per sire and dam has decreased over time.

Heritability

The heritability of PDA was calculated over the entire reference population, assuming all individuals that did not have a known PDA status were healthy, and over the phenotyped population. Using an animal model the variance components for animal effects were 3.40 for REFPOP and 2.24 for the phenotyped population. The heritability of PDA was 0.51 (±0.09) for the reference population and 0.41 (±0.10) for the phenotype population. Results of the heritability analysis are summarized in Table 2. In both cases the heritability differed significantly from zero, showing a high hereditary component to PDA in the Stabyhoun dog.

Common ancestors

Only one dog showed a significantly higher percentage of genetic contribution to the PDA cases compared to the reference population. However, this individual, coded as individual 1212 in our analyses, also contributed to all individuals in the reference population (REFPOP) to some degree. The genetic contributions of the seven most influential dogs are illustrated in Table 3. One of the limitations of this study is the fact that dogs were categorized either as positive (confirmed PDA) or negative (absence of continuous murmur and/or clinical signs). However, as described earlier, some dogs might have a blind diverticulum instead of a full PDA. This does not cause a murmur or clinical signs and, therefore, is likely to go unnoticed as it can only be diagnosed by post-mortem examination or aortic angiography. As aortic angiography was not performed in the phenotyped population the presence of blind diverticulums in some dogs considered as negative in our analysis cannot be excluded. Our pedigree analysis confirms that the inheritance of PDA is not Mendelian, with low numbers of affected sibling pairs and lack of parent-offspring transmission.

Table 2 Variance components and heritability of PDA in Stabyhoun dogs

	σ_a^2	σ_e^2	σ_{total}^2	h^2	SE (h^2)
REFPOP	3.40	3.29	6.69	0.51	0.09
Phenotyped	2.24	3.29	5.53	0.41	0.10

PDA: Patent ductus arteriosus, *REFPOP:* the total reference population of Stabyhoun dogs born between 2000 to 2013 and registered in database of the Dutch Kennel Club ($n = 7008$), *Phenotyped*: the population of Stabyhoun dogs that were confirmed to be either PDA positive ($n = 46$) or PDA negative, based on clinical examination by a resident or board certified diplomate in veterinary cardiology ($n = 213$), σ_a^2: the additive genetic variance, σ_e^2: the residual variance, σ_{total}^2 ($\sigma_a^2 + \sigma_e^2$): the phenotypic variance, h^2: narrow sense heritability, *SE* (h^2): standard error of narrow sense heritability

Table 3 The genetic contribution of most influential ancestors to positive cases and the reference population

Identification number	POSDOGS	REFPOP	Difference
1212	5.0	4.3	0.7*
411	5.0	4.8	0.2
261	28.5	28.4	0.1
72	41.5	41.5	0
196	28.9	28.9	0
71	24.5	24.6	−0.1
25	19.5	19.6	−0.1

The percentage of genetic contribution of the seven most influential ancestors is demonstrated for the PDA positive cases (POSDOGS) and the reference population (REFPOP). *significant difference ($p = 0.000$). REFPOP: Stabyhoun dogs born from 2000 to 2013 and registered in database of Dutch Kennel Club ($n = 7008$). POSDOGS: PDA positive cases, registered at databases of the Dutch Kennel Club and/or the Utrecht University Companion Animal Clinic between 2000 and 2013 ($n = 46$). Note that there is only one common ancestor to the PDA positive cases that significantly contributes more to the positive individuals than to the reference population

Conclusions

In conclusion, the results of the present study suggest that the Stabyhoun dog is a breed with a strong predisposition for PDA. Apart from the absence of a higher incidence in females, no other significant features distinguish PDA in Stabyhouns from the condition in other dog breeds. Heritability and the mean inbreeding coefficient are both very high and we, therefore, propose that the Dutch Stabyhoun breed is particularly suited to the study of inherited risk factors for PDA.

Endnotes

[1]Biogenex, Fremont, California, United States of America.
[2]Vector Laboratories, Peterborough, United Kingdom.

Abbreviations

BMH, Bavarian mountain hound; HH, Hanoverian hound; PDA, persistent ductus arteriosus; *PHENOTYPED*, the population of Stabyhoun dogs that were confirmed to be either PDA positive ($n = 46$) or PDA negative ($n = 213$), based on clinical examination by a resident or a board certified diplomate in veterinary cardiology; *POSDOGS*, PDA positive cases, registered at databases of the Dutch Kennel Club and/or the Utrecht University Companion Animal Clinic between 2000 and 2013 ($n = 46$); *REFPOP*, the total reference population of Stabyhoun dogs born between 2000 to 2013 and registered in database of the Dutch Kennel Club ($n = 7008$); TH, Tyrolean hound.

Acknowledgements

We would like to thank the Dutch Kennel Club (Raad van Beheer) and the Stabyhoun breeding clubs (Nederlandse Vereniging voor Stabij- en Wetterhounen (N.V.S.W.) and "Onze Stabyhoun") for sharing data and involving the owners. Also we would like to thank Dr. A.A. Stokhof, Dr. V.Szatmári and Dr. N. Beijerink for their assistance in the examining of the Stabyhoun dogs.

Funding

This research received no specific grant from any funding agency in the public, commercial, or not-for-profit sectors.

Authors' contributions

MDT conceived of the study, was responsible for the selection of animals, performed the clinical investigations of the dogs, revised the first draft of the manuscript and wrote the final version of the manuscript. AM participated in the acquisition and interpretation of data and wrote the first draft of the manuscript. HH supervised the interpretation and presentation of the results of the population genetics part of the study. RT was responsible for the histopathological examinations and drafted the histopathological part of the manuscript. PL and HH directed the project, obtained financial support and revised the drafts of the manuscript. All authors read and approved the final manuscript.

Competing interests

The authors declare that they have no competing interests.

Consent for publication

Not applicable.

Author details

[1]Department of Clinical Sciences of Companion Animals, Faculty of Veterinary Medicine, Utrecht University, Yalelaan 108, 3508, TD, Utrecht, The Netherlands. [2]Department of Pathobiology, Faculty of Veterinary Medicine, Utrecht University, Yalelaan 1, 3485, CL, Utrecht, The Netherlands. [3]Animal Breeding and Genomics Centre, Wageningen University, P.O. box 338, 6700, AH, Wageningen, The Netherlands.

References

1. House EW, Ederstrom HE. Anatomical changes with age in the heart and ductus arteriosus in the dog after birth. Anat Rec. 1968;160(2):289–95.
2. Coceani F, Baragatti B. Mechanisms for ductus arteriosus closure. Semin Perinatol. 2012;36(2):92–7.
3. Buchanan JW. Prevalence of cardiovascular disorders. In. Fox PR., Sisson DD. and Moise NS. eds Textbook of canine and feline cardiology Philadelphia: W.B. Saunders 1999;457–470.
4. Eyster GE, Eyster JT, Cords GB, Johnston J. Patent ductus arteriosus in the dog: characteristics of occurrence and results of surgery in one hundred consecutive cases. J Am Vet Med Assoc. 1976;168(5):435–8.
5. Stanley BJ, Luis-Fuentes V, Darke PG. Comparison of the incidence of residual shunting between two surgical techniques used for ligation of patent ductus arteriosus in the dog. Vet Surg. 2003;32(3):231–7.
6. Legendre AM, Appleford MD, Eyster GE, Dade AW. Secondary polycythemia and seizures due to right to left shunting patent ductus arteriosus in a dog. J Am Vet Med Assoc. 1974;164(12):1198–201.
7. Pyle RL, Park RD, Alexander AF, Hill BL. Patent ductus arteriosus with pulmonary hypertension in the dog. J Am Vet Med Assoc. 1981;178(6):565–71.
8. Patterson DF. Epidemiologic and genetic studies of congenital heart disease in the dog. Circ Res. 1968;23(2):171–202.
9. Patterson DF, Pyle RL, Buchanan JW, Trautvetter E, Abt DA. Hereditary patent ductus arteriosus and its sequelae in the dog. Circ Res. 1971;29(1):1–13.
10. Meijer M, Beijerink NJ. Patent ductus arteriosus in the dog: a retrospective study of clinical presentation, diagnostics and comparison of interventional techniques in 102 dogs (2003–2011). Tijdschr Diergeneeskd. 2012;137(6):376–83.
11. Reller MD, Strickland MJ, Riehle-Colarusso T, Mahle WT, Correa A. Prevalence of congenital heart defects in metropolitan Atlanta, 1998–2005. J Pediatr. 2008;153(6):807–13.
12. Samanek M, Voriskova M. Congenital heart disease among 815,569 children born between 1980 and 1990 and their 15-year survival: a prospective bohemia survival study. Pediatr Cardiol. 1999;20(6):411–7.
13. Lavoie PM, Pham C, Jang KL. Heritability of bronchopulmonary dysplasia, defined according to the consensus statement of the national institutes of health. Pediatrics. 2008;122(3):479–85.
14. Bhandari V, Zhou G, Bizzarro MJ, et al. Genetic contribution to patent ductus arteriosus in the premature newborn. Pediatrics. 2009;123(2):669–73.
15. Sletten LJ, Pierpont ME. Familial occurrence of patent ductus arteriosus. Am J Med Genet. 1995;57(1):27–30.
16. Zhu L, Vranckx R, Khau Van Kien P, et al. Mutations in myosin heavy chain 11 cause a syndrome associating thoracic aortic aneurysm/aortic dissection and patent ductus arteriosus. Nat Genet. 2006;38(3):343–9.
17. Satoda M, Zhao F, Diaz GA, et al. Mutations in TFAP2B cause char syndrome, a familial form of patent ductus arteriosus. Nat Genet. 2000;25(1):42–6.
18. Dagle JM, Lepp NT, Cooper ME, et al. Determination of genetic predisposition to patent ductus arteriosus in preterm infants. Pediatrics. 2009;123(4):1116–23.
19. Harakalova M, van der Smagt J, de Kovel CG, et al. Incomplete segregation of MYH11 variants with thoracic aortic aneurysms and dissections and patent ductus arteriosus. Eur J Hum Genet. 2013;21(5):487–93.
20. Buchanan JW, Patterson DF. Etiology of patent ductus arteriosus in dogs. J Vet Intern Med. 2003;17(2):167–71.
21. Boichard D. PEDIG: A fortran packagefor pedigree analysis suited for large populations.proceedings of the 7th world congress on genetics applied to livestock production: Montpellier, August 19-23, 2002. INRA, castanet-tolosan, france, CD-rom, comm. no. 28–13.
22. Lacy RC. Analysis of founder representation in pedigrees: founder equivalents and founder genome equivalents. Zoo Biol. 1989;8:111–123.
23. Meuwissen T, Luo Z. Computing inbreeding coefficients in large populations. Genet Select Evol. 1992;24(4):305–13.
24. Gilmour AR, Gogel BJ, Cullis BR, Thompson R. ASReml user guide release 2.0. Hemel hempstead: VSN international ltd. 2006.
25. Tidholm A. Retrospective study of congenital heart defects in 151 dogs. J Small Anim Pract. 1997;38(3):94–8.
26. Oliveira P, Domenech O, Silva J, Vannini S, Bussadori R, Bussadori C. Retrospective review of congenital heart disease in 976 dogs. J Vet Intern Med. 2011;25(3):477–83.
27. Dice JE, Bhatia J. Patent ductus arteriosus: an overview. J Pediatr Pharmacol Ther. 2007;12(3):138–46.
28. Leroy G, Rognon X, Varlet A, Joffrin C, Verrier E. Genetic variability in french dog breeds assessed by pedigree data. J Anim Breed Genet. 2006;123(1):1–9.
29. Nielen AL, van der Beek S, Ubbink GJ, Knol BW. Population parameters to compare dog breeds: differences between five dutch purebred populations. Vet Q. 2001;23(1):43–9.
30. Shariflou MR, James JW, Nicholas FW, Wade CM. A genealogical survey of Australian registered dog breeds. Vet J. 2011;189(2):203–10.
31. Voges S, Distl O. Inbreeding trends and pedigree analysis of Bavarian mountain hounds, Hanoverian hounds and Tyrolean hounds. J Anim Breed Genet. 2009;126(5):357–65.

17

Measurement of Creatine kinase and Aspartate aminotransferase in saliva of dogs

Asta Tvarijonaviciute[1], Tomas Barranco[1], Monica Rubio[2,3], Jose Maria Carrillo[2,3], Silvia Martinez-Subiela[1], Fernando Tecles[1], Juana Dolores Carrillo[1] and José J. Cerón[1*]

Abstract

Background: Muscle enzymes in saliva have been reported to be possible markers of heart and muscle damage in humans. The aim of this study was to assess if Creatine kinase (CK) and Aspartate aminotransferase (AST) activities could be measured in canine saliva, and to evaluate their possible changes in situations of muscle damage.

Results: The spectrophotometric assays for CK and AST measurement in saliva of dogs showed intra- and inter-assay imprecision lower than 1 and 16% and coefficients of correlation close to 1 in linearity under dilution tests. Healthy dogs showed activities in saliva of CK between 27 and 121 U/L and AST between 46 and 144 U/L, whereas in saliva of dogs with muscle damage CK ranged between 132 and 3862 U/L and AST between 154 and 4340 U/L. Positive moderate correlations were found between saliva and serum activities of the two enzymes (CK, $r = 0.579$; $P = 0.001$; AST, $r = 0.674$; $P = 0.001$).

Conclusions: CK and AST activities can be measured in canine saliva with commercially available spectrophotometric assays. In addition these enzymes show higher values in saliva of dogs with muscle damage and their values are moderately correlated with those of serum.

Keywords: Aspartate aminotransferase (AST), Canine, Creatine kinase (CK), Muscular damage, Saliva, Serum

Background

Saliva is a biological fluid that contains a certain number of elements common to other body fluids such as blood or urine in a sufficiently large consistency to take into interest their assays for biological analysis. Interest in saliva assays is increasing during last years [1, 2], with various scientific reviews indicating their advantages as a diagnostic medium such as its collection is safe, non-invasive, inexpensive, and simple. In addition it can be sampled repeatedly without discomfort to the patient [3].

Therefore saliva, especially in human medicine, has gained considerable attention as a possible alternate fluid to blood and urinary analysis [1] with a growing scientific literature describing the use of salivary biomarkers to determine diabetic and cardiac related risk factors, among others [4]. In dogs, analytes such as C-reactive protein [5] or cortisol [6, 7] have been measured in saliva and were found to be suitable biomarkers of inflammation and stress respectively.

Creatine kinase (CK) and Aspartate aminotransferase (AST) are two enzymes found in cytoplasm of muscle cells. They are considered to be markers of muscle cell damage, and an increase in these enzymes in serum may be an indicator of muscle stress or damage due to exercise [8–10] or muscle injuries [11, 12]. CK is primarily found in skeletal muscle, myocardium, brain and intestine [13]; although its main activity in serum is released from skeletal muscle [9]. While serum AST is less muscle specific than CK, since it is also present in liver and its activity in serum can increase due to liver damage [14]. In humans CK has been measured in saliva and it was indicated that plasma could be its main source [15].

CK and AST have been measured in serum of dogs as a marker of muscle damage under different conditions,

* Correspondence: jjceron@um.es
[1]Animal Medicine and Surgery Department, School of Veterinary Medicine, University of Murcia, Campus of Espinardo s/n, 30100 Murcia, Spain
Full list of author information is available at the end of the article

such as hemilaminectomy or ovariohysterectomy [16], exercise [10], and after anesthesia [17]. However, to the authors' knowledge no studies about CK and AST in saliva in dogs have been published previously. The knowledge about the possibility of measurement of CK and AST could be of both veterinarian and human interest, since the dog is a widely used experimental model for research.

The objective of the present study was to assess if CK and AST activities could be measured in canine saliva, and to evaluate their possible changes after processes that cause muscle damage. For this purpose, commercially available automated spectrophotometric CK and AST assays were validated in canine saliva and these two enzymes were measured in healthy dogs and in a group of dogs with increased serum CK and AST due to different causes.

Methods

All experimental procedures were approved by the Local Ethical Committee of University of Murcia, and were performed in compliance with laws RD32/2007 and RD1201/2005 concerning animal experimentation in Spain.

Assays

CK was measured by a commercial kit (Beckman Coulter, Brea, USA) based on the quantification of the NADPH formation derived from the action of CK on creatin phosphate as recommended by the International Federation of Clinical Chemistry (IFCC) [18]. AST was measured by a commercial kit (Beckman Coulter, Brea, USA) based on the quantification of the NADH consumption derived from the action of AST over aspartate and oxoglutarate as recommended by the IFCC [19]. Specimen volume used was 3 μl for CK and AST in the case of serum and 25 μl for CK and 3 μl for AST in case of saliva. A correction factor of [3/(3 + RV)]: [(25 + RV)/25] (where RV is reagent volume) was applied to the results of CK in saliva in order to take in consideration the different volume used. All the assays were performed in an automated biochemistry analyzer (Olympus AU600, Beckman Coulter, Brea, USA) at 37 °C. CK and AST assays showed an inter-assay imprecision and an inaccuracy of less than 5% in the daily quality control analysis done during the study. Manufacturer's control solutions of two different values were used for the quality control analysis (Beckman-coulter, Lot 0037 and 0038).

Analytical validation

For analytical validation of both methods the following parameters were calculated.

Precision

The intra-assay coefficient of variation (CV) was calculated after analysis of 2 saliva specimens with different CK and AST concentration 5 times in a single assay run. The inter-assay CV was determined by analyzing the same specimens in 5 separate runs, carried out on different days, being the specimens stored at −80 °C.

Accuracy

It was evaluated indirectly by linearity under dilution. For this purpose, two canine saliva specimens were serially diluted with bidistilated water.

Limit of detection

This was calculated on the basis of data from 10 replicate determinations of the zero standard (bidistilated water) as the mean value plus 3 standard deviations.

Animals

A total of 27 dogs were included in the present study. Thirteen of these animals were healthy dogs belonging to staff and students of Murcia University and were used as controls. None of the dogs presented abnormalities at physical examination, or in the CBC and biochemical profile, and did not have evidence of periodontal disease. In particular, serum activities of AST and CK were lower than 50 UI/L and 250 U/L respectively, values which represent the higher limit of the reference interval of our laboratory.

All animal were adults with a mean (range) age of 5.1 (2.0-8.0) years and a median (range) body weight (BW) of 19.3 (7.0-29.0) kg. Six dogs were mongrels, three were Beagles, two were Labrador Retrievers, one was Golden Retriever and one was Poodle.

In order to evaluate if CK and AST increased in saliva in dogs with muscle damage, fourteen dogs with increased serum CK and AST due to diverse causes such as traumas or surgery were included in the study. The saliva and blood specimens were taken at time of admission. In this group of dogs age ranged between 0.5 and 10.0 years (median 6.4 years), and BW was between 1.5 and 40.0 kg (median 25.5 kg). Seven dogs were mongrels, three were Yorkshire terriers and there was one dog of each of the following breeds: San Bernardo, Boxer, German Shepherd and Spanish water dog. In all cases, the exclusion criteria were: the saliva specimens obtained had not enough volume for measurements; and presence of periodontal disease since salivary CK and AST was shown to increase in humans with periodontal disease [20].

Saliva and blood sampling

Saliva specimens were obtained by placing a sponge in dog's mouth for 1–2 min as previously described [5, 21].

Then the sponge was placed into the Salivette (Salivette®, Sarstedt AG &Co., Nümbrecht, Germany) device for centrifugation (P Selecta®, JP Selecta S.A, Barcelona, Spain) at 3000 x g 10 min [5, 22]. After saliva collection, venous blood specimens (2 mL) were collected from the jugular vein into plain tubes (Vacutainer®, Plymouth, United Kingdom). Tubes were let to clot at room temperature for 30 min and centrifuged (2000 x g, 10 min) for careful removal of the serum.

The saliva and blood specimens were processed and measured in less than 1 h after collection, and serum and centrifuged saliva samples were keep at 4 °C until were measured.

Statistical analysis

Normality of the data distribution was evaluated with a Kolmogorov-Smirnov test and, since data was not normally distributed, non-parametric tests were used. Differences in serum and salivary CK and AST between healthy controls and dogs muscle enzymes in serum out of reference interval were evaluated using the Mann–Whitney test. Correlations between serum and saliva were calculated using the Spearman correlation coefficient. The level of significance was set at $P < 0.05$. Statistical analyses were performed with computer software (Graph Pad Prism Version 7 for Windows, Graph Pad software, La Jolla, CA).

Results

CK in saliva showed intra- and inter-assay imprecision less than 1 and 16%, respectively, while AST in saliva showed intra- and inter-assay imprecision less than 1 and 7%, respectively (Table 1). Linearity under dilution resulted in coefficient of correlation close to 1 in both cases (Fig. 1). Limit of detection for salivary CK was 6.01 U/L (mean, 2.05; SD, 1.32) and for salivary AST was 2.11 U/L (mean, 0.82; SD, 0.43).

Serum CK activity in healthy controls ranged between 57.9 and 239 U/L, whereas it was significantly higher in dogs with muscle damage ($P < 0.001$) with values between 319 and 78,650 U/L (Fig. 2a). Serum AST in healthy controls ranged between 23.8 and 36.9 U/L and dogs with muscle damage showed significantly higher activity in serum AST ($P < 0.001$) with values between 58.3 and 988 U/L (Fig. 2b).

Table 1 Intra- and interassay coefficients of variation (CV)

Assay	Comparison	Specimen	mean	Sd	CV (%)
CK, U/L	Intra	Specimen 1	64.6	0.12	0.2
		Specimen 2	293.5	1.46	0.5
	Inter	Specimen 1	49.1	7.26	14.8
		Specimen 2	182.8	27.74	15.2
AST, U/L	Intra	Specimen 1	91.8	0.36	0.4
		Specimen 2	639.3	3.19	0.5
	Inter	Specimen 1	84.7	5.75	6.8
		Specimen 2	619.1	15.47	2.5

Salivary CK in healthy controls ranged between 27 and 121 U/L, whereas dogs with muscle damage showed a significantly higher activity in saliva CK ($P < 0.001$) with values between 132 and 3862 U/L (Fig. 2c). AST in saliva in healthy controls ranged between 46.8 and 144 U/L, whereas dogs with muscle damage showed a significantly higher activity in saliva AST ($P < 0.001$) with values between 154 and 4340 U/L (Fig. 2d).

When data from healthy controls and those with muscle damage were pooled, positive correlations were observed between serum and salivary CK ($r = 0.579$; $P = 0.001$) and between serum and salivary AST ($r = 0.674$; $P < 0.001$).

Discussion

Serum activities of CK and AST reflect damage of muscle and are useful markers to determine the condition of muscle tissue both in dogs [10, 13, 23, 24] and humans [25, 26]. In particular, increases in CK following physical activity has been associated with muscle damage in both racing and hunting dogs [9] and similar findings have been described in humans [8, 25].

The assays used in our study showed an adequate intra-assay imprecision and accuracy to measure the activity of both enzymes in saliva. Therefore CK and AST can be measured in saliva in dogs with automated spectrophotometric assays available for routine use in clinical pathology laboratories. The inter-assay imprecision was higher than 15% for CK, that is considered as the acceptable limit [27]; this fact could be related with the stability of the enzyme under storage and further studies should be made to elucidate the reason. In case of using assays from a different manufacturer than those used in our study, an optimization of specimen volume and analytical validation of the assay would be recommended.

Our study reports for the first time the existence of CK and AST activities in saliva of dogs. In healthy dogs of our study CK showed lower values in saliva compared to serum which agrees with previous reports made in humans [15]. The lower values of CK in saliva could be due to the existence of a limit in the transfer of CK from plasma to saliva as it has been suggested in human for CK and other analytes such as NT-ProBNP [15, 28]. This situation seems not occur in the case of AST, that showed higher values in saliva than in serum. Additional studies should be performed to elucidate the reasons of the higher values of AST in saliva compared with serum in dogs.

Dogs with muscle damage showed significant increases in CK and AST in saliva and there was no overlap in the

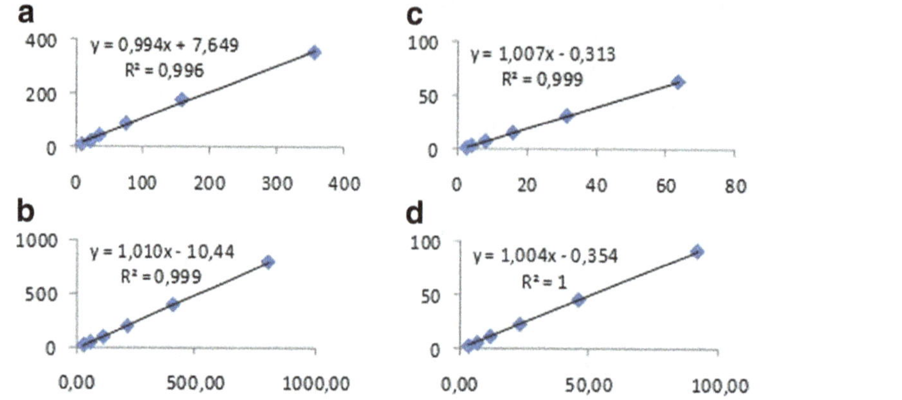

Fig. 1 Linearity under dilution of two saliva specimens with different CK and AST concentrations. CK (**a**,**b**) and AST (**c**,**d**) concentrations

values of these enzymes between healthy dogs and dogs with muscle damage. In dogs with muscle damage the values of CK in saliva did not reach the values in serum (upper value in saliva of 3862 versus 78,650 U/L in serum) and again a limit in the transfer of CK from plasma to serum could be suggested to explain this fact. On the other hand in the case of AST values in saliva of dogs with muscle damage were higher than in serum (upper value in saliva of 4340 versus 988 U/L in serum), and further studies should be undertaken to elucidate the mechanisms that can produce this effect.

Significant correlations were obtained between salivary and serum activities of CK and AST in dogs and this would indicate a possible pass of the enzymes from serum to saliva. However these correlations were moderate, similarly to what has been found in humans [15]. One cause of this moderate correlation could be due to the different dynamics after a muscle damage that the enzymes can have in serum and saliva. In addition, from the analytical point of view it should be considered the different kinetics that the enzymatic reactions had in serum and saliva, although the sample dilution and further dilution in the reagents would likely minimize the matrix effect. Further studies about the process allowing muscle enzymes to filter from plasma to saliva, as well factors that could increase or decrease this transfer, would be recommended. In addition the possibility of enzyme synthesis by the salivary glands should be explored. This would allow a better understanding of the clinical significance of muscle enzymes in saliva and their correlation with serum.

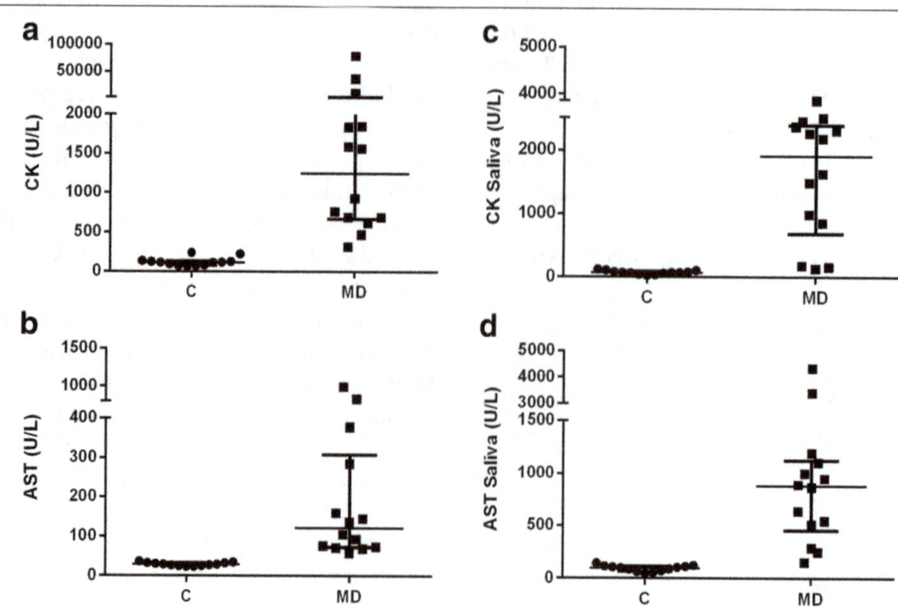

Fig. 2 Serum and saliva CK and AST in healthy dogs and dogs with muscle damage. Serum and saliva CK (**a** and **b**, respectively) and AST (**c** and **d**, respectively) in controls (C, n = 13) and dogs with muscle damage (MD, n = 14)

Saliva analysis could be a potential suitable alternative to serum due to its non-invasive collection, which could be convenient in cases where dogs are reluctant to blood sampling or in young dogs of small breeds. However, it is important to point out some limitations that the measurements of CK and AST in saliva could have from a practical point of view. The first one is that in some cases it can not be obtained enough volume for analysis, as it have been previously described for salivary cortisol measurements in dogs [29]. The second one is that the presence of gingivitis and/or dental plaque is known to produce increases in salivary CK and AST in humans [20], and therefore the interpretation of these enzymes in saliva of dogs with these diseases should be made with caution.

This is a pilot study and further studies with a larger population of dogs should be made to confirm these findings. In addition although in our study the specimens have been analyzed in the first hour after collection, it would be of interest to evaluate the influence of different storage conditions in the stability of these enzymes in saliva. Furthermore, additional studies could be of interest to evaluate the behavior of the different CK isoenzymes in saliva and also the dynamics of CK and AST in serum and saliva after an experimental induced muscle damage as well in dogs with and without periodontal disease and gingivitis.

Conclusions

Results of the present study indicate that CK and AST activities can be measured in canine saliva with commercially available spectrophotometric assays. In addition these enzymes show higher values in saliva of dogs with muscle damage compared with healthy dogs and their values have a moderate correlation with those of serum.

Acknowledgements
Isabel Rodriguez is acknowledged for her technical support.

Funding
This research was supported by the GERM programme of the Seneca Foundation of Murcia Region and the Garcia Cugat Foundation.

Authors' contributions
AT, TB and JJC conceived and designed the study. TB, MR, SM, FT and JDC collected the specimens and performed the analysis. All authors read and approved the final manuscript.

Competing interests
Jose Ceron is Section Editor for BMC Veterinary Research

Author details
[1]Animal Medicine and Surgery Department, School of Veterinary Medicine, University of Murcia, Campus of Espinardo s/n, 30100 Murcia, Spain. [2]Animal Medicine and Surgery Department, School of Veterinary Medicine, Universidad CEU Cardenal Herrera of Valencia, Valencia, Spain. [3]Garcia Cugat Foundation CEU-UCH Chair of Medicine and Regenerative 3 Surgery, Barcelona, Spain.

References

1. Pfaffe T, Cooper-White J, Beyerlein P, Kostner K, Punyadeera C. Diagnostic potential of saliva: current state and future applications. Clin Chem. 2011;57: 675–87.
2. Chiappin S, Antonelli G, Gatti R, De Palo EF. Saliva specimen: a new laboratory tool for diagnostic and basic investigation. Clin Chim Acta. 2007; 383:30–40.
3. Mirzaii-Dizgah I, Hejazi SF, Riahi E, Salehi MM. Saliva-based creatine kinase MB measurement as a potential point-of-care testing for detection of myocardial infarction. Clin Oral Investig. 2011;16:775–9.
4. Jaedicke KM, Taylor JJ, Preshaw PM. Validation and quality control of ELISAs for the use with human saliva samples. J Immunol Methods. 2012;377:62–5.
5. Parra MD, Tecles F, Subiela SM, Ceron JJ. C-reactive protein measurement in canine saliva. J Vet Diagn Investig. 2005;17:139–44.
6. Bennett A, Hayssen V. Measuring cortisol in hair and saliva from dogs: coat color and pigment differences. Domest Anim Endocrinol. 2010;39:171–80.
7. Oyama D, Hyodo M, Doi H, Kurachi T, Takata M, Koyama S, et al. Saliva collection by using filter paper for measuring cortisol levels in dogs. Domest Anim Endocrinol. 2014;46:20–5.
8. Brancaccio P, Maffulli N, Buonauro R, Limongelli FM. Serum enzyme monitoring in sports medicine. Clin Sports Med. 2008;27:1–18. vii
9. Lucas V, Barrera R, Duque FJ, Ruiz P, Zaragoza C. Effect of exercise on serum markers of muscle inflammation in Spanish greyhounds. Am J Vet Res. 2015; 76:637–43.
10. Rovira S, Munoz A, Benito M. Effect of exercise on physiological, blood and endocrine parameters in search and rescue-trained dogs. Vet Med. 2008;53:333.
11. Mokuno K, Riku S, Sugimura K, Takahashi A, Kato K, Osugi S. Serum creatine kinase isoenzymes in Duchenne muscular dystrophy determined by sensitive enzyme immunoassay methods. Muscle Nerve. 1987;10:459–63.
12. Szumilak D, Sułowicz W, Walatek B. Rhabdomyolysis: clinical features, causes, complications and treatment. PrzeglądLek. 1998;55:274–9.
13. Aktas M, Auguste D, Lefebvre HP, Toutain PL, Braun JP. Creatine kinase in the dog: a review. Vet Res Commun. 1993;17:353–69.
14. Scott-Moncrieff JC, Hawkins EC, Cook JR Jr. Canine muscle disorders. Compend Contin Educ Pract Vet. 1990;12:31 4. 36 9
15. Mirzaii-Dizgah I, Jafari-Sabet M. Unstimulated whole saliva creatine phosphokinase in acute myocardial infarction. Oral Dis. 2011;17:597–600.
16. Nevill B, Leisewitz A, Goddard A, Thompson P. An evaluation of changes over time in serum creatine kinase activity and C-reactive protein concentration in dogs undergoing hemilaminectomy or ovariohysterectomy. J S Afr Vet Assoc. 2010;81:22–6.
17. Aktas BM, Vinclair P, Autefage A, Lefebvre HP, Toutain PL, Braun JP. In vivo quantification of muscle damage in dogs after general anaesthesia with halothane and propofol. J Small Anim Pract. 1997;38:565–9.
18. Hørder M, Elser RC, Gerhardt W, Mathieu M, Sampson EJ. International Federation of Clinical Chemistry, scientific division Committee on enzymes: approved recommendation on IFCC methods for the measurement of catalytic concentration of enzymes. Part 7. IFCC method for creatine kinase (ATP: creatine N-phosphotransferase, EC 2.7.3.2). J Clin Chem Clin Biochem. 1991;29:435–56.
19. International Federation of Clinical Chemistry. IFCC methods for the measurement of catalytic concentration of enzymes. Clin Chem. 1977;23:887.
20. Todorovic T, Dozic I, Vicente-Barrero M, Ljuskovic B, Pejovic J, Marjanovic M, et al. Salivary enzymes and periodontal disease. Med Oral Patol Oral Cir Bucal. 2006;11:E115–9.
21. Luke R, Khan SN, Iqbal PS, Soman RR, Chakkarayan J, Krishnan V. Estimation of specific salivary enzymatic biomarkers in individuals with gingivitis and chronic Periodontitis: a clinical and biochemical study. J Int Oral Health. 2015;7:54–7.
22. Tvarijonaviciute A, Carrillo-Sanchez JD, García-Martinez JD, Tecles F, Martinez-Subiela S, German AJ, et al. Measurement of salivary adiponectin concentrations in dogs. Vet Clin Pathol. 2014;43:416–21.
23. de Godoy MRC, Beloshapka AN, Carter RA, Fascetti AJ, Yu Z, McIntosh BJ, et al. Acute changes in blood metabolites and amino acid profile post-exercise in Foxhound dogs fed a high endurance formula. J Nutr Sci. 2014;3:1–6.

24. McKenzie EC, Jose-Cunilleras E, Hinchcliff KW, Holbrook TC, Royer C, Payton ME, et al. Serum chemistry alterations in Alaskan sled dogs during five successive days of prolonged endurance exercise. J Am Vet Med Assoc. 2007;230:1486–92.
25. Mastaloudis A, Leonard SW, Traber MG. Oxidative stress in athletes during extreme endurance exercise. Free Radic Biol Med. 2001;31:911–22.
26. Tsubakihara T, Umeda T, Takahashi I, Matsuzaka M, Iwane K, Tanaka M, et al. Effects of soccer matches on neutrophil and lymphocyte functions in female university soccer players. Lumin J Biol Chem. 2013;28:129–35.
27. U.S. Department of Health and Human Services, Food and Drug Administration, Center For Drug Evaluation And Research (CEDER), Center for Veterinary Medicine (CVM). Guidance for industry: bioanalytical method validation. Rockville, MD: CDER; 2001.
28. Foo JYY, Wan Y, Kostner K, Arivalagan A, Atherton J, Cooper-White J, et al. NT-ProBNP levels in saliva and its clinical relevance to heart failure. PLoS One. 2012;7:e48452.
29. Wenger-Riggenbach B, Boretti FS, Quante S, Schellenberg S, Reusch CE, Sieber-Ruckstuhl NS. Salivary cortisol concentrations in healthy dogs and dogs with hypercortisolism. J Vet Intern Med. 2010;24:551–6.

18

Effect of tear collection on lacrimal total protein content in dogs and cats: a comparison between Schirmer strips and ophthalmic sponges

Lionel Sebbag[1*], Emily M. McDowell[2], Patrick M. Hepner[2] and Jonathan P. Mochel[3]

Abstract

Background: Quantification of lacrimal total protein content (TPC) is an important tool for clinical scientists to understand disease pathogenesis, identify potential biomarkers and assess response to therapy, among other applications. However, TPC is not only affected by disease state but also by the method used for tear collection. Thus, the purpose of this study is to determine the impact on TPC of two methods of tear collection in dogs and cats: Schirmer strips and polyvinyl acetal (PVA) sponges.

Methods: (i) In vivo - Ten healthy dogs and 10 healthy cats were examined. Each animal underwent two sessions, separated by 10 min, in which a Schirmer strip was placed in one randomly selected eye until the 20-mm mark was reached, while a strip of PVA sponge was placed in the other eye for 1 min. (ii) In vitro - Schirmer strips and PVA sponges were spiked with various volumes of four bovine serum albumin solutions (0.5, 4, 10, and 20 mg/mL). In both experiments, the wetted absorbent materials were centrifuged for 1 min, and the TPC was quantified on the extracted fluid using Direct Detect™ infrared spectroscopy.

Results: Lacrimal TPC in dogs and cats ranged from 5.2 to 14.6 mg/mL and from 6.2 to 20.6 mg/mL, respectively. In cats, TPC was significantly lower with Schirmer strips vs. PVA sponges ($P < 0.001$). In dogs, the volume absorbed by PVA sponges was negatively correlated with TPC ($r = -0.48$, $P = 0.033$). The inter-session coefficient of variation was significantly lower with Schirmer strips vs. PVA sponges in both species ($P \leq 0.010$). In vitro, both absorbent materials resulted in a 'concentrating effect' of the TPC obtained post-centrifugation, which was most pronounced when the volume absorbed was low, especially for Schirmer strips.

Conclusion: Schirmer strips provide a repeatable method to quantify lacrimal TPC in dogs and cats, although care should be taken to absorb sufficient volumes of tears to minimize the concentrating effect from the absorbent material.

Keywords: Total protein content, Tear fluid, Tear flow, Schirmer tear test, Ophthalmic sponge

* Correspondence: lsebbag@iastate.edu
[1]Department of Veterinary Clinical Sciences, Iowa State University, College of Veterinary Medicine, Ames, IA 50011, USA
Full list of author information is available at the end of the article

Background

Tears are a complex biological fluid composed of a mixture of substances. Proteins, one of the major classes of compounds in tear fluid, promote ocular surface health through various functions that include anti-microbial defense, anti-oxidation and modulation of wound healing [1]. Recent developments in proteomics have identified over 1500 proteins in the tear fluid [2], some being secreted by the lacrimal glands ('lacrimal-derived', e.g. lysozyme, lactoferrin, lipocalin and IgA) and some leaking into tears from the conjunctival capillaries ('serum-derived', e.g. albumin, transferring and IgG). Changes in tear protein composition have been closely associated with disease state, not only for eye-specific conditions such as dry eye [3] and allergic conjunctivitis [4], but also for systemic disorders such as diabetes mellitus [5] and cancer [6]. For instance, the expression pattern of proteins in tears is different in dogs with various cancers when compared to healthy subjects [6]. Thus, analysis of tear protein can help identify new biomarkers, better understand disease pathogenesis, and develop new diagnostic tools and therapeutics. However, it is often challenging to draw accurate conclusions and make cross-study comparisons because the protein content in tears is not only affected by disease state, but also largely by the method of tear collection used by each investigator.

The collection technique can strongly influence the protein profile in a tear sample. For instance, a higher total protein content (TPC) was found in tear samples obtained with Schirmer strips when compared to capillary tubes in humans [7] and dogs [8], largely due to a greater amount of serum-derived proteins, although these findings were not confirmed in a recent study by Posa and colleagues [9]. Direct sampling of tear fluid with capillary tubes, albeit commonly used in humans [7, 9], presents several drawbacks that limit its use in veterinary species. In particular, the collection process with capillary tubes is slow and the volume obtained is generally small, with a reported average collection time of 6–7 min to obtain ≤ 10 μL of non-stimulated tear fluid in cats [10]. Combined with the uncooperative nature of most veterinary patients, these limitations make it challenging to avoid reflex tearing or accidental trauma to the eye in a reliable and repeatable manner. The challenges of using capillary tubes also exist in human subjects, especially in individuals with reduced tear volume [11]. Thus, some investigators have encouraged the use of absorbent materials as an alternative method for tear collection: besides being safe, absorbent materials likely provide an enriched sample by retaining compounds present on the ocular surface [11]. For instance, Li and colleagues showed that defensins, key antimicrobial peptides expressed by corneo-conjunctival epithelia [12], are upregulated in Schirmer-collected tear samples of patients with Sjögren's-related dry eye [13].

The purpose of our study is to evaluate the effect of tear collection with two different absorbent materials on TPC in dogs and cats, namely Schirmer strips and polyvinyl acetal (PVA) ophthalmic sponges. The study design combines both in vivo and in vitro experiments – the former aims to capture the impact of normal ocular surface physiology (e.g. tear flow, reflex tearing) on the parameter evaluated, while the latter aims to determine the impact of various protein concentrations on the adsorptive properties of the absorbent materials, i.e. the amount of protein retained by the Schirmer strips and PVA sponge after tear extraction.

Methods

In vivo evaluation

Animals

Ten dogs and 10 cats were enrolled in the study. After obtaining informed consent from owners, all subjects were confirmed to be ophthalmoscopically healthy by slit-lamp examination,[1] indirect funduscopy,[2] tonometry,[3] Schirmer tear test,[4] and fluorescein staining. The canine population was comprised of two Labrador Retrievers, two Yorkshire terriers, and one dog of the following breeds: Greyhound, Great Pyrenees, Border Collie, English Bulldog, Poodle, and Chihuahua. The mean ± standard deviation (minimum-maximum) age and body weight of dogs were 7.7 ± 3.9 years (2–14 years) and 16.8 ± 8.7 kg (5.2–30.2 kg), respectively. The feline population was comprised of six Domestic Short Hair, two Domestic Long Hair, one Burmese and one Persian cat. The mean ± standard deviation (minimum-maximum) age and body weight of cats were 7.6 ± 3.9 years (3–15 years) and 4.9 ± 1.3 kg (3.1–6.8 kg), respectively. In both species, five subjects were castrated males and five were spayed females. The study was approved by the Institutional Animal Care and Use Committee of Iowa State University.

Tear collection

In each animal, the bent tip of a Schirmer strip[4] was placed in the ventral conjunctival fornix of one randomly selected eye (coin toss), while a 4 × 10 mm strip of PVA ophthalmic sponge[5] was placed in the ventral conjunctival fornix of the other eye, as previously described [14]. The Schirmer strip was removed when the 20-mm mark of wetness was reached, while the PVA sponge was removed after 60 s. The wetted Schirmer strip and PVA sponge were removed and placed in separate 0.2-mL Eppendorf tubes that were previously punctured at their bottom with a 18-gauge needle. The combinations were sealed into separate 1.5-mL Eppendorf tubes with adhesive tape and subsequently centrifuged at 3884 g for 1 min to extract the tear fluid.[6] Tear collection and extraction were repeated 10 min later using the same randomized eye for each absorbent material. The volume of tears absorbed (VA) and recovered in each sample were calculated by the difference of post- and pre-collection weight[7] of the 0.2-mL tubes, and the difference of post- and pre-centrifugation weight of the 1.5-mL tubes, respectively [14].

Total protein quantification

TPC was quantified in each sample using the Direct Detect™ infrared spectrometer.[8] An aliquot of 2 μL of each sample was spotted on the membrane card and analyzed using phosphate-buffered saline (PBS)[9] as blank. The card was inserted into the instrument and results were recorded in mg/mL using the included software. Since the linear range of the Direct Detect™ is 0.2–5.0 mg/mL, samples that resulted in a protein content greater than 5 mg/mL were diluted with PBS and re-analyzed. Total protein content was recorded in mg/mL, adjusting for any dilution when necessary.

In vitro evaluation

Four protein concentrations (0.5, 4, 10 and 20 mg/mL) were evaluated, representative of the range of TPC obtained in vivo in canine and feline tears (in vivo part of the present study). Solutions of 0.5 mg/mL[10] and 20 mg/mL[11] bovine serum albumin (BSA) were obtained, and the latter was used to make solutions of 4 and 10 mg/mL BSA by 5- and 2-fold dilution with PBS, respectively.

Three volumes of each BSA solution were spiked onto different sets of Schirmer strips and PVA sponges. The volumes selected were representative of the range of volume absorbed by PVA sponges from the present in vivo experiment and from a previous publication [14], while the range of volume absorbed by Schirmer strips from another experiment (unpublished data) in which Schirmer tear test values varied from 1 to 35 mm/min. This is because the present study design (i.e. standardized tear collection until the 20-mm mark was reached) had limited the range of volume absorbed by Schirmer strips.

The three volumes of BSA solutions were defined as:

- "Low volume": Representing the 10th percentile of tear volume absorbed in vivo, which is 10 μL for both absorbent materials;
- "Intermediate volume": Representing the 50th percentile of volume absorbed in vivo, which is 20 μL for STT and 25 μL for PVA sponges;
- "High volume": Representing the 90th percentile of volume absorbed in vivo, which is 30 μL for STT and 60 μL for PVA sponges.

In summary, 12 combinations were evaluated in vitro for both Schirmer strips and PVA sponges: low, intermediate and high volumes of 0.5, 4, 10, and 20 mg/mL BSA solutions.

First, each of the four BSA solutions was analyzed 10 times for its total protein content using the Direct Detect™ infrared spectrometer, and results (expressed in mg/mL) were used as 'control' for comparisons with the experimental groups. Second, each of the 12 combinations was evaluated by spotting the set volume of BSA solution in 10 separate Schirmer strips and 10 separate PVA sponges. The wetted Schirmer strips and PVA sponges were subsequently handled in a similar fashion than the in vivo study, and the TPC of fluids extracted by centrifugation was evaluated with the Direct Detect™ infrared spectrometer.

Data analysis

Normality of the data was assessed with the Shapiro–Wilk test. In each species, the Wilcoxon signed-rank test was used to compare the TPC obtained in vivo by Schirmer strips and PVA sponges, as well as the coefficients of variation (CV%) between both tear collection sessions. Associations between TPC, volume of tears absorbed, age and body weight were examined by the Spearman's rank correlation test for each species and each absorbent material. The Mann-Whitney test was used to assess differences between the TPC of each in vitro combination (volume/protein concentration) and the TPC of the corresponding BSA solution. Statistical analysis was performed using SigmaPlot version 13.0[12], and values $P < 0.05$ were considered statistically significant.

Results

In vivo evaluation

Data were not normally distributed for any parameter evaluated ($P < 0.05$), so results are presented as median and 95% range (2.5–97.5th percentiles). Median (95% range) canine TPC in tears was 8.7 mg/mL (5.2–14.6 mg/mL) with Schirmer strips and 8.8 mg/mL (5.2–14.4 mg/mL) with PVA sponges, a difference that was not statistically significant ($P = 0.898$; Fig. 1a). Median (95% range) feline TPC in tears was 9.6 mg/mL (6.2–12.1 mg/mL) with Schirmer strips and 15.9 mg/mL (6.6–20.6 mg/mL) with PVA sponges, a difference that was statistically significant ($P < 0.001$, Fig. 1b).

Inter-session comparison of TPC (initial vs. tear sample collected 10 min later) showed that the median (95% range) CV% was significantly lower ($P = 0.020$) in Schirmer strips (3.9%, 0.5–10.8%) vs. PVA sponges (10.6%, 2.2–75.0%) in canine patients. Similarly, the median (95% range) CV% was significantly lower ($P = 0.010$) in Schirmer strips (5.9%, 1.2–11.7%) vs. PVA sponges (23.7%, 0.4–57.3%) in cats.

A significant moderate negative correlation was noted between the volume of tears absorbed by the PVA sponges and the TPC quantified in tears of dogs

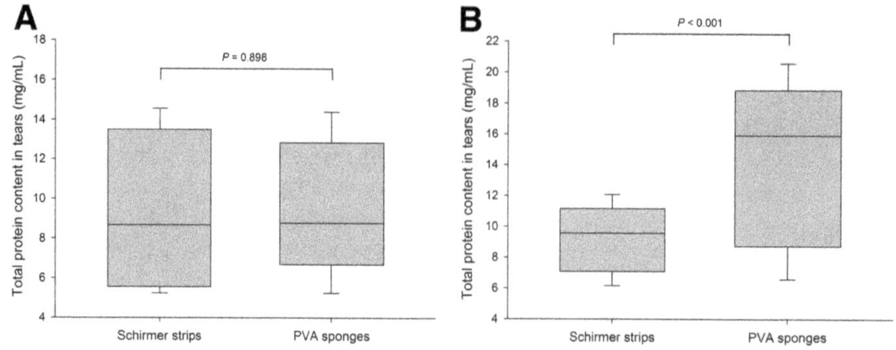

Fig. 1 Box-and-whisker plots depicting the total protein content in tear samples collected in 10 healthy dogs (**a**) and 10 healthy cats (**b**) with either Schirmer strips or PVA sponges. Median values are shown by a horizontal line. First and third quartiles (25th and 75th percentiles) are represented by the lower and upper limits of the box, respectively. The 2.5th and the 97.5th percentiles are shown as the lower and upper whiskers, respectively

(*Spearman's rho* = − 0.48, $P = 0.033$; Fig. 2), but not in cats ($P = 0.21$). No correlations were noted between the volume of tears absorbed by Schirmer strips and TPC in either species ($P \geq 0.35$). Similarly, no correlations were noted between age, body weight and TPC in either species ($P \geq 0.097$).

In vitro evaluation

Results of the in vitro experiments are summarized in Fig. 3. Each figure panel describes a different concentration of BSA (0.5, 4, 10, and 20 mg/mL), representative of the range of TPC noted in the in vivo experiments.

The fluid extracted post-centrifugation often contained a significantly higher TPC ($P \leq 0.045$) when compared to the standard BSA solution used to wet the Schirmer strips and PVA sponges. This 'concentrating effect' of the absorbent materials was variable, and depended upon two parameters (i) the volume of fluid absorbed, and (ii) the protein concentration of the solution.

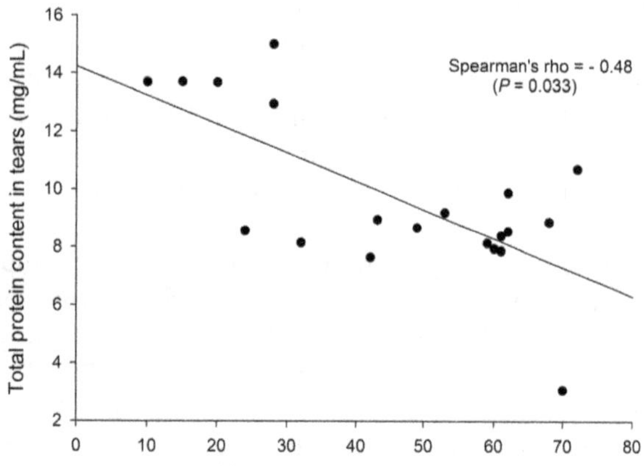

Fig. 2 Spearman's rank correlation testing for TPC and VA of tear samples collecting with PVA sponges in 10 healthy dogs. A moderate negative correlation was found (*Spearman's rho* = − 0.48, $P = 0.033$)

Indeed, the 'concentrating effect' was most pronounced when the volume absorbed was low, especially for Schirmer strips. For instance, when spiking 10 μL ('low volume') of 4 mg/mL BSA solution on Schirmer strip and PVA sponges (Fig. 3b), the recorded mean TPC of the fluid extracted post-centrifugation was 8.9 mg/mL and 6.9 mg/mL, respectively. These values represent a significant increase of TPC by 222% and 172% compared to the control BSA solution of 4 mg/mL, respectively ($P < 0.001$).

To a lesser degree, the original concentration of proteins also influenced the resulting TPC quantified in the fluid obtained post-centrifugation. For instance, when a similar 'intermediate' volume of 25 μL was spiked onto PVA sponges, the recorded mean TPC of the extracted fluid did not vary significantly from the control BSA solutions for 10 and 20 mg/mL ($P > 0.05$), but was significantly greater for 0.5 mg/mL ($P = 0.003$) and 4 mg/mL ($P < 0.001$).

Discussion

Tears collected with an absorbent material and extracted with centrifugation yielded a TPC of 5.2–14.6 mg/mL in dogs and 6.2–20.6 mg/mL in cats. These values are likely accurate estimates of the 'true' TPC for samples in which the tear volume absorbed was around 20–25 μL (i.e. median VA in vivo), but may represent an overestimation of TPC for samples with low VA and, to a lesser degree, those with high VA. Indeed, our in vitro data showed a clear 'concentrating effect' from both absorbent materials when VA was low (10 μL), which was noticeable across the entire range of protein levels tested and more pronounced with Schirmer strips than PVA sponges. Despite centrifugation, our group has previously shown that a relatively large portion of fluid was retained by ophthalmic sponges when the volume of tears absorbed was low [14], especially for cellulose-based sponges. That explains the greater concentrating

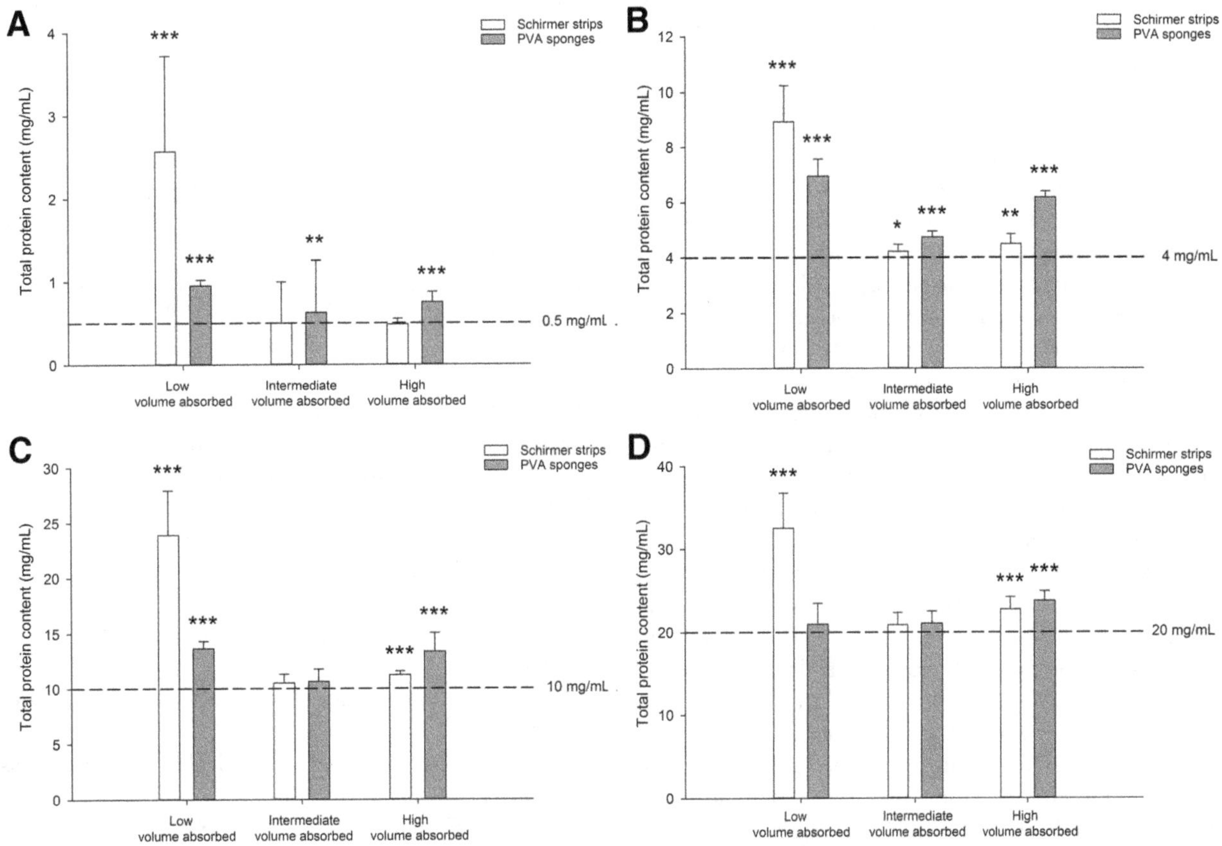

Fig. 3 Bar charts depicting the mean + standard deviation of TPC from in vitro experiments evaluating 12 combinations of volume absorbed/protein concentration in both Schirmer strips (white bars) and PVA sponges (gray bars): low, intermediate and high volumes of 0.5 mg/mL (**a**), 4 mg/mL (**b**), 10 mg/mL (**c**), and 20 mg/mL (**d**) BSA solutions. In each panel, statistical differences between the absorbent materials and the control BSA solution are shown by asterisks: * $P < 0.05$, ** $P < 0.01$, *** $P < 0.001$

effect noted in the present study for Schirmer strips, which are hydrophilic materials manufactured from cellulose filter paper [15].

Regardless, the level of proteins reported herein is superior to the one described in tear fluid collected with capillary tubes in dogs (2.6 mg/mL) [16] and cats (10.4 mg/mL) [10]. Consistent with older reports in human subjects, the higher TPC in absorbent materials such as Schirmer strips vs. capillary tubes is presumably related to an increased in serum-derived proteins due to conjunctival irritation [7, 17]. However, these findings are not consistent across the scientific literature as recent studies have described an equal [9] or inferior [18] amount of proteins in Schirmer-collected tears when compared to capillary tubes. Thus, it is likely inaccurate to compare the findings of various studies based on the tear collection method alone. Rather, one should also consider how the tears were extracted from the absorbent material - i.e. centrifugal force [9], elution with a solvent [8, 15], or a combination of both [18, 19] - as well as the method used by the investigator to quantify the protein content.

In the present study, the assay used to quantify TPC relies on infrared spectrometry that measures the amide bond absorbance across all proteins and peptides contained in the sample. This method improves the accuracy of the assay as compared to colorimetric methods [20]. Although extensively used for TPC in tear fluid because of their simplicity and sensitivity [3, 8, 16], colorimetric methods such as Lowry and Bradford have drawbacks that can result in under- or over-estimation of TPC in tears [21]. For instance, the Bradford assay highly depends on the specific protein composition in a sample [22], and this becomes a considerable disadvantage when evaluating TPC in a complex protein mixture such as tear fluid. Further, since serum albumin is not a major component of tear proteins [23, 24], using BSA as a standard likely affects the TPC obtained by the colorimetric assay; in fact, TPC in tear fluid significantly differs whether BSA or IgG is used as the standard for the method [21].

A significant negative correlation was noted between tear flow rate and TPC in dogs, consistent with findings by Fullard and colleagues [3]. In another canine study, individuals with epiphora consistently had low tear fluid protein levels while subjects with dry eye had a high protein concentration [23]. In contrast, there was no correlation between tear flow rate and TPC in our feline subjects, and a recent publication in human patients showed a positive correlation between TPC and the Schirmer readings [19]. The reason for these discrepancies remains unclear and warrants further investigation. Further, body weight and age were not correlated with TPC in either species, despite the reported positive correlation between body weight and tear volume absorbed in dogs [14]. This finding, as well as potential impact of breed on TPC, should be verified in a larger population size.

Importantly, our study found that the repeatability of protein quantification in tears was greater with Schirmer strips when compared to PVA sponges, as determined by significantly lower inter-session CV% in both species. This could be explained by the lower variability in tear volume absorbed by Schirmer strips. Indeed, the mm-marks of Schirmer strips can be used to standardize the volume of tears absorbed at each collection. In the present study, the Schirmer strips were left in the conjunctival fornices of dogs and cats until the 20-mm mark was wetted, thus reducing the variability in VA between sessions and therefore improving the repeatability of TPC measurement. On the other hand, standardizing the duration of PVA-collection to 60 s did not reduce the variability in VA obtained between sessions; for instance, the VA in one representative dog was 20 μL at the initial sampling, and 43 μL when tear collection was repeated 10 min later. Although not evaluated in the present study, the extraction of tears from Schirmer strips could be optimized by 'washing' the strip with a solvent to help retrieve any small amount of protein that remained on the absorbent material post-centrifugation [9].

The present study was limited to describing total protein content, i.e. 'gross' protein quantification in the tear fluid. Further studies could investigate which specific tear proteins (e.g. albumin, lactoferrin) are most affected by changes in tear flow rate, or by the adsorptive properties of the Schirmer strips and PVA sponges used for tear collection. A recent study in humans determined that proteins are preferentially retained by Schirmer strips based on physicochemical factors such as molecular weight and surface charge [15].

Nevertheless, results of the present study are valuable given the potential applications of total protein quantification in veterinary medicine. In a clinical setting, TPC can be used to better characterize various ocular surface diseases and assess their response to therapy, as exemplified by keratoconjunctivitis sicca in dogs [23] and corneal sequestrum in cats [25]. In a research setting, TPC can be used to standardize the amount of tear sample to be used for assessing inflammatory mediators [19], in-depth proteomics [26] and others.

Conclusion

Schirmer strips are more reliable than PVA sponges (i.e. lower inter-session CV%) for quantification of TPC in canine and feline tears. However, care should be taken to absorb sufficient volumes of tears with Schirmer strips to minimize the concentrating effect from the absorbent material.

Endnotes

[1]SL-17; Kowa Company, Ltd., Tokyo, Japan

[2]Keeler Vantage; Keeler Instruments, Inc., Broomall, PA, USA

[3]TonoVet; Icare Finland Oy, Espoo, Finland

[4]Eye Care Product Manufacturing, LLC, Tucson, AZ, USA

[5]Ultracell® Eye Wick, Beaver-Visitec International, Inc., Waltham, MA, USA

[6]VWR® Mini Centrifuge, VWR International, Radnor, PA, USA

[7]Gemini-20, American Weight Scales Inc., Norcross, GA, USA

[8]Millipore-Sigma, St Louis, MO, USA

[9]Gibco™, Thermo Fisher Scientific, Inc., Waltham WA, USA

[10]Bovine Serum Albumin, VWR International, Radnor, PA, USA

[11]Bovine Serum Albumin, Fischer Scientific, Hampton, NH, USA

[12]Systat Software Inc., San Jose, CA, USA

Acknowledgements
The authors thank the patients' owners for their support of this work.

Funding
Not applicable.

Authors' contributions
LS, EM, PH and JPM designed the study and critically revised the manuscript. LS, EM and PH carried out the sample collections and analyses. LS drafted the manuscript and created the figures. JPM assisted with the statistical analysis. All authors read and approved the final manuscript.

Consent for publication
Not applicable.

Competing interests
The authors declare that they have no competing interests.

Author details
[1]Department of Veterinary Clinical Sciences, Iowa State University, College of Veterinary Medicine, Ames, IA 50011, USA. [2]Lloyd Veterinary Medical Center, Iowa State University, College of Veterinary Medicine, Ames, IA 50011, USA. [3]Department of Biomedical sciences, Iowa State University, College of Veterinary Medicine, Ames, IA 50011, USA.

References

1. Kijlstra A, Kuizenga A. Analysis and function of the human tear proteins. In: Sullivan DA, editor. Lacrimal gland, tear film, and dry eye syndromes: basic science and clinical relevance. Boston: Springer US; 1994. p. 299–308.
2. Zhou L, Zhao SZ, Koh SK, Chen L, Vaz C, Tanavde V, et al. In-depth analysis of the human tear proteome. J Proteome. 2012;75(13):3877–85. https://doi.org/10.1016/j.jprot.2012.04.053.
3. Fullard RJ, Kaswan RM, Bounous DI, Hirsh SG. Tear protein profiles vs. clinical characteristics of untreated and cyclosporine-treated canine KCS. J Am Optom Assoc. 1995;66(7):397–404.
4. Mimura T, Usui T, Yamagami S, Miyai T, Amano S. Relation between total tear IgE and severity of acute seasonal allergic conjunctivitis. Curr Eye Res. 2012;37(10):864–70. https://doi.org/10.3109/02713683.2012.689069.
5. Csősz É, Boross P, Csutak A, Berta A, Tóth F, Póliska S, et al. Quantitative analysis of proteins in the tear fluid of patients with diabetic retinopathy. J Proteome. 2012;75(7):2196–204. https://doi.org/10.1016/j.jprot.2012.01.019.
6. de Freitas Campos C, Cole N, Van Dyk D, Walsh BJ, Diakos P, Almeida D, et al. Proteomic analysis of dog tears for potential cancer markers. Res Vet Sci. 2008;85(2):349–52. https://doi.org/10.1016/j.rvsc.2007.
7. Stuchell RN, Feldman JJ, Farris RL, Mandel ID. The effect of collection technique on tear composition. Invest Ophthalmol Vis Sci. 1984;25(3):374–7.
8. Farias E, Yasunaga KL, Peixoto RVR, Fonseca MP, Fontes W, Galera PD. Comparison of two methods of tear sampling for protein quantification by Bradford method. Pesqui Vet Bras. 2013;33:261–4. http://dx.doi.org/10.1590/S0100-736X2013000200021
9. Posa A, Bräuer L, Schicht M, Garreis F, Beileke S, Paulsen F. Schirmer strip vs. capillary tube method: non-invasive methods of obtaining proteins from tear fluid. Ann Anat. 2013;195(2):137–42. https://doi.org/10.1016/j.aanat.2012.10.001.
10. Petznick A, Evans MD, Madigan MC, Markoulli M, Garrett Q, Sweeney DF. A comparison of basal and eye-flush tears for the analysis of cat tear proteins. Acta Ophthalmol. 2011;89(1):e75–81. https://doi.org/10.1111/j.1755-3768.2010.02082.x.
11. Li S, Sack R, Vijmasi T, Sathe S, Beaton A, Quigley D, et al. Antibody protein array analysis of the tear film cytokines. Optom Vis Sci. 2008;85(8):653–60. https://doi.org/10.1097/OPX.0b013e3181824e20.
12. McDermott AM. Defensins and other antimicrobial peptides at the ocular surface. Ocul Surf. 2004;2(4):229–47. https://doi.org/10.1016/S1542-0124(12)70111-8
13. Li B, Sheng M, Li J, Yan G, Lin A, Li M, et al. Tear proteomic analysis of Sjögren syndrome patients with dry eye syndrome by two-dimensional-nano-liquid chromatography coupled with tandem mass spectrometry. Sci Rep. 2014;4:5772. https://doi.org/10.1038/srep05772.
14. Sebbag L, Harrington D, Mochel J. Tear fluid collection in dogs and cats using ophthalmic sponges. Vet Ophthalmol. 2017; https://doi.org/10.1111/vop.12502.
15. Denisin AK, Karns K, Herr AE. Post-collection processing of Schirmer strip-collected human tear fluid impacts protein content. Analyst. 2012;137(21):5088–96. https://doi.org/10.1039/c2an35821b.
16. Davidson HJ, Blanchard GL, Montgomery PC. Comparisons of tear proteins in the cow, horse, dog and rabbit. Adv Exp Med Biol. 1994;350:331–4. https://doi.org/10.1007/978-1-4615-2417-5_56
17. Berta A. Collection of tear samples with or without stimulation. Am J Ophthalmol. 1983;96(1):115–6.
18. Li K, Chen Z, Duan F, Liang J, Wu K. Quantification of tear proteins by SDS-PAGE with an internal standard protein: a new method with special reference to small volume tears. Graefes Arch Clin Exp Ophthalmol. 2010;248(6):853–62. https://doi.org/10.1007/s00417-009-1275-3.
19. Dionne K, Redfern RL, Nichols JJ, Nichols KK. Analysis of tear inflammatory mediators: a comparison between the microarray and Luminex methods. Mol Vis. 2016;22:177–88.
20. Strug I, Utzat C, Cappione A, Gutierrez S, Amara R, Lento J, et al. Development of a univariate membrane-based mid-infrared method for protein quantitation and total lipid content analysis of biological samples. J Anal Methods Chem. 2014;2014:657079. https://doi.org/10.1155/2014/657079.
21. Ng V, Cho P. The relationship between total tear protein concentrations determined by different methods and standards. Graefes Arch Clin Exp Ophthalmol. 2000;238(7):571–6. https://doi.org/10.1007/s004170000147
22. Sapan CV, Lundblad RL, Price NC. Colorimetric protein assay techniques. Biotechnol Appl Biochem. 1999;29(Pt 2):99–108. https://doi.org/10.1111/j.1470-8744.1999.tb00538.x.
23. Roberts S, Erickson O. Dog tear secretion and tear proteins. J Small Anim Pract. 1968;3(1):1–5. https://doi.org/10.1111/j.1748-5827.1962.tb04141.x.
24. Gachon AM, Richard J, Dastugue B. Human tears: normal protein pattern and individual protein determinations in adults. Curr Eye Res. 1982;2(5):301–8. https://doi.org/10.3109/02713688209000774.
25. Davidson HJ, Gerlach JA, Bull RW. Determination of protein concentrations and their molecular weight in tears from cats with normal corneas and cats with corneal sequestrum. Am J Vet Res. 1992;53(10):1756–9.
26. Winiarczyk M, Winiarczyk D, Banach T, Adaszek L, Madany J, Mackiewicz J, et al. Dog tear film proteome in-depth analysis. PLoS One. 2015;10(12):e0144242. https://doi.org/10.1371/journal.pone.0144242.

Tartrate-resistant acid phosphate as biomarker of bone turnover over the lifespan and different physiologic stages in sheep

José A. Camassa[1], Camila C. Diogo[1], João P. A. Bordelo[1], Marília de A. Bonelli[2], Carlos A. Viegas[1,3], Jorge T. Azevedo[4,5], Nuno Dourado[6] and Isabel R. Dias[1,3*]

Abstract

Background: Currently, the best resources for assessment of bone tissue using imaging techniques are expensive and available in few medical facilities, thus serum or urinary bone turnover biomarkers could be useful as early indicators of prognosis. However, there is a wide range of variability in bone turnover markers due to several factors, such as different ages and metabolic stages, thus it is important to have as much data published on the subject as possible. The aim of this study was therefore to generate a reference range for alkaline phosphatase (ALP) and tartrate-resistant acid phosphatase (TRAP) and validate the already published data.

Results: Serum alkaline phosphatase decreased with age, with statistical difference between the 1 month old and the other groups and between the over 8 years and the 6 months old groups. There was also a statistical difference in the ALP levels between the 3 to 5 years old gestation and lactation groups. For serum tartrate-resistant acid phosphatase, there was a statistical difference mainly between the 1 month old and the 6 months old, 6–8 years old, and above 8 years old groups.

Conclusions: The results obtained could represent a useful tool for future studies using sheep as an animal model for orthopedic research. The different groups presented a wide variation of serum ALP and TRAP levels, however, these variations are entirely explained by known physiology. Therefore, this detailed study confirms the prediction that unexplained changes in these bone turnover markers do not occur during the lifespan of sheep.

Keywords: ALP, Bone tissue, Serum minerals, Sheep, Tartrate-resistant acid phosphatase

Background

Currently, skeletal and bone tissue assessment is performed by diagnostic imaging such as radiography, computed tomography, magnetic resonance and densitometry techniques, or invasive methods, such as bone biopsy, although these methods are still limited in many situations. Therefore, determination of the serum levels or urinary bone turnover biomarkers (BTMs) could be a good noninvasive analytical method for evaluation of bone metabolism, as it allows predicting bone cell activity in a quick and real time manner [1].

At present, some studies have been performed on BTMs in animal models for orthopedic research not only to improve the knowledge in animal and veterinary sciences, but also in human orthopedic research of metabolic bone diseases, such as post-menopausal osteoporosis. BTMs could be useful in diagnosing early-stage bone diseases, and helping to monitor evolution and efficiency of treatment.

BTMs are generally divided in two groups: the formation and the bone resorption markers, although there is a third group that is still poorly studied, the osteoclast

* Correspondence: idias@utad.pt
[1]Department of Veterinary Sciences, Agricultural and Veterinary Sciences School (ECAV), University of Trás-os-Montes and Alto Douro (UTAD), Quinta de Prados, P.O. Box 1013, 5001-801 Vila Real, Portugal
[3]CITAB – Centre for the Research and Technology of Agro-Environmental and Biological Sciences, UTAD, Vila Real, Portugal
Full list of author information is available at the end of the article

regulatory protein [2]. During the metabolic process of bone formation by osteoblasts, formation markers are represented by serum alkaline phosphatase (ALP) and its bone-specific isoform (BALP), serum osteocalcin, and two other molecules that are released during synthesis of the type I collagen molecule – serum procollagen type I carboxy- and amino-terminal propeptides [3].

The ALP is a glycoprotein that is connected to the surface of cells. In humans ALP are expressed in four gene loci code: nonspecific, intestinal, placental and germ cells [4]. Nonspecific gene is synthesized in a variety of tissues (bone, kidney, liver and early placenta) [4]. BALP has been used due to its high sensitivity as a bone formation marker [4]. It is produced by osteoblasts [5] and is involved in the calcification of bone matrix [6].

In the bone resorption process, there is a breakdown of type I collagen, so resorption markers are represented by serum C-terminal telopeptide of type I collagen, urinary collagen type I cross-linked C- and N-telopeptide, urinary hydroxyproline, total and free urinary pyridinoline and deoxypyridinoline, as well as by the serum tartrate-resistant acid phosphatase (TRAP), which is produced by active osteoclasts [7].

TRAP is a glycoprotein produced by mature osteoclasts, activated dendritic cells, and macrophages, therefore TRAP is an indicator of osteoclast and macrophage activity [8, 9]. There are two known isoforms (TRAP5a,b). TRAP5b is a specific biomarker of osteoclastic resorption activity, while TRAP5a is a non-osteoclastic form [10]. In the future, the latter may be useful in clinical evaluation since it is expressed in bone pathologies, such as fracture healing in different mammals or osteoporosis in women [9, 11, 12].

The use of sheep as animal models in orthopedic research, also in studies focusing on BTMs, is based on different aspects such as easy handling [13, 14] and possibility of blood sample collection several times per day [15] due to a high blood volume when compared to other laboratory animal species. Nevertheless, bone markers in small ruminants are influenced by circadian and seasonal variation [16], among other possible factors causing serum and urinary variability such as diet, exercise, skeletal growth, as well as intra-individual variability [4]. As such, BTMs undergo variations throughout a lifetime, namely with age and different metabolic states. It is therefore important to assess BTMs variation during these phases and establish a reference range for BTMs in this species, to which the greatest limitation is the inter-individual variability [17].

Therefore, the aim of this study was to generate a reference range for some of the main BTMs – ALP and TRAP, throughout the lifespan and different physiological states in sheep and to evaluate possible correlations of these parameters with serum minerals.

Methods

Animals

Ninety ewes (Churra-da-Terra-Quente sheep) from the same flock, located in Carrazeda de Ansiães, a municipality in the district of Bragança in northern Portugal were used. Average minimum temperature was 1.9 °C and average maximum temperature 10.2 °C in December at Bragança. Sheep were kept in a natural pasture during the day and housed overnight. The barn is easily approachable and spacious, dry, well-drained, well-ventilated and bedding composed by hay and straw. These animals were chosen among a flock according to their age or physiologic state and divided into 9 groups of 10 animals each. The groups were as follows: 1 month old (mean weight 9.3 kg), 6 months old (mean weight 22.2 kg), 1 year old (mean weight 40.7 kg), 2 years old (mean weight 50.2 kg), 3 to 5 years old dry (mean weight 52.4 kg), 3 to 5 years old with 2 or 3 months of pregnancy (mean weight 55.3 kg), 3 to 5 years old with 2 or 3 months of lactation (mean weight 51.5 kg), 6 to 8 years old (mean weight 52.1 kg), and the last group with animals over 8 years old (mean weight 48.1 kg). The diet was composed by grass hay, supplemented with 0.250 kg of concentrate feed per animal per day and water provided ad libitum. Dry matter and chemical composition of grass hay is made up of dry matter per kg feed (88.5 g), ash per kg dry matter (5.9 g), neutral detergent fiber per kg (73.3 g) dry matter and crude protein per kg dry matter (6.1 g). Dry matter and chemical composition of feed concentrate is made up of dry matter per kg feed (90.4 g), ash per kg dry matter (8.5 g), neutral detergent fiber per kg (31.6 g) dry matter and crude protein per kg dry matter (20.7 g).

All animal handling practices followed Directive 2010/63/EU of the European Parliament and of the Council on the protection of animals used for scientific purposes.

Blood sampling

Blood was drawn in December during the European winter. Blood samples were drawn from the jugular vein and placed into serological tubes (S-Monovette®, SARSTEDT, Nümbrecht, Germany). Samplings were performed between 9:00 a.m. and 10:00 a.m. and the blood carried in a thermal box to laboratory facilities immediately. Blood was centrifuged (3000 rpm for 10 min) and the serum stored in Eppendorf tubes at −20 °C until analyses.

Serum biochemical analysis

Following the manufacturer's instructions, the assays were always performed in duplicate to achieve higher accuracy.

Determination of ALP (Alkaline Phosphatase, Beckman Coulter, Ref. OSR6004, CA, USA) and TRAP (ACP, Ref. 17,617; Sentinel Diagnostics, Milan, Italy) were performed via an enzymatic method and molecular absorption spectrophotometry using commercially available kits. Calcium (Ca) (Calcium, Beckman Coulter, Ref. OSR60117, CA, USA), phosphorus (P) (Phosphorus, Beckman Coulter, Ref. OSR6122, CA, USA) and magnesium (Mg) (Magnesium, Beckman Coulter, Ref. OSR6189, CA, USA) were also determined using commercially available kits, via chemical method and molecular absorption spectrophotometry.

Statistical analysis

Statistical normality was checked using the Shapiro-Wilk W-Test for all groups. Serum BTMs and mineral values are presented as median ± interquartile range (IQR), minimum (Min) and maximum (Max). Spearman's correlation was obtained between the serum biochemical markers. The Kruskal - Wallis Test was used for testing the non-parametric statistical hypothesis and the Kruskal – Wallis pairwise method for multiple comparisons. Statistical analysis was performed using SPSS software (version 23.0, SPSS, Inc., IBM Company, NY, USA). The level of significance was set at $P < 0.05$.

Results

All parameters in this study revealed a non-normal distribution for age analysis. The median and interquartile range for each marker in different ages are shown in Table 1.

Figure 1a shows a significant difference between the 1 month old group and all the other groups, and a significant difference between animals of 6 months of age and over 8 years for ALP (Fig. 1). For TRAP, the 1 month old and 1 year old groups were the ones with a significant statistical difference from the other groups (Fig. 1b).

Calcium and phosphorus both suffer a slight decrease throughout the animal's life, with a statistical difference seen in the 1 month old and over 8 years old groups for Ca (Fig 1c), and 6 months old and 1 month old groups for P (Fig. 1d), with the latter showing a significant difference when compared to all other groups except the 6 months old group. Magnesium had a slight increase with age (Fig. 1e), with the most significant difference observed between the 1 month old group and the other groups. The degrees of correlation are shown in Table 2. The results expressed a fair correlation between markers, with the highest correlation observed between ALP and P ($r < 0.60$; $P < 0.01$).

In the analyses of the groups with animals between 3 and 5 years of age in different physiologic stages, ALP had a significant difference between the gestation and lactation groups (Fig. 2a) and TRAP (Fig. 2b) had a significant difference between the dry and lactation groups. Normality analyses of the groups with 3 to 5 years of age had a normal distribution for Ca and P (Fig. 2c and d), ALP, TRAP and Mg (Fig. 2e) had a non-normal

Table 1 Values of serum biochemical markers and serum minerals by ages

		Median ± IQR	Range (Min–Max)
ALP (U/L)	1 month	849.5 ± 270.7	520–1354
	6 months	269.5 ± 136.2	89–454
	1 year	220.0 ± 135.0	138–583
	2 years	200.5 ± 90.25	116–295
	3–5 years gestation	104.5 ± 116.0	66–350
	3–5 years lactation	330.5 ± 159.2	105–390
	3–5 years dry	181.0 ± 133.5	108–363
	6–8 years	197.0 ± 127.0	63–444
	>8 years	119.0 ± 177.0	35–277
TRAP (U/L)	1 month	3.15 ± 0.45	2.9–3.7
	6 months	2.65 ± 0.10	2.5–2.9
	1 year	3.10 ± 0.50	2.4–3.6
	2 years	2.95 ± 0.60	2.2–3.2
	3–5 years gestation	2.80 ± 0.25	2.6–3.0
	3–5 years lactation	2.55 ± 0.37	2.3–2.8
	3–5 years dry	2.80 ± 0.25	2.0–3.3
	6–8 years	2.50 ± 0.07	2.4–2.7
	>8 years	2.65 ± 0.47	1.6–3.3
Calcium (mmol/L)	1 month	2.83 ± 0.12	2.57–2.90
	6 months	2.59 ± 0.23	2.35–2.75
	1 year	2.63 ± 0.10	2.55–2.83
	2 years	2.53 ± 0.20	2.33–2.68
	3–5 years gestation	2.49 ± 0.16	2.18–2.68
	3–5 years lactation	2.49 ± 0.18	2.38–2.65
	3–5 years dry	2.54 ± 0.13	2.35–2.65
	6–8 years	2.61 ± 0.10	2.50–2.68
	>8 years	2.33 ± 0.21	1.85–2.48
Magnesium (mmol/L)	1 month	0.91 ± 0.07	0.78–1.03
	6 months	0.96 ± 0.04	0.96–1.04
	1 year	1.02 ± 0.14	0.92–1.29
	2 years	1.04 ± 0.09	0.95–1.12
	3–5 years gestation	1.08 ± 0.17	0.92–1.29
	3–5 years lactation	1.03 ± 0.03	1.02–1.08
	3–5 years dry	0.97 ± 0.07	0.93–1.13
	6–8 years	1.05 ± 0.13	0.89–1.32
	>8 years	1.12 ± 0.26	0.88–1.56
Phosphorous (mmol/L)	1 month	3.21 ± 0.27	3.10–3.52
	6 months	2.21 ± 0.53	1.06–2.87
	1 year	1.87 ± 0.46	1.58–2.29
	2 years	1.59 ± 0.25	1.23–1.81
	3–5 years gestation	1.42 ± 0.63	1.13–1.98
	3–5 years lactation	1.45 ± 0.30	1.16–1.81
	3–5 years dry	1.36 ± 0.24	0.90–1.90
	6–8 years	1.56 ± 0.36	1.10–2.06
	>8 years	1.64 ± 0.05	1.06–2.42

ALP: alkaline phosphatase; TRAP: tartrate-resistant acid phosphatase; IQR: interquartile range; Min: minimum; Max: maximum

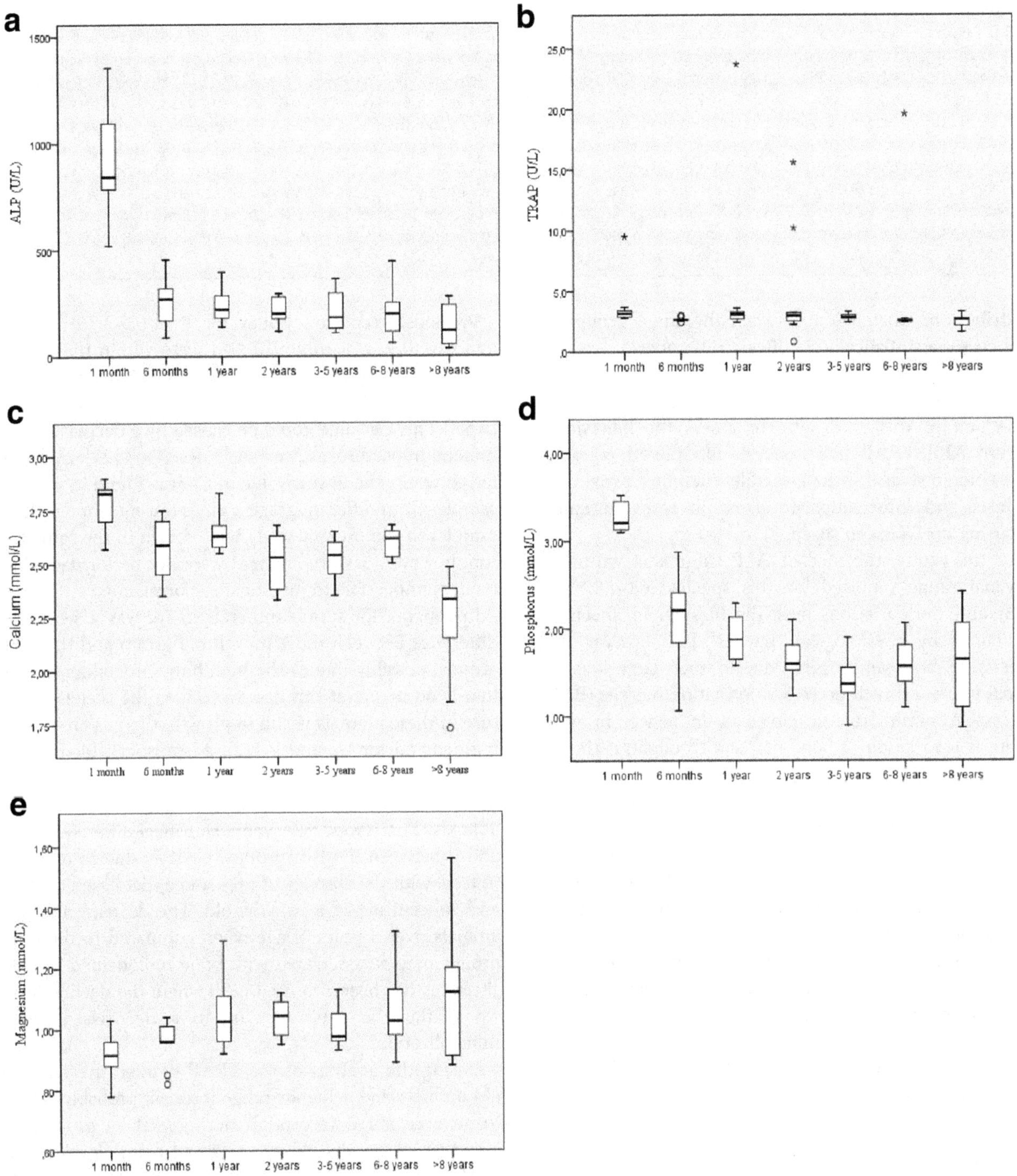

Fig. 1 (See legend on next page.)

(See figure on previous page.)
Fig. 1 Box plot presentations of serum concentrations of biomarkers of bone metabolism by age. **a** Serum ALP activity presented significant difference between 1 month vs. 6 months ($P < 0.01$), between 1 month vs. 1 year, 2 years, 3–5 years, 6–8 years and >8 years ($P < 0.001$), between 6 months vs. >8 years ($P < 0.05$). **b** Serum TRAP activity presented significant difference between 1 month vs. 6 months, >8 years ($P < 0.01$), between 1 month vs. 6–8 years ($P < 0.001$), between 1 year vs. 6 months, >8 years ($P < 0.05$), between 1 year vs. 6–8 years ($P < 0.01$), between 2 years vs. 6–8 years ($P < 0.05$). **c** Serum calcium activity presented significant difference between 1 month vs. 6 months, 6–8 years ($P < 0.05$), between 1 month vs. 2 years and 3–5 years ($P < 0.01$), between 1 month vs. >8 years ($P < 0.001$), between >8 years vs. 2 years and 3–5 years ($P < 0.05$), between >8 years vs. 6 month and 6–8 years ($P < 0.01$) and between >8 years vs. 1 year ($P < 0.001$). **d** Serum ALP activity presented significant difference between 1 month vs. 6 months ($P < 0.05$), between 1 month vs. 1 year ($P < 0.01$), between 1 month vs. 2 years, 3–5 years, 6–8 years and >8 years ($P < 0.001$), between 6 months vs. 2 years, 3–5 years, 6–8 years and >8 years ($P < 0.05$) and between 1 year vs. 3–5 year ($P < 0.05$). **e** Serum Magnesium activity presented significant difference between 1 month vs. 3–5 years ($P < 0.05$) and between 1 month vs. 1 year, 2 years, 6–8 years and >8 years ($P < 0.01$). Outliers are identified with small circle for out values and star for extreme values

distribution. Correlation between the three groups did not reveal a statistically significant difference.

Discussion

The aim of this study was to assess the behavior of serum ALP, TRAP, and minerals in different ages and physiologic stages of the ewes life, therefore providing a dataset and information to assist in research studies focusing on BTMs in sheep.

In this study, the median ALP value was within the normal range reported for this species (68–387 U/L) [18] and the variations over the lifespan in sheep can explained by physiological changes. The interval range was wide, however, possibly due to such factors as seasonal influence, with decreased formation marker (BALP) during Autumn [16], or circadian influence, in which there is a variation of bone markers throughout the day. Because of the latter, blood samples sampling must be drawn at a standardized time [15]. Age was another influencing factor, with a higher level of ALP found in 1-month old animals, possibly due to synthesis in a variety of tissues, not only due to the bone isoenzyme [4], and high juvenile metabolism [19]. Lower levels of ALP were found in sheep over 8 years of age, possibly due to the influence of age in decreasing bone formation. In another study, Haversian remodelling in the caudal aspect of the femur, diaphysis of the radius and humerus was observed in sheep between 7 and 9 years of age [20], which justifies a link between advanced age and bone loss.

Table 2 Correlation between serum biochemical markers and serum minerals

	ALP	TRAP	Ca	P	Mg
ALP	-	$r = 0.44^b$	$r = 0.514^b$	$r = 0.581^b$	$r = 0.229$
TRAP	-	-	$r = 0.379^b$	$r = 0.261^a$	$r = -0.066$
Ca	-	-	-	$r = 0.492^b$	$r = -0.322^b$
P	-	-	-	-	$r = -0.289^a$
Mg	-	-	-	-	-

[a]*correlation* coefficient is *significant* at the *0.05* level
[b]*correlation* coefficient is *significant* at the *0.01* level

Previously reported values for P (1.62–3.36 mmol/L) and Mg (0.9–1.31 mmol/L) [18] were within the interval found in the present study, although Ca levels (2.88–3.2 mmol/L) [18] were higher in the aforementioned paper. This Ca value could be caused by a decrease in this mineral in pasture, as previously described [21]. In the referred works the lowest value of Ca was found in different samples from different grazing areas during Winter. Blood samples in the present study were drawn in the same season, however, pasture analyses were not performed which renders impossible to investigate a correlation.

In general, for serum minerals, there was a significant difference between the 1 month old group and the other groups, possibly due to the high bone modelling process that is occurring at this age. In fact, as the skeletal structure in these animals is still in growth, there is an increasing demand for Ca and P [22]. A statistical difference in serum minerals between 1-month-old and 6-months-old groups was not expected since both groups have growing animals. There was, however, a statistical difference in Ca and P between the two groups, possibly due to a change in feed, with the absence of milk and a diet based on grass and concentrate at 6 months old. The decrease in Ca in animals over 8 years of age when compared to the other groups may be associated with bone remodelling in older sheep, as has been reported [20], where the decline in Ca would thus be expected due to a decrease in bone mineralization.

During the analysis of the TRAP marker, the 1-month old animals had a higher range interval, probably related to an accelerated resorption during skeletal growth [9]. However, 6-months-old animals had a low level of this marker even though the sheep were undergoing skeletal growth, possibly because of a difference in diet, as previously mentioned. This marker showed an inversely proportional relationship with age, thus the animals with 6 to 8 years of age had lower values among all the groups. However, those over 8 years old had an increased TRAP, possibly due to osteoclastic activity [9] in geriatric animals. An explanation for this increase has not been investigated in this study in older sheep. Nevertheless, in older women, it is associated to osteoporosis [23]. Therefore, there may

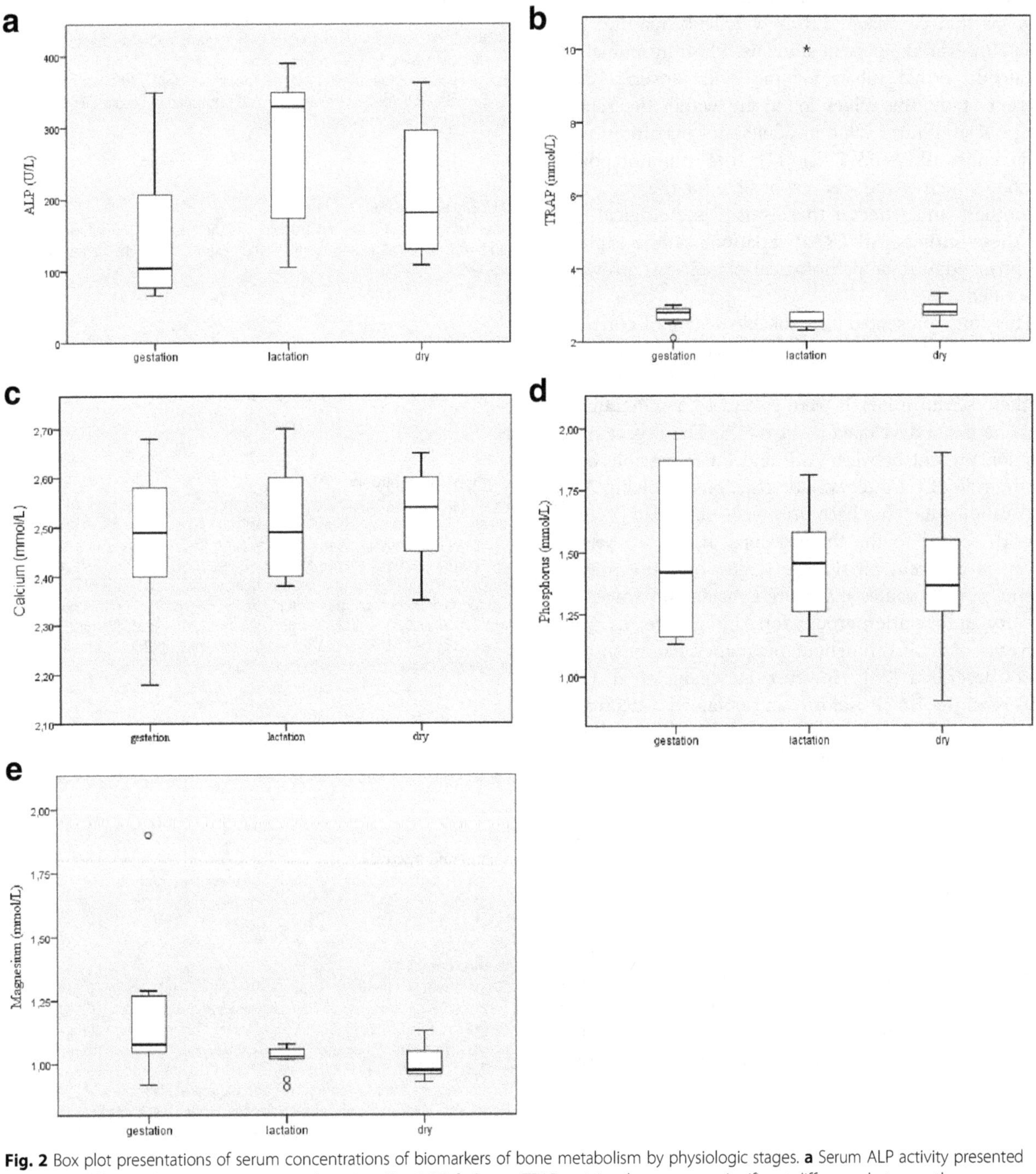

Fig. 2 Box plot presentations of serum concentrations of biomarkers of bone metabolism by physiologic stages. **a** Serum ALP activity presented significant difference between gestation vs. lactation ($P < 0.05$). **b** Serum TRAP activity, there was no significant difference between the groups. **c** Serum Calcium activity, there was no significant difference between the groups. **d** Serum Phosphorus activity, there was no significant difference between the groups. **e** Serum Magnesium activity, there was no significant difference between the groups. Outliers are identified with small circle for out values and star for extreme values

be an osteopenia in old animals related to an increase of this marker, but analyses of the bone, such as bone densitometry, would be necessary to prove that.

It should also be mentioned that the ideal TRAP markers to assess bone metabolism should determine the TRAP5b isoform by itself, since it has an osteoclastic origin, resulting from resorption activity, whereas the TRAP5a isoform is nonosteoclastic [24]. The occurrence of seven outliers (three in 6 months old, one in the 2 years and three in 8 years old group) in the determination of TRAP could be justified in this study by the marker being expressed in different tissues, such as muscles and heart, or pathological conditions. There are published studies in humans that correlated TRAP with leukemia and AIDS [25]. However, the present study used healthy animals and obtained normal values for the ovine species. In the present study, the values found are within the reported range of minimum value in adults and maximum values in juveniles (0,14–5,9 U/L) [11]. It is thus not possible to state which tissue was responsible for the occurrence of outliers and whether there was a pathological cause for these outliers. All TRAP variations can be explained by physiological or pathological changes as previously described.

This study presented a reasonable degree of correlation between P and Ca, previously described in sheep as being involved in bone mineralization [26]. In rats, the increase of these serum minerals were essential for mineralization of bone tissue developed in vitro [27]. The degree of correlation present between ALP and Ca is possibly caused by the role of Ca in enzymatic reactions involving ALP, a correlation which has been previously described [3, 12].

With regard to the three groups of 3- to 5-year old sheep in different physiologic stages, only the pregnant group showed values that were considerably lower than the dry and lactation groups for ALP analyses. A similar increase of ALP throughout pregnancy has been previously described [28]. However, Liesegang et al. (2006) [29] used the BALP isoform and obtained a decrease of the marker during gestation. Therefore, when the animals become pregnant, there is a significant reduction of ALP, which then increases between gestation and lactation, and is slightly decreased in dry sheep [28]. In this study, the same marker variation was observed among the three described physiologic states, as has been previously described. However, during the analysis of TRAP, the lactating group showed lower values when compared to the dry ones. This could be due to the abrupt drop in bone resorption during the 2 to 3 months of lactation, with values going back to basal values in dry animals. Another greatly important factor would be that the maximum peak of TRAP would occur closer to parturition, as described [28].

Conclusions

This study provided information on the variation of two of the most used BTMs – ALP and TRAP, throughout the different stages of life and metabolic stages in sheep. These bone turnover markers variations can be entirely explained by known physiology, confirming that unexplained changes do not occur during the lifespan of sheep. This information may be a useful tool in clinical orthopedic research studies both in animal and veterinary sciences, as well as when using sheep as an animal model for translational studies for humans.

Abbreviations

ALP: Alkaline phosphatase.; BALP: Bone-specific isoform alkaline phosphatase.; BTMs: Bone turnover biomarkers.; Ca: Calcium; IQR: Interquartile range; Kg: Kilogram; Max: Maximum; Mg: Magnesium; Min: Minimum; P: Phosphorus; rpm: Revolutions per minute; TRAP5a: Tartrate-resistant acid phosphatase isoform 5a; TRAP5b: Tartrate-resistant acid phosphatase isoform 5b; TRAP: Tartrate-resistant acid phosphatase

Acknowledgements

José Arthur de A. Camassa acknowledges the National Council for Scientific and Technological Development (CNPq - Brazil) for his PhD scholarship 202248/2015-1.

Funding

National Council for Scientific and Technological Development (CNPq - Brazil) PhD scholarship 202248/2015–1.

Authors' contributions

All authors of this paper have read and approved the final version of the manuscript submitted, they also agree to be accountable for all aspects of the work in ensuring that questions relating to the accuracy or integrity of any part of the work ate appropriately investigated and resolved and all of them have made substantive contributions to the work, namely: Substantially contributed to conception or design (JA, CC, CA, ND, IR). Contributed to acquisition, analysis, or interpretation of data (JA, CC, JP, MA, JT, IR). Drafted the manuscript (JA, CC, IR). Critically revised the manuscript for important intellectual content (JP, MA, JT, CA, ND, IR).

Consent for publication

Not applicable.

Competing interests

The authors declare that they have no competing interests.

Author details

[1]Department of Veterinary Sciences, Agricultural and Veterinary Sciences School (ECAV), University of Trás-os-Montes and Alto Douro (UTAD), Quinta de Prados, P.O. Box 1013, 5001-801 Vila Real, Portugal. [2]Federal Rural University of Pernambuco (UFRPE), R. Dom Manoel de Medeiros, s/n, Dois Irmãos, Recife, PE 52171-900, Brazil. [3]CITAB – Centre for the Research and Technology of Agro-Environmental and Biological Sciences, UTAD, Vila Real, Portugal. [4]Department of Animal Sciences, ECAV, UTAD, Vila Real, Portugal. [5]CECAV – Centre for Animal Sciences and Veterinary Studies, UTAD, Vila Real, Portugal. [6]CMEMS-UMinho, Department of Mechanical Engineering, University of Minho, Campus de Azurém, 4804-533 Guimarães, Portugal.

References

1. Allen MJ. Biochemical markers of bone metabolism in animals: uses and limitations. Vet Clin Pathol. 2003;32:101–13.
2. Baharuddin NA, Coates DE, Cullinan M, Seymour G, Duncan W. Localization of rank, rankl and osteoprotegerin during healing of surgically created periodontal defects in sheep. J Periodont Res. 2015;50:211–9.
3. Dias IR, Viegas CA, Azevedo JT, Costa EM, Lourenco P, Rodrigues A, Cabrita AS. Assessment of markers of bone formation under controlled environmental factors and their correlation with serum minerals in adult sheep as a model for orthopaedic research. Lab Anim. 2008;42:465–72.

4. Cremers S, Garnero P, Seibel MJ. Biochemical markers of bone metabolism. In: Bilezikian JP, Raisz LG, Martin TJ, editors. Bone biology. San Diego: Academic Press; 2008. p. 1857–81.
5. Millan JL. Alkaline Phosphatases: structure, substrate specificity and functional relatedness to other members of a large superfamily of enzymes. Purinergic Signal. 2006;2:335–41.
6. Masrour Roudsari J, Mahjoub S. Quantification and comparison of bone-specific alkaline phosphatase with two methods in normal and paget's specimens. Caspian J Intern Med. 2012;3:478–83.
7. Seibel MJ. Nutrition and molecular markers of bone remodelling. Curr Opin Clin Nutr Metab Care. 2002;5:525–31.
8. Schleicher I, Lips KS, Sommer U, Schappat I, Martin AP, Szalay G, Hartmman S, Schnettler R. Biphasic scaffolds for repair of deep osteochondral defects in a sheep model. J Surg Res. 2013;183:184–92.
9. Leeming DJ, Alexandersen P, Karsdal MA, Qvist P, Schaller S, Tanko LB. An update on biomarkers of bone turnover and their utility in biomedical research and clinical practice. Eur J Clin Pharmacol. 2006;62:781–92.
10. Halleen JM, Alatalo SL, Suominem H, Cheng S, Janckila AJ, Väänänen HK. Tartrate-resistant acid phosphatase 5b: a novel serum marker of bone resorption. J Bone Miner Res. 2000;15:1337–45.
11. Seebeck P, Bail HJ, Exner C, Schell H, Michel R, Amthauer H, Bragulla H, Duda GN. Do serological tissue turnover markers represent callus formation during fracture healing? Bone. 2005;37:669–77.
12. Sousa C, Abreu H, Viegas C, Azevedo J, Reis R, Gomes ME, Dias I. Serum total and bone alkaline phosphatase and tartrate-resistant acid phosphatase activities for the assessment of bone fracture healing in dogs. Arq Bras Med Vet Zootec. 2011;63:1007–11.
13. O'Loughlin PF, Morr S, Bogunovic L, Kim AD, Park B, Lane JM. Selection and development of preclinical models in fracture-healing research. J Bone Joint Surg Am. 2008;90:79–84.
14. Reichert JC, Saifzadeh S, Wullschleger ME, Epari DR, Schutz MA, Duda GN, Schell H, van GM RH, Hutmacher DW. The challenge of establishing preclinical models for segmental bone defect research. Biomaterials. 2009; 30:2149–63.
15. Liesegang A, Sassi M-L, Risteli J. Diurnal variation in concentrations of various markers of bone metabolism in growing female goats and sheep. Anim Sci. 2003;77:197–203.
16. Arens D, Sigrist I, Alini M, Schawalder P, Schneider E, Egermann M. Seasonal changes in bone metabolism in sheep. Vet J. 2007;174:585–91.
17. Souberbielle JC, Cormier C, Kindermans C. Bone markers in clinical practice. Curr Opin Rheumatol. 1999;11:312–9.
18. Kahn CM. Reference guides: the Merck veterinary manual. 10th ed. New Jersey: Whitehouse Station; 2010.
19. Chai J, Diao Q, Wang H, Tu Y, Tao X, Zhang N. Effects of weaning age on growth, nutrient digestibility and metabolism, and serum parameters in Hu lambs. Animal Nutrition. 2015;1:344–8.
20. Newman E, Turner AS, Wark JD. The potential of sheep for the study of osteopenia: current status and comparison with other animal models. Bone. 1995;16:277–84.
21. Metson AJ, Saunders WMH. Seasonal variations in chemical composition D of pasture. New Zeal J Agr Res. 1978;21:341–53.
22. Clarke B. Normal bone anatomy and physiology. Clin J Am Soc Nephrol. 2008;3:S131–9.
23. Blumer MJ, Hausott B, Schwarzer C, Hayman AR, Stempel J, Fritsch H. Role of tartrate-resistant acid phosphatase (TRAP) in long bone development. Mech Dev. 2012;129:162–76.
24. Halleen JM, Ylipahkala H, Alatalo SL, Janckila AJ, Heikkinen JE, Suominen H, Cheng S, Väänänen HK. Serum tartrate-resistant acid phosphatase 5b, but not 5a, correlates with other markers of bone turnover and bone mineral density. Calcif Tissue Int. 2002;1:20–5.
25. Hayman AR, Bune AJ, Bradley JR, Rashbass J, Cox TM. Osteoclastic tartrate-resistant acid phosphatase (Acp 5): its localization to dendritic cells and diverse murine tissues. J Histochem Cytochem. 2000;48:219–28.
26. Sousa CP, Azevedo JT, Silva AM, Viegas CA, Reis RL, Gomes ME, Dias IR. Serum total and bone alkaline phosphatase levels and their correlation with serum minerals over the lifespan of sheep. Acta Vet Hung. 2014; 62:205–14.
27. Chang YL, Stanford CM, Keller JC. Calcium and phosphate supplementation promotes bone cell mineralization: implications for hydroxyapatite (HA)-enhanced bone formation. J Biomed Mater Res. 2000;52:270–8.
28. Khatun A, Wani GM, Bhat JIA, Choudhury AR, Khan MZ. Biochemical indices in sheep during different stages of pregnancy. Asian J Anim Vet Adv. 2011; 6:175–81.
29. Liesegang A, Risteli J, Wanner M. The effects of first gestation and lactation on bone metabolism in dairy goats and milk sheep. Bone. 2006;38:794–802.

20

The effect of storage at ambient temperature on the feline fecal microbiota

Moran Tal[1], Adronie Verbrugghe[1*], Diego E. Gomez[2,3], Charlotte Chau[1] and J. Scott Weese[2]

Abstract

Background: Feline fecal microbiota analyses can potentially be impacted by a variety of factors such as sample preparation, sequencing method and bioinformatics analyses. Another potential influence is changes in the microbiota from storage of samples prior to processing. This study examined the effect of ambient temperature exposure on the feline fecal microbiota composition.

Fecal samples were collected from 12 healthy cats, within 15 min after defecation. Samples were aliquoted and the first aliquot was frozen at −80 °C within 1 hour of defecation. Remaining aliquots were maintained at ambient temperature (20 to 23 °C) and frozen at −80 °C at 6, 12, 24, 36, 48, 72 and 96 h after collection. DNA was extracted from all aliquots, and polymerase chain reaction (PCR). The PCR products were sequenced with next-generation sequencing (Illumina MiSeq).

Results: No significant differences were observed in alpha and beta biodiversity indexes, as well as relative abundance of different taxa over time ($P > 0.05$ for all tests between time points). Principal coordinate analyses demonstrated that samples cluster mainly by cat, with no significant differences between time points (AMOVA, $P > 0.05$; HOMOVA, $P > 0.05$). Linear discriminant analysis effect size method was performed and failed to detect any enriched taxa, between time points. Random forest algorithm analysis indicated homogeneity across time points.

Conclusions: Although existing evidence from human fecal storage studies is contradictory, a recent study in companion animals agreed with the current study, demonstrating that maintenance of feline fecal samples at ambient temperature for up to 4 days has no effect on the bacterial membership and structure.

Keywords: Gastrointestinal, Fecal, Microbiota, Storage, Temperature, Ambient

Background

The human gastrointestinal (GI) microbial community (the 'microbiota') is extremely complex in composition, and very high in concentration, reaching 10^{12}–10^{14} cell/g of intestinal content. The microbiota is dominated by bacteria, but also consists of Archaea, viruses, fungi and parasites. The bacterial concentration progresses from the stomach to the colon, with the highest concentration found in the colon [1–4]. Similar numbers are found in dogs and cats, although composition and bacterial species dominance are different from humans [5, 6]. Increased evidence exists in humans and companion animals for the health implications and clinical importance of the commensal or symbiotic relationship between the intestinal bacteria and their host. The intestinal microbiota plays a crucial role in the development of the host immune system, protection against pathogens, toxins and mutagens and utilization of excess nutrients or nutrients that are unavailable to the host [7]. The microbiota produces short chain fatty acids (SCFAs) that serve as energy sources to the colonocytes, produces vitamins, and aids in mineral absorption and intestinal integrity, along with a myriad of other effects, many of which remain to be properly defined [5, 8, 9].

Any deviation from the 'normal' microbiota is referred to as intestinal dysbiosis [5, 10]. In humans, animal models and companion animals, dysbiosis can be associated with a range of disease states, particularly inflammation [11–14]. Alterations of the normal gut microbiota balance [15, 16], due to inherent, environmental or immunological factors can be involved in the pathogenesis of intestinal inflammatory diseases [11, 17–

* Correspondence: averbrug@uoguelph.ca
[1]Department of Clinical Studies, Ontario Veterinary College, University of Guelph, Guelph, ON N1G 2W1, Canada
Full list of author information is available at the end of the article

19], or with other organ-related diseases, such as diabetes mellitus, obesity or asthma [2, 20–22].

In order to characterize the human or animal microbiota, a variety of methods can be used. In the past, the use of bacterial cultivation techniques dominated, but results are limited because of the inability to grow a large percentage of the microbiota using standard culture methods [23, 24]. Recently developed high-throughput techniques, such as Illumina MiSeq, are capable of quick massive parallel sequencing, providing more into-depth understanding of human and companion animal microbiome, and are considered as the preferred analytical method nowadays [25].

Aside to the effects of DNA extraction methods [26] or molecular tools, fecal sampling technique and sample storage conditions can potentially influence phylogenetic identification. The effects of different sampling and storage methods on the fecal bacterial population of healthy and diseased human subjects were examined [27]. Fecal samples were aliquoted within 10 min of defecation and stored at different temperatures: -80 °C, at -20 °C for a week, at +4 °C for 24 h and at ambient temperature for 24 h. No significant differences were found in the number of operational taxonomic units (OTUs), diversity or richness between the different storage temperatures [27]. This study agreed with the results of previous studies [28], but is in contradiction with others, that reported a mild gradual difference in the fecal bacterial composition when samples were stored at ambient temperature for 24 h compared to the composition assessed around defecation [29, 30]. Studies evaluating the impact of storage conditions on fecal microbiota in companion animals are scarce. One study in dogs and cats identified limited change in the microbiota from short term (<2 week) refrigeration [31]. However, the impact of room temperature storage was not assessed. This is an important aspect to understand for field studies, particularly of species such as cats. Fecal collections for microbiota-related studies in client-owned cats are often challenging, as significant time may pass between defecation, sample collection, and submission for analyses. During this time the sample may be left at room temperature (e.g. overnight in the litter box) before proper storage. The objective of this study was to determine the effect of ambient temperature exposure on the feline fecal microbiota.

Methods

Sample collection

Fresh fecal samples were collected from 12 healthy cats located at a cat boarding facility in Guelph, Ontario from June to July 2016. The subjects were determined to be healthy based on information provided to the facility manager by cat owners prior to boarding. Cats were observed closely by facility personnel and fecal samples were collected within 15 min of defecation. Samples were maintained unrefrigerated until arrival at the laboratory. Upon arrival, samples were weighed,[1] manually homogenized and aliquoted into 200 mg samples. One aliquot was frozen at −80 °C within 1 hour of defecation (time point (T) 0). The remaining aliquots were kept at ambient temperature (20 to 23 °C) in a biosafety cabinet.[2] Aliquots were frozen at −80 °C at the following time points: 6, 12, 24, 36, 48, 72, 96 h. Downstream processing was then performed on samples that had all undergone the same freeze-thaw cycle and were processed as a batch.

DNA extraction

For DNA extraction, a commercial stool extraction kit[3] was used according to the manufacturer's instructions. The DNA was collected in 1.5 ml micro-centrifuge tubes, and stored at −80 °C until further analysis.

Polymerase chain reaction (PCR)

The quantity of extracted DNA was assessed using a spectrophotometer,[4] with readings ranging from 33 to 661 ng/ml. To prepare the 16S rRNA gene amplicons for the Illumina MiSeq system,[5] all DNA samples were diluted (if needed) to a range of 30 to 100 ng/ml. The V4 region of the 16S rRNA gene was amplified using the forward primer S-D-Bact-0564-a-S-15 (5′-AYTGGGYDTAAAGNG-3′), reverse primer S-D-Bact-0785-b-A-18 (5′-TACNVGGGTATCTAATCC-3′), KAPA HiFi ReadyMix,[6] and PCR grade water. The PCR cycles were conducted in a thermal cycler.[7] The purified PCR products were evaluated with 1.5% agarose gel for gel electrophoresis and DNA was measured using spectrophotometry.

DNA sequencing

Using an Illumina MiSeq system, the samples were amplified by bridge amplification and sequenced with terminator nucleotides [32]. At least 100,000 reads/sample with sequences of approximately 500 bp in length from 2 × 250 paired end reads were obtained [32].

Bioinformatics analyses and statistics

Mothur v1.36.1 was used for bioinformatics analyses, as well as some of the statistical analyses [33, 34]. Additional statistical analyses were performed using JMP 13.0.[8] Paired end reads were assembled and filtered to remove sequences greater than 250 base pairs (bp) in length. Sequences with any ambiguous base calls or runs of homopolymers greater than 8 bp were removed. Sequences were aligned to the Silva16S rRNA reference database [35], and those that did not align with the correct region were removed. In addition, chimeras were identified using uchime [36] and removed. Sequences were classified using the RDP classifier (v14) [37], and those taxonomic assignments were used to create OTUs using a closed (database-dependent) OTU picking approach. Archeae were removed. Subsampling was performed based on the smallest number of sequences from a sample, to standardize sequence number used for analysis [38].

Alpha-diversity indexes (Shannon diversity [39], Simpson diversity [40] and Chao1 [41]) were calculated to assess evenness, diversity and richness, respectively, and compared between time points using a nonparametric multiple comparisons test (Wilcoxon Each Pair). Relative abundances were calculated for the different taxonomic levels, at each time point. Differences in relative abundance of taxa accounting for ≥1% of sequences within phyla and ≥0.1% within genera were evaluated using nonparametric multiple comparison test (Wilcoxon Each Pair), with *p*-values adjusted using the Benjamini-Hochberg correction to control for the false discovery rate [42]. Beta-diversity was assessed, using the classical Jaccard index [43] and Yue & Clayton index of dissimilarity [44] to examine community membership and population structure, respectively. For visualisation of differences in membership and structure between cats and time points, dendrograms were created, and significance of clustering according to time point was determined using parsimony and unifrac unweighted [45]. Beta-diversity was visualized using principal coordinate analyses (PCoA) and further assessed using analysis of molecular variance (AMOVA) and homogeneity of molecular variance (HOMOVA). Linear discriminatory analysis (LDA) effective size (LefSe) [46] was conducted as well for the identification of genomic features between time points. Random forest algorithm analysis was used to assess the ability to predict group classification, by cat or by time point [47].

Results

Ninety-three samples were processed from the 12 cats. Three aliquots (two at T96, and one at T72) were not obtained due to small fecal samples size from two cats. A total of 9,118,609 sequences passed all filters, with a median of 93,909 sequences per sample, and a range of 50,315 to 207,127 sequences per sample. A random subsample of 50,315 sequences per sample was used to normalize samples for analysis.

There were no significant differences in evenness, diversity and richness between the different time points (all $P > 0.05$) (Fig. 1). Median bacterial relative abundance accounting for ≥1% of phyla and ≥0.1% of genera, are presented in Figs. 2 and 3 respectively. No significant differences in relative abundances were noted at any taxonomic level (all adjusted $P > 0.05$). There was a numerical decrease in *Megasphaera* (Fig. 3); however, this was not statistically significant (unadjusted $P = 0.06$, adjusted $P = 0.81$).

No differences in community membership (Classical Jaccard index – unifrac $P = 0.74$; parsimony $P > 0.05$ for all comparisons) or population structure (Yue & Clayton – unifrac $P = 0.83$; parsimony $P > 0.05$ for all comparisons) were observed. Clustering by cat, but not time point, was apparent on the dendrograms for both community membership and structure (Fig. 4). Principal coordinate analyses indicated that fecal microbiota mainly clustered by cat, with no significant differences in community membership (Fig. 5a and b) or structure between time points (AMOVA $P > 0.05$ and HOMOVA $P > 0.05$ for all comparisons).

Linear discriminant analysis (LDA) effect size (LEfSe) analysis failed to identify enriched taxa between time points. Random forest algorithm analysis was performed both to evaluate the ability to differentiate between time points and between cats. When random forest was analysed according to time point, 92% error rate was established, indicating homogeneity across time points, and a very poor ability to separate samples into their appropriate groups. However, when "cat" was analysed as the group, the error rate was only 15%, indicating a much stronger ability to assign samples to the appropriate cat.

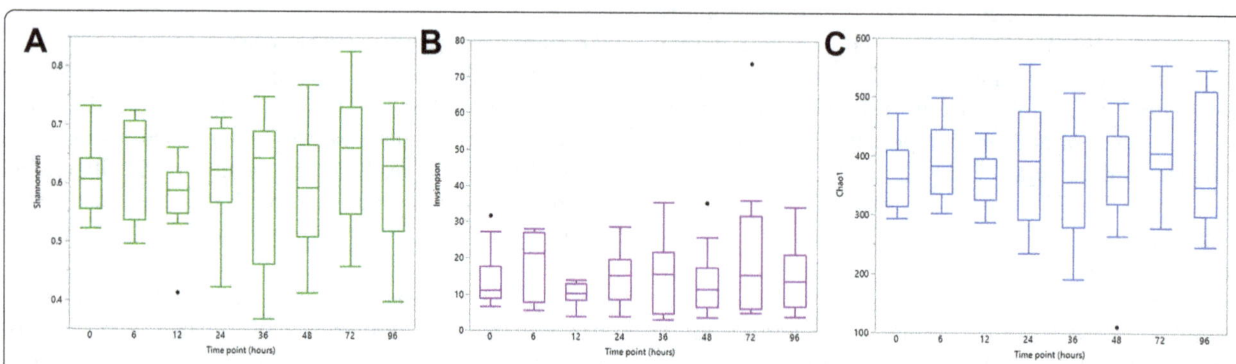

Fig. 1 Comparison of fecal bacterial population evenness (**a**), diversity (**b**) and richness (**c**) in 12 healthy cats between time points 0, 6, 12, 24, 36, 48, 72 and 96 h

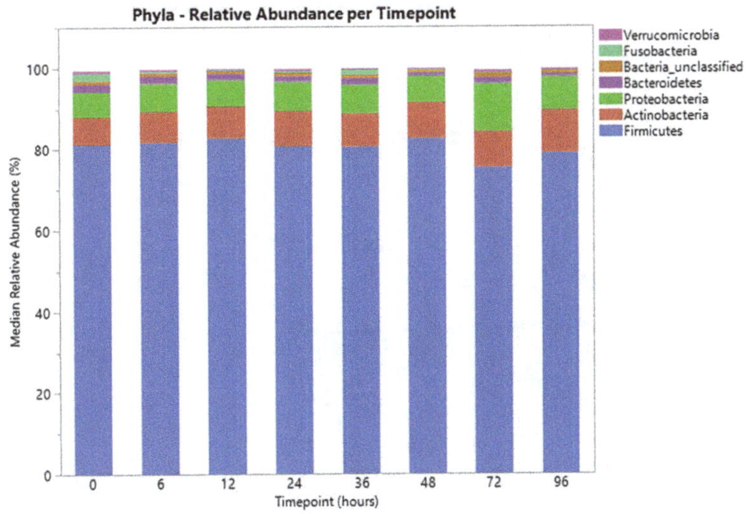

Fig. 2 Comparison of median relative abundances of predominant phyla originating from fecal samples of 12 healthy cats, between time points 0, 6, 12, 24, 36, 48, 72 and 96 h

Discussion

The results from the study imply that there are no significant changes in feline fecal microbiota evenness, diversity and richness, as well as community membership and structure over 96 h, while fecal samples are kept at ambient temperature.

Microbiota assessment in feline fecal samples can provide important insight. However, multiple variables can impact the results. It is important to understand potential external influences or biases that might affect the ability to properly define the microbiota and detect true biological differences. The potential impact of sample storage is one potential concern, particularly in studies that involve collection of samples from the community and inherent delays until processing. Understanding the potential influences of sample storage is important for proper design and interpretation of studies.

A variety of ecological indices can be used to assess microbial biodiversity. Despite the use of a range of methods, including assessment of relative abundances and alpha and beta diversity indices, no significant impact of storage on the fecal microbiota was identified. In addition to statistical analyses, clear numerical, non-statistically significant, differences were evident. While

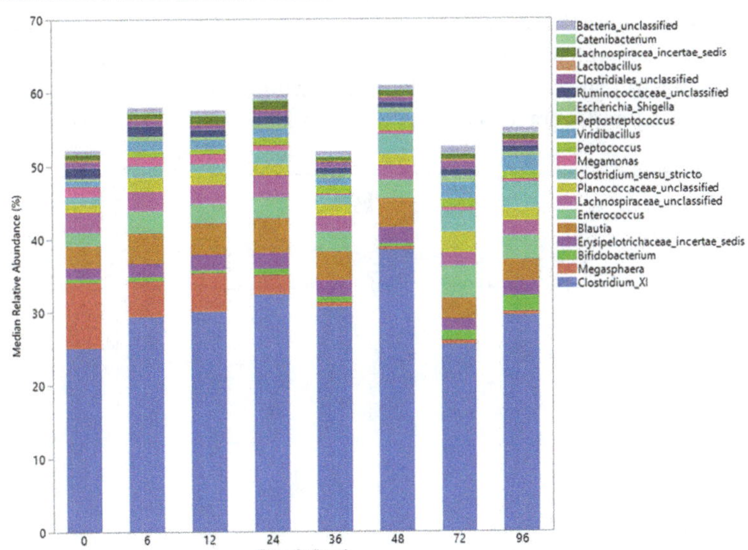

Fig. 3 Comparison of median relative abundances of predominant genera originating from fecal samples of 12 healthy cats, between time points 0, 6, 12, 24, 36, 48, 72 and 96 h

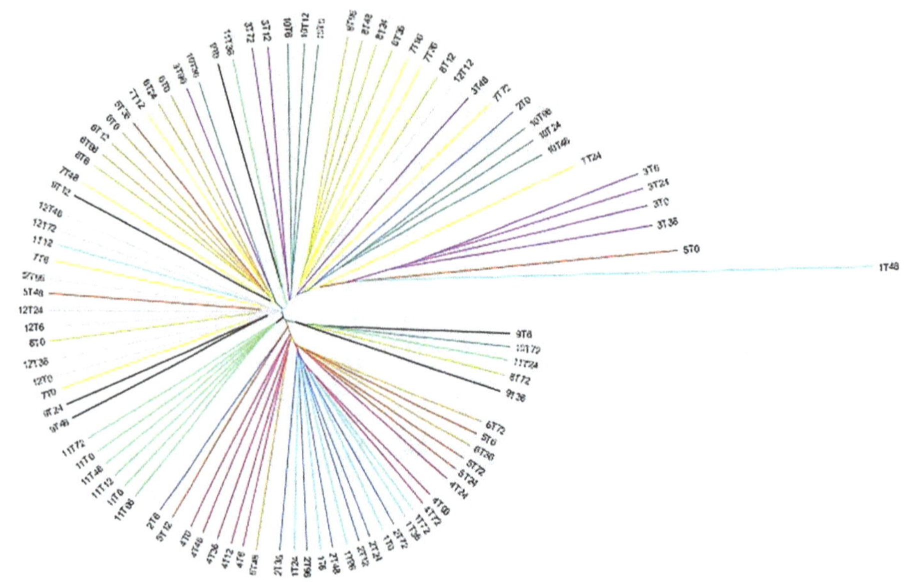

Fig. 4 Dendrogram of the Classical Jaccard index representing the community membership of the fecal microbiota in 12 healthy cats, compared between time points 0, 6, 12, 24, 36, 48, 72 and 96 h. Each cat is represented with a different colour

care must be taken when considering any non-significant results, these results should not be completely dismissed as statistical differences can be clouded by the degree of inter-sample variation and power limitations. The most readily apparent numerical difference was a decrease in the relative abundance over time of *Megasphaera,* a genus of relatively fastidious anaerobes [48]. Therefore, the trend for decreased *Megasphaera* abundance over time could correspond to air exposure during storage, something that might have been accentuated by manual homogenization during preparation of fecal samples. However, since the methods used in this study do not depend on viable microorganisms, it is unclear whether poor aerotolerance can accurately explain these results. *Megasphaera* was shown to play a dominant role in bacterial composition of the feline GI tract [49]. It is associated with ruminal fermentation of lactate into short-chain fatty acids (SCFA), and is especially related to butyrate formation [50]. Due to its fermentation capacity, the bacterium was shown to have beneficial effects on the GI health of some monogastric mammals [51, 52]. However, further research is required for the understanding of the underlined role of *Megasphaera* in the cat, an obligate carnivore [49], especially when increased protein content may promote a steep decrease in *Megasphaera* abundance, as well as jeopardise the GI microbiota health [53].

While the extent of studies investigating the impact of storage on feline fecal microbiota has been limited, the results of this study are similar to other studies that have shown limited or no impact of short-term storage. One study investigated the effect of storage at 4 °C on fecal

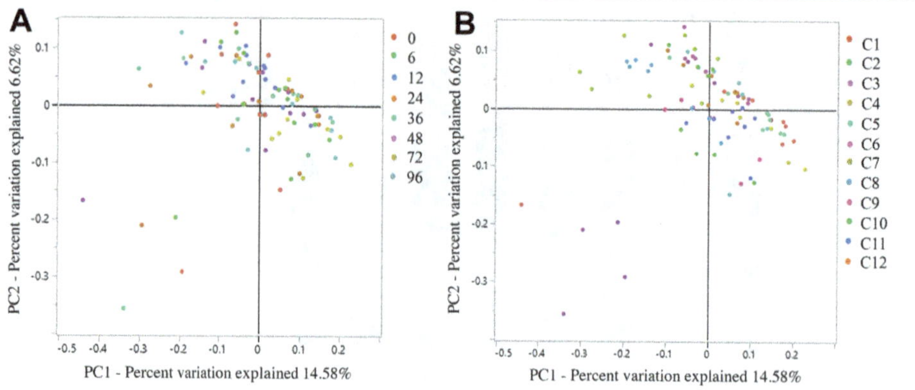

Fig. 5 Two dimensional principal coordinate analysis of population membership of the fecal microbiota of 12 healthy cats, assessed at time points 0, 6, 12, 24, 36, 48, 72 and 96 h. (**a**) By time point; (**b**) By cat

samples from seven dogs and ten cats, after 0, 3, 7 and 14 days [31]. Only a couple of significant changes were observed in the feline fecal microbiota, such as a decrease in the relative abundance of Erysipelotrichaceae *incertae sedis* after 7 days, or enrichment with *Psychrobacter* and *Arthrobacter* (Proteobacteria and Actinobacteria respectively) after 14 days [31]. In comparison to this refrigeration study, it would be expected that changes would occur prior to 7 days of storage at ambient temperature, which was not observed in the current study. A human study involving fecal samples from four healthy children, kept at room temperature for 12, 24, 48 and 72 h, reported a minor change in community structure over time [29]. A small but significant increase in diversity was identified after 12 h along with a decrease in strains of *Ruminococcus* and *Faecalibacterium* [29]. Corresponding changes were not noted in the present study, with possible explanations being differences in sample preparation as well as inter-species variation in fecal microbiota composition. In contrast to the study by Roesch et al. (2009), non-sterile containers were used for sample preservation in the current study and fecal samples were homogenised, as performed similarly by Weese et al. (2014) [29, 31]. Homogenization of stool assists in standardization of aliquots [4, 31, 54]. However, some researchers opt not to homogenise samples as it also causes increased oxygen exposure, which can influence the microbiota membership and structure over time [27]. Additional methodological parameters that can contribute to differences in sample membership and population structure are freeze-thaw cycles [55], differences in extraction methods [56] as well as sequencing methods. Regardless, while there have been variable results from studies in different species using different storage conditions, changes noted over the short time-frame of this study have been mild or absent, consistent with these data.

In general, changes in membership or population structure would correlate to either degradation of microbial DNA or bacterial growth. Dietary ingredients may include microbial metabolic inhibitors. Most feline diets are composed of both animal products and plants ingredients. Plant ingredients contain chlorophyll metabolites such as pheophorbide *a* and pyropheophorbide *a* [57], which inhibit bacterial efflux pumps [58]. The inhibitory effect of these metabolites could be one potential explanation for the lack of bacterial growth in the current study. Nonetheless, the dietary history of the cats was unavailable and further tests were not conducted to confirm this assumption.

Fecal samples in the current study were stored only for four days. This should be sufficient time in field studies to transport samples to better storage conditions, such as refrigeration or freezing. The sample size was relatively small, but it was based on a recent storage study in companion animals [31], as well as on human storage studies, that used a similar smaller sample size. Nonetheless, it is possible that with a larger sample size numerical trends in microbiota composition would become significant. Since very little research exists on the effects of storage on fecal samples in general, and even more so in cats, more research is warranted prior to solid conclusions in regards to short-term fecal storage recommendations.

Conclusions

This study demonstrate that several-day-storage of healthy cats' feces at ambient temperature, has no effect on microbial biodiversity. Although sample freezing at −80 °C is recommended for long term storage, the current study suggests that short term storage, up to 4 days, at ambient temperatures can be appropriate, especially when field studies are performed.

Endnotes

[1]Denver MAXX, Denver Instrument, Bohemia, New York, USA

[2]Class II, Type A2 Biosafety 283 Cabinet, Thermo Fischer Scientific, Waltham, Massachusetts, USA

[3]E.Z.N.A. Stool DNA Kit, 284 Omega Bio-Tek Inc., Doraville, Georgia, USA

[4]NanoDrop 1000 Spectrophotometer, Nano 285 Drop Technologies Inc. (Thermo Fisher Scientific), Waltham, Massachusetts, USA

[5]Illumina, San Diego, California, USA

[6]Kapa Biosystems, Wilmington, Massachusetts, USA

[7]Mastercycler Pro, Eppendorf Canada Ltd., Mississauga, Ontario, Canada;

[8]SAS Campus Drive, Cary, North Carolina, USA

Acknowledgements

We wish to thank Amanda Santarossa for assisting with sample collection, Joyce Rousseau for her technical assistance with the laboratory work and Dr. Alex zur Linden for assistance with electronic artwork.

Funding

The research was supported by a Natural Sciences Engineering Research Council of Canada, Discovery Grant.

Authors' contributions

MT, JSW and AV designed the study. MT coordinated fecal collection, and CC collected the samples. MT and CC were responsible for fecal samples extraction and analyses. MT, JSW and DEG performed bioinformatics and statistical analyses. MT drafted the manuscript. All authors contributed to manuscript preparation and approved the final manuscript.

Authors' information

The study is within the scope of the graduate studies, Doctor Veterinary Science (DVSc) degree, of MT, who received a DVSc scholarship from the Ontario Veterinary College, University of Guelph.

Consent for publication

Not applicable

Competing interests

All authors declare no conflict of interest. A.V. is the Royal Canin Veterinary Diets Endowed Chair in Canine and Feline Clinical Nutrition at the Ontario Veterinary College.

Author details

[1]Department of Clinical Studies, Ontario Veterinary College, University of Guelph, Guelph, ON N1G 2W1, Canada. [2]Department of Pathobiology, Ontario Veterinary College, University of Guelph, Guelph, ON N1G 2W1, Canada. [3]College of Veterinary Medicine, University of Florida, Gainesville, Florida, USA.

References

1. Whitman WB, Coleman DC, Wiebe WJ. Prokaryotes: the unseen majority. Proc Natl Acad Sci U S A. 1998;95(12):6578–83.
2. Ley RE, Turnbaugh PJ, Klein S, Gordon JI. Microbial ecology: human gut microbes associated with obesity. Nature. 2006;444(7122):1022–3.
3. Manson JM, Rauch M, Gilmore MS. The commensal microbiology of the gastrointestinal tract. Adv Exp Med Biol. 2008;635:15–28.
4. Carroll IM, Ringel-Kulka T, Siddle JP, Klaenhammer TR, Ringel Y. Characterization of the Fecal Microbiota Using High-Throughput Sequencing Reveals a Stable Microbial Community during Storage. PLoS One. 2012;7(10):e46953.
5. Minamoto Y, Hooda S, Swanson KS, Suchodolski JS. Feline gastrointestinal microbiota. Anim Health Res Rev. 2012;13(1):64–77.
6. Swanson KS, Dowd SE, Suchodolski JS, Middelbos IS, Vester BM, Barry KA, Nelson KE, Torralba M, Henrissat B, Coutinho PM, et al. Phylogenetic and gene-centric metagenomics of the canine intestinal microbiome reveals similarities with humans and mice. ISME J. 2011;5(4):639–49.
7. Wagner RD. Effects of microbiota on GI health: Gnotobiotic research. In: Huffnagle GB, Noverr MC, editors. GI microbiota and regulation of the immune system. New York: Springer New York; 2008. p. 41–56.
8. McBain AJ, Macfarlane GT. Ecological and physiological studies on large intestinal bacteria in relation to production of hydrolytic and reductive enzymes involved in formation of genotoxic metabolites. J Med Microbiol. 1998;47(5):407–16.
9. Macfarlane S, Steed H, Macfarlane GT. Intestinal bacteria and inflammatory bowel disease. Crit Rev Clin Lab Sci. 2009;46(1):25–54.
10. Dore J, Corthier G. The human intestinal microbiota. Gastroenterol Clin Biol. 2010;34:S7–S15.
11. Elson CO, Sartor RB, Tennyson GS, Riddell RH. Experimental models of inflammatory bowel disease. Gastroenterology. 1995;109(4):1344–67.
12. Palm NW, De zoete MR, Cullen TW, Barry NA, Stefanowski J, Hao L, Degnan PH, Hu J, Peter I, Zhang W, et al. Immunoglobulin A coating identifies Colitogenic bacteria in inflammatory bowel disease. Cell. 2014;158(5):1000–10.
13. Gevers D, Kugathasan S, Denson LA, Vázquez-Baeza Y, Van Treuren W, Ren B, Schwager E, Knights D, Song SJ, Yassour M, et al. The treatment- naive microbiome in new- onset Crohn's disease. Cell Host Microbe. 2014;15(3):382–92.
14. Allenspach K, House A, Smith K, McNeill FM, Hendricks A, Elson-Riggins J, Riddle A, Steiner JM, Werling D, Garden OA, et al. Evaluation of mucosal bacteria and histopathology, clinical disease activity and expression of toll-like receptors in German shepherd dogs with chronic enteropathies. Vet Microbiol. 2010;146(3):326–35.
15. Pathmakanthan S. Mucosally associated bacterial flora of the human colon: quantitative and species specific differences between normal and inflamed colonic biopsies. Microb Ecol Health Dis. 1999;11(3):169–74.
16. Matsuda H, Fujiyama Y, Andoh A, Ushijima T, Kajinami T, Bamba T. Characterization of antibody responses against rectal mucosa- associated bacterial flora in patients with ulcerative colitis. J Gastroenterol Hepatol. 2000;15(1):61–8.
17. Inness VL, McCartney AL, Khoo C, Gross KL, Gibson GR. Molecular characterisation of the gut microflora of healthy and inflammatory bowel disease cats using fluorescence in situ hybridisation with special reference to Desulfovibrio spp. J Anim Physiol Anim Nutr. 2007;91(1–2):48–53.
18. Suchodolski JS, Markel ME, Garcia-Mazcorro JF, Unterer S, Heilmann RM, Dowd SE, Kachroo P, Ivanov I, Minamoto Y, Dillman EM, et al. The fecal microbiome in dogs with acute diarrhea and idiopathic inflammatory bowel disease. PLoS One. 2012;7(12):e51907.
19. Minamoto Y, Otoni CC, Steelman SM, Büyükleblebici O, Steiner JM, Jergens AE, Suchodolski JS. Alteration of the fecal microbiota and serum metabolite profiles in dogs with idiopathic inflammatory bowel disease. Gut Microbes. 2015;6(1):33–47.
20. Caricilli AM, Picardi PK, de Abreu LL, Ueno M, Prada PO, Ropelle ER, Hirabara SM, Castoldi Â, Vieira P, Camara NOS, et al. Gut microbiota is a key modulator of insulin resistance in TLR 2 knockout mice (TLR2, gut microbiota, and insulin resistance). PLoS Biol. 2011;9(12):e1001212.
21. Bisgaard H, Li N, Bonnelykke K, Chawes BLK, Skov T, Paludan-Müller G, Stokholm J, Smith B, Krogfelt KA. Reduced diversity of the intestinal microbiota during infancy is associated with increased risk of allergic disease at school age. J Allergy Clin Immunol. 2011;128(3):646–52.
22. van Nimwegen FA, Penders J, Stobberingh EE, Postma DS, Koppelman GH, Kerkhof M, Reijmerink NE, Dompeling E, van Den Brandt PA, Ferreira I, et al. Mode and place of delivery, gastrointestinal microbiota, and their influence on asthma and atopy. J Allergy Clin Immunol. 2011;128(5):948–55.
23. Johnston KL, Swift NC, Forster-van Hijfte M, Rutgers HC, Lamport A, Ballèvre O, Batt RM. Comparison of the bacterial flora of the duodenum in healthy cats and cats with signs of gastrointestinal tract disease. J Am Vet Med Assoc. 2001;218(1):48.
24. Goodman AL, Kallstrom G, Faith JJ, Reyes A, Moore A, Dantas G, Gordon JI. Extensive personal human gut microbiota culture collections characterized and manipulated in gnotobiotic mice. Proc Natl Acad Sci U S A. 2011; 108(15):6252–7.
25. Liu L, Li Y, Li S, Hu N, He Y, Pong R, Lin D, Lu LH, Law M. Comparison of Next- Generation Sequencing Systems. J Biomed Biotechnol. 2012. doi:10. 1155/2012/251364.
26. Mathay C, Hamot G, Henry E, Georges L, Bellora C, Lebrun L, de Witt B, Ammerlaan W, Buschart A, Wilmes P, et al. Method optimization for fecal sample collection and fecal DNA extraction. Biopreserv Biobank. 2015;13(2): 79–93.
27. Tedjo DI, Jonkers DMAE, Savelkoul PH, Masclee AA, van Best N, Pierik MJ, Penders J. The effect of sampling and storage on the fecal microbiota composition in healthy and diseased subjects. PLoS One. 2015;10(5):e0126685.
28. Lauber CL, Zhou N, Gordon JI, Knight R, Fierer N. Effect of storage conditions on the assessment of bacterial community structure in soil and human- associated samples. FEMS Microbiol Lett. 2010;307(1):80–6.
29. Roesch LFW, Casella G, Simell O, Krischer J, Wasserfall CH, Schatz D, Atkinson MA, Neu J, Triplett EW. Influence of fecal sample storage on bacterial community diversity. Open Microbiol J. 2009;3:40–6.
30. Cardona S, Eck A, Cassellas M, Gallart M, Alastrue C, Dore J, Azpiroz F, Roca J, Guarner F, Manichanh C. Storage conditions of intestinal microbiota matter in metagenomic analysis. BMC Microbiol. 2012;12(1):158.
31. Weese JS, Jalali M. Evaluation of the impact of refrigeration on next generation sequencing-based assessment of the canine and feline fecal microbiota. BMC Vet Res. 2014;10:230.
32. Sturgeon A. Analysis of the Oral and Fecal Microbiota of Companion Animals Using Next-Generation Sequencing of the 16S rRNA Gene. MSc Thesis. Edited by Weese JS; 2014.
33. Schloss PD, Westcott SL, Ryabin T, Hall JR, Hartmann M, Hollister EB, Lesniewski RA, Oakley BB, Parks DH, Robinson CJ, et al. Introducing mothur: open-source, platform-independent, community-supported software for describing and comparing microbial communities. Appl Environ Microbiol. 2009;75(23):7537–41.
34. Kozich JJ, Westcott SL, Baxter NT, Highlander SK, Schloss PD. Development of a dual- index sequencing strategy and Curation pipeline for analyzing

amplicon sequence data on the MiSeq Illumina sequencing platform. Appl Environ Microbiol. 2013;79(17):5112.
35. Quast C, Pruesse E, Yilmaz P, Gerken J, Schweer T, Yarza P, Peplies J, Glockner FO. The SILVA ribosomal RNA gene database project: improved data processing and web-based tools. Nucleic Acids Res. 2013;41(D1):D590–6.
36. Edgar RC, Haas BJ, Clemente JC, Quince C, Knight R. UCHIME improves sensitivity and speed of chimera detection. Bioinformatics. 2011;27(16):2194–200.
37. Cole JR, Wang Q, Fish JA, Chai BL, McGarrell DM, Sun YN, Brown CT, Porras-Alfaro A, Kuske CR, Tiedje JM. Ribosomal database project: data and tools for high throughput rRNA analysis. Nucleic Acids Res. 2014;42(D1):D633–42.
38. Gihring T, Green S, Schadt CW. Massively parallel rRNA gene sequencing exacerbates the potential for biased community diversity comparisons due to variable library sizes. Environ Microbiol. 2011;14(2):285–90.
39. Shannon CE. A mathematical theory of communication. Bell Syst Tech J. 1948;27(3):379–423.
40. Simpson E. Measurement of Diversity. Nature. 1949;163:688.
41. Chao A. Nonparametric estimation of the number of classes in a population. Scand J Stat. 1984;11(4):265–70.
42. Benjamini Y, Hochberg Y. Controlling the false discovery rate: a practical and powerful approach to multiple testing. J R Stat Soc Ser B Methodol. 1995;57(1):289–300.
43. Smith E. Nonparametric estimation of species richness. Biometrics. 1984; 40(1):119–29.
44. Yue J, Clayton M. A similarity measure based on species proportions. Commun Stat Theory Methods. 2005;34(11):2123–31.
45. Lozupone C, Hamady M, Knight R. UniFrac – an online tool for comparing microbial community diversity in a phylogenetic context. BMC Bioinform. 2006;7:371.
46. Segata N, Izard J, Waldron L, Gevers D, Miropolsky L, Garrett WS, Huttenhower C. Metagenomic biomarker discovery and explanation. Genome Biol. 2011;12(6):R60.
47. Weese JS, Nichols J, Jalali M, Litster A. The rectal microbiota of cats infected with feline immunodeficiency virus infection and uninfected controls. Vet Microbiol. 2015;180(1–2):96–102.
48. Fernandez VM, Rao KK, Fernandez MA, Cammack R. Activation and deactivation of the membrane-bound hydrogenase from Desulfovibrio Desulfuricans. Norway strain Biochimie. 1986;68(1):43–8.
49. Deusch O, Flynn C, Colyer A, Morris P, Allaway D, Jones PG, Swanson KS. Deep Illumina-based shotgun sequencing reveals dietary effects on the structure and function of the fecal microbiome of growing kittens. PLoS One. 2014;9(7):e101021.
50. Counotte GH, Prins RA, Janssen RH, Debie MJ. Role of Megasphaera elsdenii in the fermentation of dl- 2-Clactate in the rumen of dairy cattle. Appl Environ Microbiol. 1981;42(4):649.
51. Yoshida Y, Tsukahara T, Ushida K. Oral administration of lactobacillus plantarum Lq80 and Megasphaera elsdenii iNP- 001 induces efficient recovery from mucosal atrophy in the small and the large intestines of weaning piglets. Anim Sci J. 2009;80(6):709–15.
52. Hashizume K, Tsukahara T, Yamada K, Koyama H, Ushida K. Megasphaera elsdenii JCM1772^T normalizes hyperlactate production in the large intestine of fructooligosaccharide- fed rats by stimulating butyrate production1. J Nutr. 2003;133(10):3187–90.
53. Hooda S, Vester Boler BM, Kerr KR, Dowd SE, Swanson KS. The gut microbiome of kittens is affected by dietary protein:carbohydrate ratio and associated with blood metabolite and hormone concentrations. Br J Nutr. 2013;109(9):1637.
54. Ott SJ, Musfeldt M, Timmis KN, Hampe J, Wenderoth DF, Schreiber S. In vitro alterations of intestinal bacterial microbiota in fecal samples during storage. Diagn Microbiol Infect Dis. 2004;50(4):237–45.
55. Rossmanith P, Röder B, Frühwirth K, Vogl C, Wagner M. Mechanisms of degradation of DNA standards for calibration function during storage. Appl Microbiol Biotechnol. 2011;89(2):407.
56. Albertsen M, Karst SM, Ziegler A, Kirkegaard RH, Nielsen P. Back to basics - the influence of DNA extraction and primer choice on Phylogenetic analysis of activated sludge communities. PLoS One. 2015;10(7):e0132783.
57. Ma L, Dolphin D. The metabolites of dietary chlorophylls. Phytochemistry. 1999;50(2):195–202.
58. Tegos G, Stermitz FR, Lomovskaya O, Lewis K. Multidrug pump inhibitors uncover remarkable activity of plant antimicrobials. Antimicrob Agents Chemother. 2002;46(10):3133.

Mixed-method tutoring support improves learning outcomes of veterinary students in basic subjects

María J. García-Iglesias[1*], Claudia Pérez-Martínez[1], César B. Gutiérrez-Martín[2], Raquel Díez-Laiz[3] and Ana M. Sahagún-Prieto[3]

Abstract

Background: Tutoring is a useful tool in the university teaching-learning binomial, although its development is impaired in large classes. Recent improvements in information and communication technologies have made tutoring possible via the Internet. The aim of this study was to evaluate the efficacy of mixed-method academic tutoring in two basic subjects in Veterinary Science studies at the University of León (Spain) to optimize the usefulness of tutoring support in the college environment. This quasi-experimental study was firstly carried out as a pilot study in a small group of tutored students of "Cytology and Histology" (CH) (47/186; 25.3%) and "Veterinary Pharmacology" (VP) (33/141; 23.4%) subjects, and was implemented in a large class of CH the next academic year (150 students) while comparing the results with those obtained in a previous tutorless course (162 students). Tutored students were given access to online questionnaires with electronic feedback on each subject. In addition to traditional tutoring carried out in both tutored and tutorless students, the pilot study included three sessions of face-to-face tutoring in order to monitor the progress of students. Its efficacy was assessed by monitoring students' examination scores and attendance as well as a satisfaction survey.

Results: Although the examination attendance rate in the pilot study was not significantly different between tutored and tutorless groups in both subjects, an increase for numerical scores in tutored groups was observed, with a significant higher final score in VP ($p = 0.001$) and in the CH practice exams (first term, $p = 0.009$; final, $p = 0.023$). Good and merit scores were also better in tutored students with significant differences in VP ($p = 0.005$). Students felt comfortable with the tutoring service (100% in CH; 91.7% in VP). Implementation of this additional support in CH also resulted in a significant increase of attendance at the final exam in tutored courses (87.3% versus 77.2%; $p = 0.026$), scaled ($p = 0.001$) and numerical scores (final score, $p = 0.001$).

Conclusions: Online tutoring support, together with conventional teaching methods, may be a useful method to incorporate student-centered learning in basic subjects in Veterinary Science.

Keywords: Online tutoring support, Large class, Cytology and Histology, Veterinary Pharmacology, Learning strategy, Veterinary Science Degree

* Correspondence: mjgari@unileon.es
[1]Department of Animal Health, Faculty of Veterinary Science, Institute of Biomedicine (IBIOMED), University of León, Campus de Vegazana, s/n, 24071 León, Spain
Full list of author information is available at the end of the article

Background

Implementing the policies of the European Higher Education Area (EHEA) has resulted in significant changes in the learning process. Under the EHEA, teachers are not mere suppliers of knowledge but facilitators who help students receive integral training combining knowledge, attitudes and skills. The target is to place students at the core of the learning process [1].

This new approach considers tutoring as a methodological tool with great potential within the EHEA framework. Research suggests that tutoring has a positive effect in different areas of knowledge including Health Science at High School [2]. One of the tutorial areas that must be particularly enhanced is the academic tutoring [3], which should be conceived as a support for academic, professional and personal development of all college students. Its tools should not only facilitate the monitoring of the learning process by teachers but also serve as a corrective feedback mechanism for the students themselves. At Spanish University, where every teacher is by law obliged to dedicate 6 h a week to tutoring activities, time allocated to this practice has long been used to solve students' queries [4]. It is usually carried out in face-to-face settings in which tutor and students meet at an agreed time and location. However, tutoring should not be simply reduced to "six office hours a week" but rather be seen as a more complex and global process. It is a fact, at least in Spain, that most students do not benefit from tutoring hours as they do not find them helpful and they do not match their needs.

Recent improvements in information and communication technologies (ICTs) have enabled online tutoring [5–7]. Therefore, additional online learning support to students could be a useful tool independent of space and time. Furthermore, it could increase student participation since the use of electronic resources could represent a less pressurized environment than face-to-face communication and taking into account their popularity among students [8]. Moreover, students can identify their strengths and weaknesses, which leads to a better performance and understanding of the subject [7] and promotes life-long learning activities [9].

Published literature in this field relies on subjective interpretation of cases to demonstrate tutorial success; however, there is a lack of objective research demonstrating its usefulness after implementation [10, 11]. There should be more studies on how online tutoring support quantitatively enhances learning outcomes and student motivation to participate in the learning process, mainly in overcrowded classes of Health Science subjects. Monitoring a tutoring program is important for several reasons [12]: a) ongoing evaluation of progress can motivate both the students and the tutor; b) feedback on student performance can be used to highlight effective methods and improve on ineffective ones; and c) evaluation results can also be used as an example to demonstrate the value of the program to interested parties. To our knowledge, only one pilot study providing effective experience on how online tutoring influences the learning process has been reported in veterinary studies in Spain, namely in "Microbiology" [13].

Taking the above into account, the aim of this study was to evaluate the usefulness of mixed-method tutoring (face-to-face and online) support conducted in two basic subjects of Veterinary Science to optimize the efficacy of tutoring support in the college environment.

Methods

Context

In Spain, students may register at the Faculty of Veterinary Sciences after graduating from high school and passing a national selective test. Only 120 students are admitted to the faculty each year based on their scores. The veterinary education programme lasts 5 years.

This study was possible thanks to students enrolled in two basic subjects taught at the Faculty of Veterinary Sciences of the University of León (Spain): "Cytology and Histology" (CH) and "Veterinary Pharmacology" (VP). Students can follow CH during the second semester of the Degree, whereas VP is taught in the fourth semester. CH is worth a total of 6 European credits (ECTS) and consists of theory (12 h) and practical training (40 h). This subject focuses on the morphological study of healthy cells (Cytology) and the association among cells to form tissues (Histology), organs and systems (Microscopic Anatomy). Examination methods include the assessment of practical and theoretical knowledge in both first term and final exams. In the first one, Cytology and Histology contents are evaluated by a written theoretical exam with short answers and another written practical exam in which students must identify cells and tissues using overhead digital images. The final exam evaluates microscopic anatomy contents and follows the same method described above together with another practical examination in which the identification and description of organs under light microscope is assessed. This final exam includes also a second-chance exam for those students who failed the first term one.

VP is also worth 6 ECTS and consists of 32 theoretical hours, 10 h focused on working groups and 18 h of practical training. VP focuses on the safe, effective and rational use of veterinary drugs, including general concepts on Pharmacology (Pharmacokinetics and Pharmacodynamics), as well as on the main pharmacological groups used to treat and prevent animal diseases. Exams consist of a multiple choice test and several short questions. As far as practical knowledge is concerned, students are subjected to continuous assessment, and only need to sit an exam in case they have failed this assessment.

Pilot study

Participants

The number of participants (tutored group) was 47 out of 186 (25.3%) students (female/male: 35/12) in CH and 33 out of 141 (23.4%) (female/male: 17/16) in VP. Their age ranged approximately from 18 to 20 years old.

Study design and procedures

A quasi-experimental design including online and face-to-face tutoring was assessed in both subjects during 2012–2013 academic year. All the students enrolled in CH and VP received an electronic mail inviting them to take part in the pilot study described below. Moreover, details about this pilot study were provided in the lecture-rooms at the beginning of the academic year. The students chose to participate on a voluntary basis after being explicitly informed in the information sessions. No incentives were offered for participation. The proposed protocol was first reviewed by peers within the Teaching Innovation Project Office, and its implementation was authorized as pilot study in both basic subjects. Besides, it was approved by each department (Animal Health and Biomedical Sciences) and the Dean of the Faculty of Veterinary Science The research design is shown in Fig. 1.

Both tutorless and tutored students received tutoring in which the tutor answered to spontaneous requests from students by electronic mail and individual face-to-face meetings. In addition, the tutored group received three one-hour sessions of face-to-face tutoring in a small group. The first one was scheduled after admission of students to inform them about the timetable and methodology before the pilot study began. The second face-to-face tutoring session was carried out after the first online questionnaire and the first term exam for progress monitoring purposes, and the third session was held at the end of the semester in order to solve doubts related to online questionnaires, the subject itself and the results of examinations.

The questionnaires consisted of different types of exercises such as embedded (gap fill), true/false, multiple choice and matching answers (Fig. 2a–c and Additional file 1). Only the tutored group had access to the three questionnaires through the online course management system (Moodle). The availability of these questionnaires was limited to a certain period of time, and the students were only able to access the questionnaires once. Students received scores immediately after the first and third questionnaires had been fulfilled, and corrective feedback was provided once the tool was closed. As far as the second questionnaire is concerned, students took part in the correction of the test themselves by reviewing the results of one of their colleagues and giving the score. Further correction was also performed by the teachers at a later stage. After closing the questionnaires, a two-day period was established in order to answer and solve the doubts of the students via electronic mail.

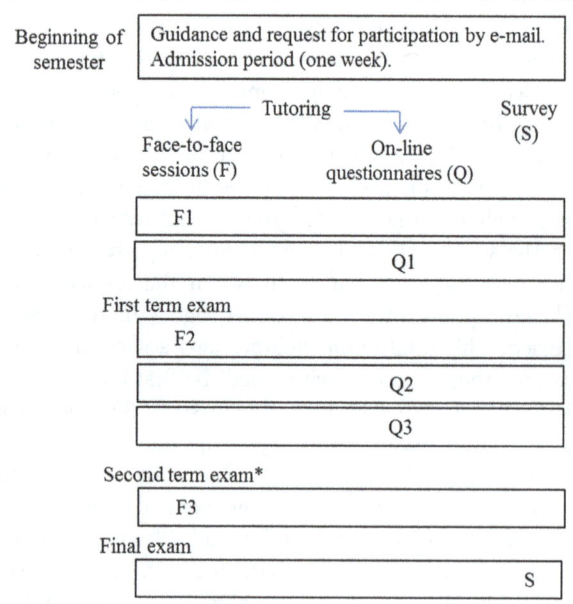

Fig. 1 Schedule of the pilot study. CH, Cytology and Histology. VP, Veterinary Pharmacology. * only in Veterinary Pharmacology

Achievement criteria for study evaluation

The utility of the online tutoring support was assessed in three ways:

1. Student attendance to exams
2. Acquisition of content-specific knowledge evaluated through standard written exams in both tutored and unsupervised groups. The efficacy of this tutoring support on the learning process was assessed by monitoring exam scores based on a 10-point scale where 0 stands for the lowest score. Another parameter used for this matter was a scaled score obtained by grouping the 10-point scale into 4 categories as follows: <5 stands for "fail", 5 to 6.9 stands for "pass", 7 to 8.9 stands for "good" and ≥9 stands for "merit" [14].
3. An anonymous satisfaction survey including 7 items was designed to evaluate the student perception on the utility of combined tutoring and teacher skills. It was conducted via Moodle at the end of the learning innovation experience (Fig. 1). The items were valued on a four-level scale ("strongly agree", "agree", "neutral" and "disagree"). It also included a "free comment" section.

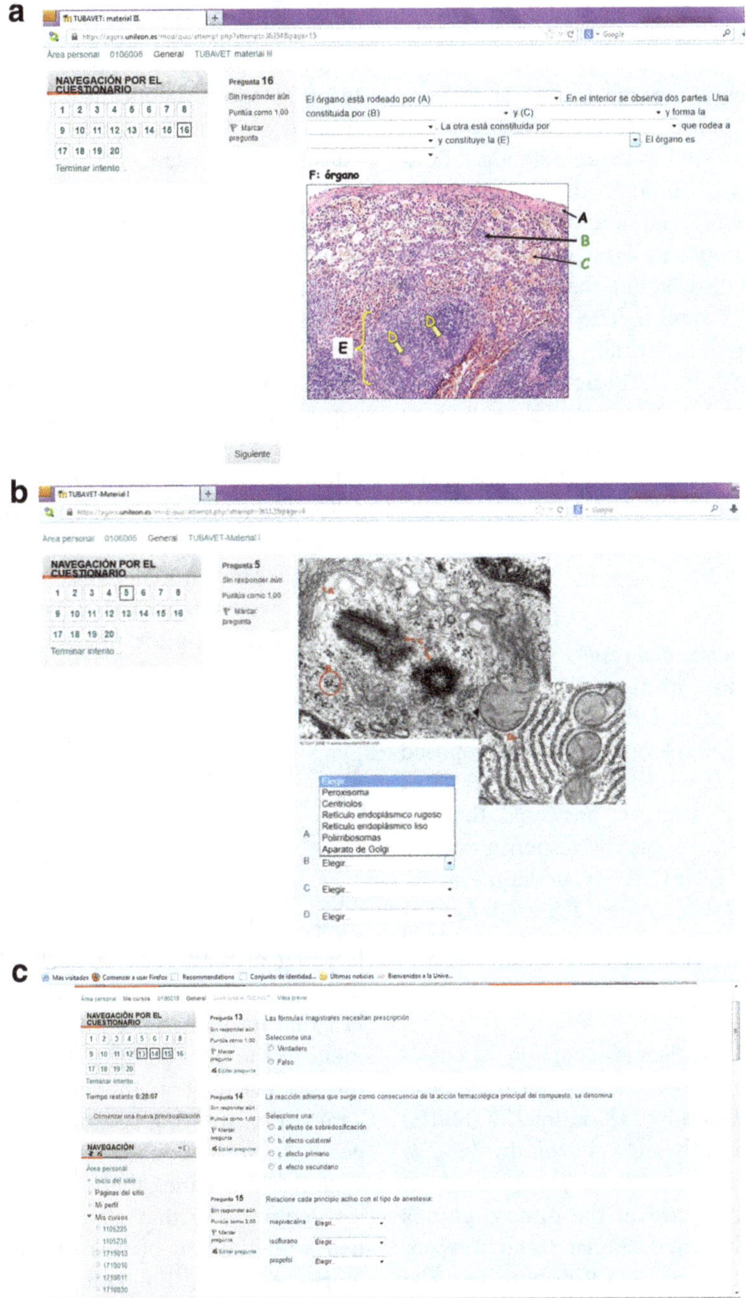

Fig. 2 Different types of online questionnaires. **a** Embedded answers (gap fill). **b** matching. **c** true/false, multiple choice and matching tests

Implementation study

The use of online tutoring was implemented in CH the next academic year (2013–2014). A similar design to the one described in the pilot study for online tutoring was followed. No face-to-face sessions in small groups were held due to the difficulty in scheduling this type of tutoring in overcrowded classes. Both tutored and tutorless courses had access to tutoring by electronic mail and individual face-to-face support, being online tutoring the main difference between both groups. This online activity was not mandatory in the tutored course, but was included in the evaluation criteria as continuous assessment and represented 4% of the overall score. The usefulness of this online service was assessed by comparing the learning outcomes between 150 (female/male: 102/48) tutored and 162 (female/male: 100/62) tutorless students enrolled in 2013–2014 and 2011–2012 academic courses respectively. Factors such as staff, specific content and timetable did not vary in both academic years.

Statistical analysis

The qualitative variables (student attendance at exams, pass rates, and scale scores) were compared between tutored and tutorless groups through Chi-square test or Fisher's exact test when appropriate. Numerical scores of written examinations, expressed as mean ± standard deviation (SD), were analysed through the Kolmogorov-Smirnov test for normal distribution. When data had normal distribution, the unpaired t-test was used. When data follow a non-normal distribution, the non-parametric Mann-Whitney U test was applied. The value of $p \leq 0.05$ (two-tailed) was considered statistically significant. SPSS software version 21 (SPSS Inc., Chicago, IL, USA) for Windows was used to conduct the statistical analyses of the data. All data were used anonymously and treated confidentially according to the EU Data Protection Directive 95/46/EC.

Results

Pilot study

Answer to online questionnaires and results

The highest response rates of tutored students were reached in CH for the first and third online questionnaires, reaching 87.2 and 83.0% respectively as opposed to the second one, which was only answered by 53.2% of undergraduates. In VP, all students answered the two first online questionnaires, whereas the response rate for the third one dropped to 81.8% of undergraduates. Table 1 shows the numerical scores achieved for the three questionnaires in both subjects.

Attendance at exams

A total of 117 out of 139 tutorless (84.2%) and 43 out of 47 tutored (91.5%) students took the first term exam in CH. The final exam was taken by 118 out of 137 (86.1%) unsupervised students and by 44 out of 46 (95.7%) tutored undergraduates. As a result, a rising trend attendance at exams was observed in the tutored groups in CH (Table 2). Nevertheless, a similar trend was not seen in the attendance at exams in VP in both first (32 out of 33, 97.0% in tutored students versus 107 out of 108, 99.1% in unsupervised group) and second (30 out of 33, 91.0% versus 104 out of 108, 96.3%, respectively) term exams (Table 2).

Influence of experimental design tutoring on learning outcomes

Evaluation of the exam pass rates (Table 2) revealed that tutoring tools significantly improved the outcomes in tutored students compared with those who followed a conventional instruction in all examinations conducted in CH for the first term exam. Regarding the exam pass rate in VP, a rising trend has been observed in all the examinations done (Table 2).

In VP, an important and significant improvement associated with the use of the experimental design tutoring system was also observed for scaled scores which, as expected, were better in tutored students than in the unsupervised group for "good" and "merit" scores. A similar trend was observed in CH subject although significant differences were not found.

The comparison of the numerical scores in both subjects for the tutored and tutorless groups is shown in Table 3. The tutored group in CH reached significantly higher scores than the unsupervised one in practical exams. Regarding the first term exam and overall evaluation in VP, scores were significantly higher in the tutored than in the unsupervised groups.

Student satisfaction survey

The satisfaction survey conducted after the final exam was completed by 25 out of the 47 tutored students (53.2%) in CH and by 12 out of 33 students (36.4%) in VP. Most of them agreed or strongly agreed with the utility of these innovative methodologies to improve the learning of both basic subjects (Table 4). Amongst students' opinions, special attention should be drawn to the fact that tutors had been heavily engaged in the development of the pilot study and with the use of this tutoring tool as teaching methodology (Table 4). Students also agreed that tutoring sessions proved to be very advantageous to solve doubts about the subjects, prepare the exams and enhance the students' motivation. In all, it is also noteworthy that almost all participants were satisfied with the use of this tutoring as learning methodology. Amongst the comments received, the greatest utility of online tests to improve the practice training in CH, the positive attitude of tutors and the satisfaction with the high level and quality of the online tutoring tool may be highlighted.

Table 1 Pilot study. Online questionnaires: percentage of tutored students that completed them and their numerical scores achieved

Online questionnaires	Cytology and Histology		Veterinary Pharmacology	
	Percentage of students	Scores (mean ± SD)	Percentage of students	Scores (mean ± SD)
First	87.2	8.87 ± 1.06	100	9.39 ± 0.74
Second	53.2	8.99 ± 0.96	100	7.36 ± 0.22
Third	83.0	8.72 ± 1.20	81.8	8.99 ± 1.16

Table 2 Pilot study. Attendance, pass rates and scaled scores of tutored and tutorless students in exams

	Percentage of students		*p* value
	Tutorless group	Tutored group	
Cytology and Histology			
First term exam			
Attendance	84.2	91.5	0.157
Pass rate			
Practice	75.2	90.7	0.044
Theory	56.0	76.7	0.018
Total	50.4	74.4	0.007
Final exam			
Attendance	86.1	95.7	0.061
Pass rate			
Practice	88.0	93.2	0.406
Theory	76.3	77.3	1.000
Total	75.4	75.0	1.000
Scaled score			0.361
Fail	24.6	25.0	
Pass	39.8	27.3	
Good	33.9	43.2	
Merit	1.7	4.5	
Veterinary Pharmacology			
First term exam			
Attendance	99.1	97.0	0.074
Pass rate	78.7	84.8	0.619
Second term exam			
Attendance	96.3	91.0	0.212
Pass rate	45.4	60.6	0.164
Final exam[a]			
Pass rate	81.5	90.1	0.284
Scaled score			0.005
Fail	18.5	9.1	
Pass	54.6	30.3	
Good	22.2	48.5	
Merit	4.6	12.1	

[a] Final examination only for students who failed previous exams

Implementation study

The pilot study revealed positive outcomes after using this learning methodology, justifying thus its implementation in teaching large classes of undergraduates. For this reason, an online tutoring system was developed in CH the following academic year (2013–2014). When comparing the attendance of undergraduates at the first term exam, no significant differences were found between the tutorless (2011–2012) and tutored (2013–2014) courses, while a rising trend was observed in the

Table 3 Pilot study. Numerical scores achieved by tutored and tutorless students in exams

	Scores (Mean ± SD)		*p* value
	Tutorless group	Tutored group	
Cytology and Histology			
First term exam			
Practice	6.50 ± 1.91	7.37 ± 1.62	0.009
Theory	5.38 ± 1.73	5.95 ± 1.67	0.067
Final exam			
Practice	6.76 ± 1.67	7.42 ± 1.48	0.023
Theory	5.72 ± 1.46	6.03 ± 1.49	0.244
Final score	6.32 ± 1.45	6.76 ± 1.43	0.084
Veterinary Pharmacology[a]			
First term exam	5.73 ± 1.88	6.74 ± 1.66	0.038
Second term exam	4.58 ± 1.94	5.63 ± 1.80	0.100
Final exam	6.56 ± 1.14	7.38 ± 1.08	0.001

[a] Theory exam

pass rates (including theoretical exam and overall evaluation) (Table 5). With regard to the final examination, attendance was significantly higher in the tutored than in the tutorless courses and the percentage of students passing both practical and theoretical exams reflected a rising trend when online tutoring was carried out.

Tables 5 and 6 show the learning results achieved by the undergraduates enrolled in tutorless (2011–2012) and tutored (2013–2014) courses. Percentage scaled scores significantly differed between both courses, showing higher scores for "good" and "merit" marks in the tutored course. When numerical scores were compared, students of the course in which the tutoring tool was implemented got significantly higher scores than those tutorless enrolled 2 years before.

Discussion

Bologna Process has had an impact on methodological tools used in higher education in the last decades. It has changed the teaching scene from a system mainly based on passive teacher's lectures to one based on self-student learning. In this new framework, students have to assume new responsibilities to become autonomous and self-sufficient [15]. On the other hand, educators, more than being perceived as a source of knowledge, are expected to teach students how to study as well as to be initiative-oriented behavior and take their own decisions [16]. Undergraduates perceive as good teachers those that are close to students and active as motivators of the learning process. Tutoring is a methodological teaching tool with an enormous potential in the EHEA context. However, it is not easy to design new stimulating strategies that can be implemented in large classes of undergraduates. The use of Internet seems a way to solve this

Table 4 Pilot study. Online satisfaction survey on the experimental design tutoring support

Questions and subjets	Four-level scale Percentage of students			
	Disagree	Neutral	Agree	Strongly agree
1. The number of face-to-face tutoring sessions has been appropriate				
Cytology and Histology	4.0	16.0	40.0	40.0
Veterinary Pharmacology	0.0	16.7	8.3	75.0
2. The number of online tutoring sessions has been appropriate				
Cytology and Histology	4.0	8.0	36.0	52.0
Veterinary Pharmacology	0.0	0.0	33.3	66.7
3. The degree of involvement of tutors has been high				
Cytology and Histology	0.0	0.0	12.0	88.0
Veterinary Pharmacology	0.0	0.0	33.3	66.7
4. The tutoring sessions help to solve doubts about the matter				
Cytology and Histology	0.0	12.0	48.0	40.0
Veterinary Pharmacology	8.3	8.3	33.3	50.0
5. The tutoring sessions help to prepare for exams				
Cytology and Histology	0.0	12.0	40.0	48.0
Veterinary Pharmacology	0.0	33.3	25.0	41.7
6. The tutoring sessions have improved the motivation-related factors				
Cytology and Histology	0.0	16.0	44.0	40.0
Veterinary Pharmacology	0.0	33.3	58.3	8.3
7. Overall, I am glad with the use of tutoring as a teaching methodology				
Cytology and Histology	0.0	0.0	32.0	68.0
Veterinary Pharmacology	0.0	8.3	41.7	50.0
8. Free comments:				
Cytology and Histology	- Online questionnaires are more useful to improve the practical training than the theory knowledge. - A positive attitude of tutors during online service increases the motivation of students. - Satisfaction with the level and quality of online tutoring.			
Veterinary Pharmacology	- I am really satisfied with the pilot study. It is useful to prepare the exams. - I think it has been an interesting activity.			

problem through online tutoring [17, 18], and Moodle is considered a powerful and flexible tool employed for monitoring and diagnosing the student work [19]. This method may be designed in different ways depending on the type of university degree and subject to be implemented such as: access to an online resource by addressing student questions [18], online problem-based learning [20] and online questionnaires for assessing the skills acquired by veterinary students [21].

The tutoring model presented in this study comprised two environments. One of them was represented by three online content-specific questionnaires proposed at different times during the development of both basic subjects and their feedback, which can be considered as instructional tutoring in which the tutor initiates or intervenes in the students' learning process [22]. The second component of this study, also known as *reactive tutoring* [23], was represented by face-to-face settings in which the tutor answers to spontaneous requests for help from tutored students. The use of periodical online questionnaires to evaluate the acquisition of new knowledge by undergraduates is currently being carried out in subjects of Health Sciences. However, few research studies on its qualitative and quantitative usefulness have been undertaken to determine its real value at university level. For this reason, the novelty of our research is to have shown the quantitative and qualitative efficacy of a tool that is far from conventional tutoring and applicable to large classes of undergraduates. This has been first demonstrated in a small group pilot study and then confirmed after its implementation in an overcrowded class. To our knowledge, only one systematic investigation had been previously reported in a basic subject of Veterinary Science providing information on the influence of this

Table 5 Implementation study in Cytology and Histology. Attendance, pass rates and scaled scores of veterinary students from tutorless (2011-2012) and tutored (2013-14) courses

	Percentage of students		*p* value
	Tutorless group	Tutored group	
First term exam			
Attendance	95.1	93.3	0.629
Pass rate			
Practice	91.5	90.0	0.690
Theory	81.5	85.6	0.429
Total	79.7	85.6	0.218
Final exam			
Attendance	77.2	87.3	0.026
Pass rate			
Practice	87.9	91.6	0.409
Theory	86.4	89.3	0.566
Total	86.2	87.8	0.713
Scaled score			0.001
Fail	15.3	12.2	
Pass	56.5	26.0	
Good	25.8	57.3	
Merit	2.4	4.6	

type of online tutoring on the learning process, although it is to be noted that the study was only developed within a small group of students [16].

The poor opinion that undergraduates have on tutorial support was evidenced by the relatively low engagement to take part in the pilot study. However, those students who participated considered this experimental design tutoring as a very useful methodological tool. The high participation maintained over time is a good success indicator of this learning strategy. Slight decreases in response rates to complete the online content-specific questionnaires could be explained because of the long time passed between the activity itself and the examination of the subjects and/or the heavy workload at the end of the semester.

Table 6 Implementation study in Cytology and Histology. Numerical scores achieved by veterinary students from tutorless (2011-2012) and tutored (2013-2014) courses

	Scores (Mean ± SD)		*p* value
	Tutorless group	Tutored group	
First term exam			
Practice	6.69 ± 1.60	7.08 ± 1.75	0.044
Theory	5.59 ± 1.55	6.21 ± 1.67	0.001
Final exam			
Practice	6.47 ± 1.80	7.14 ± 1.61	0.002
Theory	5.82 ± 1.69	6.57 ± 1.57	0.001
Final score	6.33 ± 1.53	7.08 ± 1.42	0.001

As mentioned above, several face-to-face tutoring sessions were also developed as a way to guide and help students to overcome any difficulties they could find with the methodological tool or the subject taught. Students considered these extra tutoring sessions as a positive and rewarding experience, in which teachers became learning guiders and motivators, and they thanked and greatly appreciated their implication. The information obtained in these sessions and in the satisfaction surveys was very useful for the implementation of this learning strategy in large classes. In this respect and taking into account the students' comments in CH subject, the design of online questionnaires was modified to increase the motivation in theoretical training, compared with the pilot study by including more questions on theoretical knowledge. This modification might have contributed to the significant improvement in scaled and numerical scores achieved by the veterinary students during the implementation phase. Our experience supports the importance of students' surveys for teaching enhancing, as previously cited [24]. However, the scarce participation of students in this sort of surveys suggests an absence of motivation since they consider that their opinions will not be taken into account. In addition, these surveys are usually tedious. For these reasons, higher education needs to make significant progress for undergraduates to perceive that their voices are heard as part of quality assurance [25].

The assessment of several parameters related to practical and theoretical training suggests that this mixed-method tutoring support was beneficial for the learning outcomes of veterinary students in the pilot study. However, it is to be noted that the results were not significant, probably due to the small size of the samples. These positive findings were supported by higher attendance at final exam and better numerical and scaled scores achieved after implementation in CH, even though overall pass rates did not raise. This improvement could be attributed to online questionnaires whose feedback may enhance students' motivation and confidence to succeed in their examinations. Besides, this online support helped to maintain a daily work done by students on specific contents allowing them to identify shortcomings that could be solved at an early stage. Thus, online quizzes may indirectly induce the use of reactive tutoring in which the tutor answers to spontaneous requests by electronic mail or in individual face-to-face sessions. Hence, the effect of both tutoring systems (online and traditional) could be associated with an improvement in student outcomes and the poor opinion undergraduates have on tutoring support.

Limitations of the study

Results reported above must be interpreted within the limits of the pilot and implementation studies. First of all, success may be partially attributed to the motivated students who voluntarily participated in this innovative strategy, which may also be related to the positive effects found in the pilot study, as other authors have mentioned [26]. However, statistically significant higher participation in final exam and better scores achieved by veterinary students when this learning tool was implemented in CH supports its positive impact. Secondly, the use of year-to-year comparisons in the implementation study may differ mainly as far as students are concerned, since other factors such as staff, contents and timetable did not vary from one academic year to the other. Finally, another potential influencing factor could be related to prior knowledge of questions and examination formats in tutored groups as opposed to tutorless ones.

Conclusions

The results of this study reveal that an online tutoring tool in overcrowded classes with specific-content questionnaires, together with conventional teaching methods, results in (a) improved outcomes in terms of numerical and scaled scores, (b) a high satisfaction of undergraduates with the learning process and an increase in their motivation, and (c) a better theoretical and practical acquisition of knowledge. For all these reasons, the future implementation of this methodology in basic subjects in higher education with large numbers of students is strongly advised. It should logically be adapted to the particular idiosyncrasy of each subject.

Abbreviations

CH: Cytology and Histology; ECTS: European credit transfer and accumulation system; EHEA: European Higher Education Area; ICTs: Information and communication technologies; SD: Standard deviation; VP: Veterinary Pharmacology

Acknowledgments

The authors express their sincere thanks to all students who voluntarily participated in the pilot study.

Funding

This study was funded by a grant from the University of León (Spain) from the Teaching Innovation Project Office titled "La tutoría presencial y *on line* como herramienta para la adaptación y mejora en el rendimiento académico de asignaturas básicas en el Grado en Veterinaria (TUBAVET)".

Authors' contributions

MJGI, CPM and AMSP conceived and carried out the different studies, as well as the statistical analysis; in addition, they drafted and revised the manuscript for important intellectual content. CBGM and RDL drafted and revised the manuscript for important intellectual content. All authors read and approved the final manuscript.

Authors' information

Dr. med. vet. MJGI and Dr. med. vet. CPM are lecturers in "Histology and Anatomical Pathology" of the Department of Animal Health (Faculty of Veterinary Science) as well as researchers at the Institute of Biomedicine (IBIOMED) of the University of León.
Dr. med. vet. CBGM is a lecturer in "Microbiology and Immunology" of the Department of Animal Health (Faculty of Veterinary Science) of the University of León.
Dr. med. vet. AMSP and Dr. pharm. RDL are lecturers in "Pharmacology" of the Department of Biomedical Sciences (Faculty of Veterinary Science) as well as researchers at the Institute of Biomedicine (IBIOMED) of the University of León.
All authors are involved in education research with a strong interest in implementing and researching education technologies.

Ethics approval and consent to participate

No ethical approval from a research ethics committee is required for this type of educational study as stated by the Ethics Committee of the University of León (Spain). Peer review of the proposed experimental design was carried out in order to take part in the Teaching Innovation Program at the University of León. Its development was authorized as a pilot study and funded by the University of León (Spain). This tutoring resource was also approved by each department (Animal Health and Biomedical Sciences) and the Dean of the Faculty of Veterinary Science. Participation was granted on a voluntary basis, as mentioned above, and the pilot study was explained in detail to all students. Students' replies indicating their willingness to participate by electronic mail were considered as written consent. Students not participating in the pilot study faced no disadvantages with respect to tutored ones.

Consent for publication

Not applicable.

Competing interests

All authors declare that they have no competing interests.

Author details

[1]Department of Animal Health, Faculty of Veterinary Science, Institute of Biomedicine (IBIOMED), University of León, Campus de Vegazana, s/n, 24071 León, Spain. [2]Department of Animal Health, Faculty of Veterinary Science, University of León, Campus de Vegazana, s/n, 24071 León, Spain. [3]Department of Biomedical Sciences, Faculty of Veterinary Science, Institute of Biomedicine (IBIOMED), University of León, Campus de Vegazana, s/n, 24071 León, Spain.

References

1. Álvarez P, Álvarez D, González M. Evaluación de la implantación de un plan de tutoría en la Universidad. X Congreso Nacional de modelos de investigación educativa: Investigación y evaluación educativa en la sociedad del conocimiento. La Coruña, Spain. 2001.
2. Mastropieri MA, Scruggs TE, Gaetz J. Cognition and learning in inclusive high school chemistry classes. In: Scruggs TE, Mstropieri MA, editors. Cognition and learning in diverse settings: advances in learning and behavioral disabilities. Oxford: Elsevier; 2005. p. 99–110.

3. Cano R. Tutoría universitaria y aprendizaje por competencias. ¿Cómo lograrlo? Rev Elect Interuniv Form Prof (REIFOP). 2009;12:181–204.
4. Molina JM. The academic tutoring at the university level: development and promotion methodology through project work. Procedia Soc Behav Sci. 2013;106:2594–601.
5. Fleisher P. Help is on the way: on-line tutoring services expand students' options. Technol Learn. 2006;26:14.
6. Lin H-T, Lee P-M, Hsiao T-C. On line pedagogical tutorial tactics optimization using genetic-based reinforcement learning. Sci World J. 2015;352895. doi: https://doi.org/10.1155/2015/352895.
7. Lull ME, Mathews JL. Online self-testing resources prepared by peer tutors as a formative assessment tool in pharmacology courses. Am J Pharm Educ. 2016;80:124. doi: https://doi.org/10.5688/ajpe807124.
8. Kistantas A, Chow A. College students' perceived threat and preference for seeking help in traditional, distributed, and distance learning environments. Comp Educ. 2007;48:383–95.
9. Stewart D, Panus P, Hagemeier N, Thigpen J, Brooks L. Pharmacy student self-testing as a predictor of examination performance. Am J Pharm Educ. 2017;78:32. doi: https://doi.org/10.5688/ajpe78232.
10. O'Donovan J, Maruthappu M. Distant peer-tutoring of clinical skills, using tablets with instructional videos and Skype: a pilot study in the UK and Malaysia. Med Teacher. 2015;37:463–9.
11. Maxwell M. Does tutoring help? A look at the literature. Rev Res Develop Educ. 1994;7:3–7.
12. Tansy M, de Barona M. Peer and cross-age tutoring programs: counselor contribution to student achievement. Guid Counc. 1996;12:21–5.
13. Gutiérrez Martín CB, García Iglesias MJ, Pérez Martínez C, Sahagún Prieto AM, Martínez Martínez S, Díez Láiz R, López Cadenas C, Rodríguez Lago JM, Fernández Martínez N, Sierra Vega M, García Viéitez JJ, Rodríguez Ferri EF. Implementación de tutorías académicas en línea en una asignatura básica del Grado en Veterinaria. REDU Rev Doc Univ. 2015;13:97–121.
14. Ministerio de Educación, Cultura y Deporte. Real Decreto 1125/2003, de 5 de septiembre, por el que se establece el sistema europeo de créditos y el sistema de calificaciones en las titulaciones universitarias de carácter oficial y validez en todo el territorio nacional. BOE. 2003;224:34355–6.
15. Del Rincón B. Tutorías personalizadas en la universidad. Toledo: Servicio de Publicaciones de la Universidad de Castilla-La Mancha; 2000.
16. Torrego JC. Resolución de conflictos desde la acción tutorial. Madrid: Dirección General de Ordenación Académica, Comunidad de Madrid; 2003.
17. Turrentine P, MacDonald L. Tutoring online: increasing effectiveness with best practices. NADE Digest. 2006;2:1–10.
18. Kersaint G, Dogbey J, Barber J, Kephart D. The effect of access to an on-line tutorial service on college algebra student outcomes. Mentor Tutor: Partner Learn. 2011;19:25–44.
19. Cole J, Foster H. Using Moodle: teaching with the popular open source course management system. 2nd ed. O'Reilly Media Inc: Sebastopol; 2007.
20. Chen JY, Lee MC, Lee HS, Wang YC, Lin LY, Yang JH. An on-line evaluation of problem-based learning (PBL) in Chung Shan Medical University, Taiwan – a pilot study. Ann Acad Med. 2006;35:624–33.
21. Rösch T, Schaper E, Tipold A, Fischer MR, Dilly M, Ehlers JP. Clinical skills of veterinary students - a cross-sectional study of the self-concept and exposure to skills training in Hannover, Germany. BMC Vet Res. 2014;10:969. doi: https://doi.org/10.1186/s12917-014-0302-8.
22. Hock MF, Deshler DD, Schumaker JB. Tutoring programs for academically underprepared college students: a review of the literature. JCRL. 1999;29:101–22.
23. De Lievre B, Depover C, Dillenbourg P. The relationship between tutoring mode and learners' use of help tools in distance education. Instr Sci. 2006; 34:97–129.
24. Strydom JF, Basson N, Mentz M. Enhancing the quality of teaching and learning: using student engagement data to establish a culture of evidence. Pretoria: Council on Higher Education; 2012.
25. Shah M, Nair CS. Using student voice to improve student satisfaction: two Australian universities the same agenda. JIRSEA. 2009;7:43–55.
26. Keim J, McWhirter JJ, Bernstein BL. Academic success and university accommodation for learning disabilities: is there a relationship? J Coll Student Dev. 1996;37:502–9.

Pharmacokinetic and urinary profiling reveals the prednisolone/cortisol ratio as a valid biomarker for prednisolone administration

Lieven Van Meulebroek[1†], Nathalie De Clercq[1†], Julie Vanden Bussche[1], Mathias Devreese[2], Eric Fichant[3], Philippe Delahaut[3], Siska Croubels[2] and Lynn Vanhaecke[1*]

Abstract

Background: In Europe, synthetic corticosteroids are not allowed in animal breeding for growth-promoting purposes. Nevertheless, a high prevalence of non-compliant urine samples was recently reported for prednisolone, however, without any indication of unauthorized use. Within this context, 20β-dihydroprednisolone and the prednisolone/cortisol ratio have been suggested as potential tools to discriminate between exogenous and endogenous urinary prednisolone. In this study, the validity of these strategies was verified by investigating the plasma pharmacokinetic and urinary excretion profiles of relevant glucocorticoids in bovines, subjected to exogenous prednisolone treatment or tetracosactide hexaacetate administration to induce endogenous prednisolone formation. Bovine urine and plasma samples were analysed by liquid chromatography and mass spectrometry.

Results: Based on the plasma pharmacokinetics and urinary profiles, 20β-dihydroprednisolone was confirmed as the main prednisolone-derived metabolite, being detected in the biological fluids of all 12 bovines (plasma $AUC_{0\text{-}inf}$ of 121 h μg L^{-1} and urinary concentration > 0.695 μg L^{-1}). However, this metabolite enclosed no potential as discriminative marker as no significant concentration differences were observed upon exogenous prednisolone treatment or tetracosactide hexaacetate administration under all experimental conditions. As a second marker tool, the prednisolone/cortisol ratios were assessed along the various treatments, taking into account that endogenous prednisolone formation involves the hypothalamic-pituitary-adrenal axis and is associated with an increased cortisol secretion. Significantly lower ratios were observed in case of endogenous prednisolone formation (i.e. ratios ranging from 0.00379 to 0.129) compared to the exogenous prednisolone treatment (i.e. ratios ranging from 0.0603 to 36.9). On the basis of these findings, a discriminative threshold of 0.260 was proposed, which allowed classification of urine samples according to prednisolone origin with a sensitivity of 94.2% and specificity of 99.0%.

Conclusion: The prednisolone/cortisol ratio was affirmed as an expedient strategy to discriminate between endogenous and exogenous prednisolone in urine. Although the suggested threshold value was associated with high specificity and sensitivity, a large-scale study with varying experimental conditions is designated to optimize this value.

Keywords: Glucocorticoids, Prednisolone, Screening tools, Prednisolone/cortisol ratio, 20β-dihydroprednisolone, Adrenocorticotropic hormone, Urinary profiling

* Correspondence: Lynn.Vanhaecke@ugent.be
[†]Equal contributors
[1]Faculty of Veterinary Medicine, Department of Veterinary Public Health & Food Safety, Laboratory of Chemical Analysis, Ghent University, Salisburylaan 133, 9820 Merelbeke, Belgium
Full list of author information is available at the end of the article

Background

Synthetic glucocorticoids are extensively employed in cattle for therapeutic purposes because of their well-recognized anti-inflammatory and immunosuppressive properties. Among these glucocorticoids, the most commonly used are dexamethasone methylprednisolone, and prednisolone. For example, the latter is frequently used in cattle, including dairy cows, for the treatment of allergic dermatitis, otitis, pruritus and musculoskeletal inflammation [1, 2]. Apart from the therapeutic applications, synthetic glucocorticoids may also be administered unauthorized to promote the growth of veal calves, finishing bulls and cows at the end of their production cycle [3]. Glucocorticoids tend to increase live weight gain, improve feed intake, reduce the feed conversion ratio, reduce nitrogen retention, increase the fat content and promote water retention [4]. As such, growth-promoting effects have been demonstrated for beef cattle after oral administration of prednisolone acetate (15–30 mg per animal per day) for 30–35 days [5]. Because of the strong pharmacological activity, the residues of most synthetic corticosteroids might impose a risk for food safety. Therefore, to protect consumer's health, the administration of synthetic glucocorticoids in livestock is restricted to therapeutic applications only and should be done by a licensed veterinarian [6]. Moreover, appropriate withdrawal times have been defined for glucocorticoid treatment in order to comply with the maximum residue limits (MRLs), as they have been established for bovine edible tissues [6, 7].

In the past few years, the European Commission reported a higher prevalence of non-compliant urine samples for prednisolone [8–11], without any direct evidence of unauthorized use. Therefore, in order to account for potential endogenous prednisolone, the European Reference Laboratories have proposed a threshold level for urinary prednisolone in bovine urine of 5 μg L^{-1} [12, 13]. However, such an artificial cut-off value may still leave the possibility for false accusations or legalization of low-level prednisolone abuse. In this regard, alternatives to discriminate between exogenous and endogenous prednisolone have been suggested, i.e. usage of the prednisolone/cortisol urinary concentration ratio and analysis of 20β-dihydroprednisolone [14–17], although both have not been confirmed or validated yet. Therefore, in this study, to verify the applicability and validity of these screening tools, the pharmacokinetics and urinary excretion profiles of prednisolone, prednisone, 20α- and 20β-dihydroprednisolone were assessed during a growth-promoting and therapeutic prednisolone treatment (Additional file 1). Moreover, also a pharmacologically-induced stress treatment was considered as it has recently been evidenced that stress induction with a synthetic analogue of the adrenocorticotropic hormone (ACTH), i.e. tetracosactide hexaacetate, leads to the presence of endogenous prednisolone in bovine urine. In addition, the overall cortisol secretion during growth-promoting, therapeutic prednisolone, and ACTH treatment was assessed by profiling natural urinary glucocorticoid metabolites, i.e. cortisone, dihydrocortisone, corticosterone, deoxycorticosterone, allotetrahydrocortisol, tetrahydrocortisone, urocortisol, α-cortolone and 6β-hydroxycortisol. To date, only a few studies have been dedicated to correlate endogenous (e.g. cortisol) and exogenously administered glucocorticoids (e.g. dexamethasone, prednisolone) as a means to estimate the degree of glucocorticoid resistance or super sensitivity [18–20]. Nevertheless, a deepened knowledge on these correlations is believed to support the understanding of endogenous formation mechanisms and might yield an adequate screening tool.

Methods

Test animals

Twelve clinically healthy cows of a mixed breed were housed under controlled experimental conditions at the animal facilities of Centre d'Economie Rurale (CER, Marloie, Belgium). These cows were 2 to 6 years of age and had a body weight between 370 and 600 kg. They were fed a commercial diet, with ad libitum access to water and hay. During the entire study, animals were kept in three separate groups (4 animals per group), all housed in a half-covered pen. Prior to the in vivo study, an initial acclimatization period of 10 days was foreseen, allowing adaptation to the environmental and feeding conditions. This study was approved by CER's Ethical Committee (CE/Sante/ET/004).

Experimental protocol

After acclimatization (Fig. 1A), animals were subjected to a similar oral (per os, PO) and intramuscular (IM) prednisolone treatment sequence. First, a growth-promoting treatment (long-term, 40 mg per cow a day, PO and IM) was applied, followed by a therapeutic treatment (short-term, 0.5 mg per kg bodyweight a day, PO and IM) (Fig. 1A). Then, a washout period of 11 weeks was incorporated, after which tetracosactide hexaacetate (2 mg per day) was administered intramuscularly for 4 days to mimic stress (Fig. 1B). All types of treatment were executed at 8 h in the morning.

Phase I: Prednisolone treatments

The growth-promoting treatment started with 30 consecutive days of PO administration of 40 mg per day of prednisolone in capsules (prednisolone, Fagron, Belgium) (Day + 1 till Day + 30), followed by a washout period of 10 days. Next, IM injections of 40 mg per day of Solu-Delta-Cortef® (prednisolone sodium succinate, Zoetis, Belgium) were given for 30 consecutive days

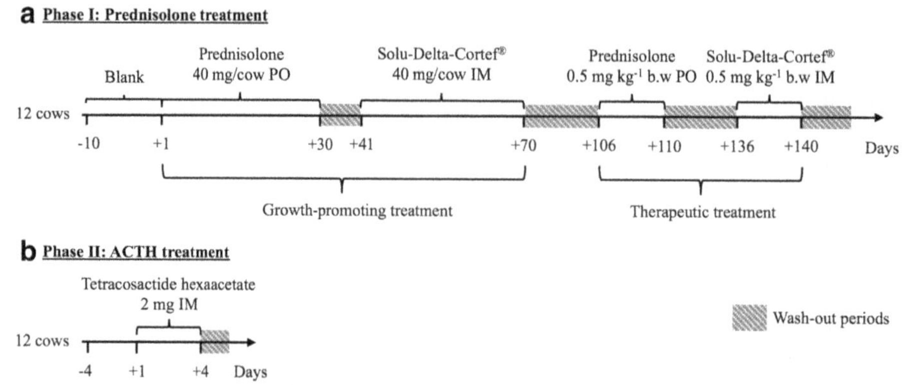

Fig. 1 Schematic representation of the in vivo study. The various experimental treatments include oral (PO) and intramuscular (IM) prednisolone administration (**a**) and the treatment with tetracosactide hexaacetate, a synthetic analogue of ACTH (**b**). The wash-out periods are indicated in blue. This experimental procedure was implemented to each of the test animals ($n = 12$)

(Day + 41 till Day + 70). Before the start of the therapeutic prednisolone treatment, a washout period of 35 days was foreseen.

During the therapeutic treatment, a similar experimental set-up was implemented. First, the animals received 0.5 mg prednisolone per kg body weight PO for 5 days (Day + 106 till Day + 110), which was followed by a washout period of 25 days. Next, IM injections of 0.5 mg of Solu-Delta-Cortef® per kg body weight were given during 5 consecutive days (Day + 136 till Day + 140). Until 32 days (Day + 141 till Day + 172) after the last prednisolone administration, urine samples were collected in order to monitor the reconversion to the natural glucocorticoid body state.

Phase II: ACTH treatment

After phase I, a washout period of 11 weeks was considered. Subsequently, all animals received IM injections of 2 mg tetracosactide hexaacetate (Utrecht University, Faculty of Veterinary Medicine, Utrecht, The Netherlands), corresponding to 200 I.U. of ACTH, during 4 consecutive days.

Sample collection

During prednisolone treatments, urine samples were each time collected in the morning, prior to prednisolone administration. These samples were obtained by a veterinarian using a probe (to prevent faecal contamination) and were immediately portioned into 15-mL tubes, which were then stored in the dark at −80 °C until analysis. During the growth-promoting treatment, samples were collected every five days whereas during the therapeutic treatment, urine samples were collected the first, third and last day. In addition, samples were also collected every day during the acclimatization period and every five days during the washout periods. Also, urine samples were collected twice a day during the ACTH treatment period, whereby samples were collected prior to and at 4 h (Day + 1 and Day + 2) or at 6 h (Day + 3 and Day + 4) after tetracosactide hexaacetate administration.

Blood samples were collected in the morning, thereby applying a similar sampling strategy as for urine. In addition, blood samples for pharmacokinetic analysis were collected at the beginning and end of each treatment period at time 0 (just before administration), 15 min, 30 min, 45 min, 1 h, 2 h, 4 h, 6 h, 8 h, and 24 h (post-administration). With each collection, 5 mL of blood was sampled into heparin tubes. One hour after collection, blood was centrifuged at 600 x g during 15 min at 4 °C and divided into 2-mL plasma aliquots, which were then immediately stored at −20 °C until analysis.

Reagents and chemicals

Standards of prednisolone, prednisone, cortisone, cortisol, dihydrocortisone, aldosterone, allotetrahydrocortisol, urocortisol, tetrahydrocortisone, corticosterone, deoxycorticosterone, α-cortolone and 6β-hydroxycortisol were purchased from Sigma-Aldrich (St. Louis, MO, USA). Internal standards were prednisolone-d_8 (TRC, Canada), cortisol-d_4 and prednisolonde-d_4 (Sigma-Aldrich). Reagents were of analytical grade (Merck, Darmstadt, Germany) when used for extraction purposes and of liquid chromatography-mass spectrometry (LC-MS) Optima grade (Fisher Scientific, Loughborough, UK) for ultra-high performance LC (UHPLC) tandem MS (MS/MS) and high-resolution MS (HRMS) applications. Ultrapure water was obtained by usage of a purified-water system (Sartorius AG, Goettingen, Germany). Stock solutions were prepared in ethanol at a concentration of 200 μg mL^{-1} and stored in dark glass bottles at −20 °C.

Sample preparation

Urine

A detailed description of the analytical procedure, which was used for glucocorticoid extraction from urine, has been given in earlier work [21]. In brief, 5 mL of urine was enriched with the internal standards cortisol-d_4 and prednisolone-d_8 to reach final concentration of 10 μg L $^{-1}$. Next, a twofold liquid-liquid extraction with tert-butyl methyl ether was applied, whereby the organic phases were collected, pooled and dried under a gentle stream of nitrogen at 50 °C. The residue was then dissolved in 100 μL of initial mobile phase conditions and transferred into an LC- vial.

Plasma

Two mL of vortexed plasma was spiked with the internal standards cortisol-d_4 and prednisolone-d_4 to obtain final concentrations of 10 μg L^{-1}. Glucocorticoids were extracted by liquid-liquid extraction, thereby using 5 mL acetonitrile. After 30 min of extraction, samples were centrifuged at 3760 x g for 10 min at 10 °C. Then, the supernatants were collected and evaporated under a gentle stream of nitrogen at 40 °C. The residue was suspended in 200 μL of water-acetonitrile (80/20, *v*/v) and transferred into an LC-vial.

Mass spectrometric detection

UHPLC-Orbitrap MS for urine

Glucocorticoid analysis of urine was performed by UHPLC-Orbitrap MS, according to the method of De Clercq et al. (2013) [21]. Chromatographic separation of the target analytes was thereby achieved using an Accela UHPLC system (Thermo Fisher Scientific, San José, USA), equipped with a Nucleodur Isis C18 column (1.8 μm, 100 mm × 2 mm, Macherey-Nagel, Düren, Germany). High-resolution mass spectrometric analysis was performed with an Exactive™ single-stage Orbitrap mass spectrometer (Thermo Fisher Scientific), equipped with a heated electrospray ionization probe (HESI II), operating in polarity switching mode. Instrument control and data processing were carried out by Xcalibur 2.1 software (Thermo Fisher Scientific, San José, USA).

UHPLC-MS/MS analysis for plasma

The chromatographic analysis of glucocorticoids in plasma was performed by a Waters Acquity system (Waters, Manchester, UK) according to Delahaut et al. (2014) [16]. Chromatographic separation of the target analytes was thereby achieved using an Acquity C18 column (1.7 μm, 125 × 3 mm). Mass spectrometric analysis was performed with a Xevo TSQ tandem mass spectrometer (Waters Corporation, Manchester, UK), operating in the positive ion electrospray mode and applying multiple reaction monitoring (MRM). For each target compound, two transitions were monitored (Additional file 2), the first being the quantifier and the second being the qualifier. For quantification, two internal standards were used: prednisolone-d_4 and cortisol-d_4. Instrument control and data processing were carried out by MassLynx and QUANLYNX software (Waters Corporation, Manchester, UK) respectively.

A brief validation of the newly developed method for glucocorticoid analysis of plasma was performed based on Commission Decision 2002/657/EC guidelines [22]. The method performance in terms of repeatability, within-laboratory reproducibility, recovery, CC_α and specificity was thereby assessed. Plasma samples that were used for validation were obtained from non-medicated cows (n = 3), which were housed at the animal facilities of CER. Linearity was evaluated based on eight-point matrix-matched calibration curves with concentration levels ranging from 0.25 to 20 μg L^{-1} for prednisolone, prednisone, 20α-dihydroprednisolone, and 20β-dihydroprednisolone and from 0.5 to 40 μg L^{-1} for cortisol, cortisone, and dihydrocortisone. Repeatability was determined by analysis of samples that were spiked with the target compounds, thereby considering seven replicates for two different concentration levels, i.e. 0.50 and 5 μg L^{-1} for prednisolone, prednisone, 20α-dihydroprednisolone, and 20β-dihydroprednisolone and 1 and 10 μg L^{-1} for cortisol, cortisone, and dihydrocortisone. For evaluation of the within-laboratory reproducibility, the specified analyses were performed on two different occasions, with a different operator on the second occasion. The CC_α was derived from chromatograms and corresponded to a concentration giving a peak with a signal-to-noise ratio of 3. Specificity was evaluated by analyzing a potential interfering substance (methylprednisolone) to verify potential cross-talk during analysis.

Quantitation and normalization

Due to the broad concentration range expected in the urine samples during the different prednisolone treatments, quantitation of the various urinary glucocorticoid compounds was based on two eight-point calibration curves (using area ratios), which were prepared in urine matrix. Samples were thereby fortified with all glucocorticoid standards to reach concentrations from 0.50 to 75 ng mL^{-1} and from 100 to 200 ng mL^{-1} for cortisol, cortisone, dihydrocortisone, prednisolone, prednisone, methylprednisolone, 20α-dihydroprednisolone, and 20β-dihydroprednisolone. The employed urine matrix was previously verified to contain no residues of prednisolone, prednisone, 20α-dihydroprednisolone and 20β-dihydroprednisolone, but the other glucocorticoids were found to be endogenously present. Therefore, the endogenous concentration levels of cortisol, cortisone, and dihydrocortisone were determined as the average of five non-fortified urine samples and taken into account during quantitation. In addition, since urine is a matrix prone to dilution, normalization by means of the specific gravity (Pocket Refractometer™, Atago, Tokyo) was applied using the Levine-Fahy eq. [23].

Pharmacokinetic analysis

Pharmacokinetic analysis was performed with WinNonlin 6.3 (Pharsight Corporation, St-Louis, USA). Plasma concentration-time profiles were modeled using a one-compartmental model for PO and a two-compartmental model for IM prednisolone administration. The most important pharmacokinetic parameters were the peak plasma concentration (C_{max}), time to reach the peak plasma concentration (T_{max}), area under the plasma concentration-time curve from time 0 to time inf (AUC_{0-inf}), absorption rate constant (k_a), absorption half-life ($T_{1/2a}$), apparent clearance (Cl/F) and apparent volume of distribution (Vd/F). Additionally, for two-compartmental methods, the distribution rate constant ($k_{el\alpha}$), the elimination rate constant ($k_{el\beta}$) and elimination half-life ($T_{1/2el\beta}$) were also determined. The coefficient of determination (R^2) was hereby used as an indicator for the goodness-of-fit. For the main metabolites, only C_{max}, T_{max}, AUC_{0-inf}, k_{el} en $T_{1/2el}$ were calculated.

Statistical analysis

All pharmacokinetic parameters were compared between administration routes according to dose (therapeutic and growth-promoting), thereby using one-way analysis of variance (ANOVA) (p-value ≤ 0.05) (SPSS 21, IBM, USA). Urinary concentrations were statistically evaluated using Student's t-test and one-way ANOVA with post-hoc Tukey's multiple comparisons test.

Results

Method validation

For each of the targeted compounds, the determination coefficient (R^2) was above 0.99 for all three calibration curves, established in plasma and analyzed on three different days. The other performance characteristics of the validation are presented in Additional file 3. Recoveries ranged from 92 to 107%. Repeatability and within-laboratory reproducibility were evaluated based on the coefficients of variation (RSD) and were below the 15%-tolerance level, specified in CD 2002/657/EC [22], except for 20α-dihydroprednisolone (22.3% at 0.5 μg L^{-1}), which was nevertheless considered acceptable because of the low target concentration.

Pharmacokinetics of prednisolone and its metabolites

The pharmacokinetic parameters were determined for plasma prednisolone during the growth-promoting and therapeutic treatments (Fig. 2. A), thereby using a one- (PO) or two-compartmental (IM) model. A growth-promoting (40 mg day^{-1}) and therapeutic (0.5 mg kg^{-1} day^{-1}) PO administration of prednisolone in cattle resulted in a relatively fast absorption with C_{max} being reached within 2.95 h and 3.85 h (T_{max}), respectively (Table 1). Evidently, prednisolone absorption in case of IM administration was much faster, with T_{max} ranging from 0.168 to 0.866 h. The absorption ($T_{1/2a}$) and elimination half-life ($T_{1/2el}$) for unbound prednisolone after PO and IM administration was considered rather independent of dose, although the highest IM dose (0.5 mg kg^{-1} day^{-1}) showed a somewhat increased $T_{1/2el}$. The Vd/F for oral administered prednisolone increased from 11.95 to 30.06 L kg^{-1} during, respectively, growth-promoting and therapeutic treatment. The same effect was noticed during the two types of IM prednisolone administration.

Pharmacokinetic parameters (one-compartmental) of the main prednisolone metabolites, i.e. prednisone, 20α-, and 20β-dihydroprednisolone, were only considered for the IM therapeutic prednisolone treatment (Table 2) as plasma concentration levels were below the associated CC_α for all these metabolites during oral therapeutic treatment and growth-promoting treatments (PO and IM). Based on the AUC_{0-inf}, it was determined that 20β-dihydroprednisolone is the most abundant prednisolone-derived metabolite in plasma. Additionally, 20β-dihydroprednisolone could be detected already 15 min after IM prednisolone administration. Maximum plasma concentration levels for this metabolite were reached about 2 h after start of the treatment (Fig. 2. B). For prednisone, a similar T_{max} was observed as for prednisolone (0.857 h and 0.866 h, respectively), indicating a very fast conversion of prednisolone into prednisone by the 11β-hydroxysteroid dehydrogenase type 2 enzyme in the liver [24].

During tetracosactide hexaacetate administration, traces of prednisolone in plasma could be detected, but were below CC_α. As reliable quantification is hereby not possible, pharmacokinetic parameters were not determined.

Urinary excretion profile of prednisolone and its metabolites

Growth-promoting treatment

Based on the analysis of the urine samples that were collected prior to prednisolone administration, it was verified that prednisolone, prednisone, 20α-, and 20β-dihydroprednisolone were not endogenously present at detectable concentration levels. After five days of oral prednisolone treatment (40 mg day^{-1}), urinary prednisolone reached an average concentration of 0.832 ± 0.38 μg L^{-1}. When animals were given a same dose by intramuscular injection, an average prednisolone concentration of 1.16 ± 1.08 μg L^{-1} was reached. These urinary prednisolone concentrations are below the threshold of 5 μg L^{-1}, suggested by the EURL. During the following 25 days, the urinary prednisolone concentrations remained rather constant for both treatments.

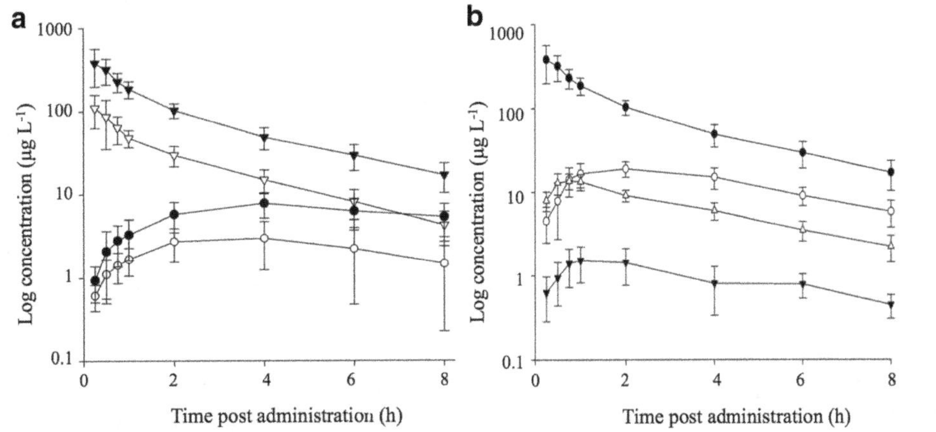

Fig. 2 **a** Plasma concentration profile for prednisolone, as observed after growth-promoting or therapeutic prednisolone administration. Results are expressed as mean plasma concentration levels ± SD (n = 12). The growth-promoting and therapeutic treatment are represented by black and white symbols, respectively. Hereby, a distinction is made between oral (circle) and intramuscular (triangle) prednisolone administration. **b** Plasma concentration profile for prednisolone, 20β-dihydroprednisolone, prednisone, and 20α-dihydroprednisolone as observed after intramuscular therapeutic administration. Results are expressed as mean plasma concentration levels ± SD (n = 12). Prednisolone is represented by black circles, 20β-dihydroprednisolone by white circles, prednisone by white triangles and 20 α-dihydroprednisolone by black triangles

Eventually, 24 h after the growth-promoting treatment was ended, prednisolone concentrations started to decrease. Undetectable levels were reached after 5 days, which appeared to be independent of the administration route.

During growth-promoting treatment, prednisolone and 20β-dihydroprednisolone were detected in all urine samples, whereas 20α-dihydroprednisolone was only present in the urine of 8 out of 12 animals (Table 3. A). Prednisone was not detected in any urine sample when prednisolone was administered orally, being in contrast with intramuscular injection where prednisone was detected in the urine samples from 4 animals. The major prednisolone metabolite, i.e. 20β-dihydroprednisolone, was found until 24 h after the end of the IM treatment, with undetectable levels after five days.

Therapeutic treatment

After three days of PO and IM therapeutic administration of prednisolone, mean urinary prednisolone concentrations of respectively 0.922 µg L^{-1} and 20.1 µg L^{-1} were retrieved. After two more days of IM injection, the urinary average prednisolone concentration further increased to 42.4 µg L^{-1}, whereas the concentration remained rather constant in case of oral treatment. After ending the PO treatment, the urinary excretion profile of prednisolone revealed a very strong decrease. Indeed, within 40 h after final administration, prednisolone concentration levels were diminished with almost 80%. Eventually, after 5 days, no more prednisolone could be detected at concentration levels above the CC_α. For IM injection, prednisolone concentrations above the CC_α were observed in two animals up to 10 days after final treatment.

Table 1 Pharmacokinetic parameters for prednisolone after oral and intramuscular administration during growth-promoting and therapeutic treatment

	Oral treatment		Intramuscular treatment	
	40 mg day^{-1}	0.5 mg kg^{-1} day^{-1}	40 mg day^{-1}	0.5 mg kg^{-1} day^{-1}
C_{max} (µg L^{-1})	2.96 ± 1.50	7.01 ± 1.52	117 ± 25.8	156 ± 78.1
T_{max} (h)	2.95 ± 0.820	3.85 ± 0.909	0.168 ± 0.063	0.866 ± 0.273
$AUC_{0\text{-}tinf}$ (h µg L^{-1})	26.1 ± 19.1	75.5 ± 25.0	232 ± 17.5	678 ± 11.5
k_a (h^{-1})	0.363 ± 0.099	0.307 ± 0.129	17.1 ± 11.2	1.93 ± 0.395
$T_{1/2a}$ (h)	2.05 ± 0.588	2.53 ± 0.854	0.064 ± 0.052	0.370 ± 0.083
k_{el} (h^{-1})	0.362 ± 0.091	0.245 ± 0.053	0.325 ± 0.046	0.132 ± 0.092
$T_{1/2el}$ (h)	2.04 ± 0.553	2.97 ± 0.728	2.16 ± 0.308	3.80 ± 0.499
Vd/F (L kg^{-1})	11.9 ± 4.89	30.1 ± 9.98	0.503 ± 0.215	2.47 ± 1.61
Cl/F (L h^{-1} kg^{-1})	4.66 ± 2.68	7.15 ± 1.97	0.346 ± 0.026	0.737 ± 0.012

Average parameter values and SD were determined on the basis of 12 samples. Therapeutic treatment concerned the administration of 0.5 mg prednisolone kg $^{-1}$ day^{-1}, whereas during growth-promoting treatment 40 mg day^{-1} was administered

Table 2 Pharmacokinetic parameters for prednisone, 20α-dihydroprednisolone and 20β-dihydroprednisolone after intramuscular administration during therapeutic prednisolone treatment

	Prednisone	20α-dihydroprednisolone	20β-dihydroprednisolone
C_{max} (μg L^{-1})	13.3 ± 2.56	1.64 ± 0.677	19.2 ± 4.31
T_{max} (h)	0.857 ± 0.136	1.42 ± 0.413	2.17 ± 0.571
$AUC_{0\text{-}inf}$ (h μg L^{-1})	58.5 ± 12.1	7.07 ± 3.33	121 ± 26.9
k_{el} (h^{-1})	0.307 ± 0.101	0.553 ± 0.184	0.349 ± 0.086
$T_{1/2el}$ (h)	2.43 ± 0.649	1.53 ± 1.02	2.09 ± 0.522

Average parameter values and SD were determined on the basis of 12 samples. Intramuscular therapeutic treatment concerned the injection of 0.5 mg prednisolone kg^{-1} day^{-1}

During PO administration of prednisolone, all urine samples contained prednisolone and 20β-dihydroprednisolone, whereas prednisone and 20α-dihydroprednisolone could only be detected in 2 and 8 animals, respectively. For IM prednisolone injection, all target glucocorticoids were detected in the urine samples of all animals (Table 3B). At the end of the therapeutic treatment, 20β-dihydroprednisolone could be detected in urine up to 24 h and 5 days for PO and IM prednisolone treatment, respectively. The other metabolites were not found after ending PO administration and only until 24 h after ending the IM treatment.

ACTH treatment

The synthesis of various glucocorticoids may be induced by treatment with tetracosactide hexaacetate, affecting

Table 3 Urinary prednisolone, prednisone, 20α-dihydroprednisolone and 20β-dihydroprednisolone concentrations during growth-promoting and therapeutic prednisolone treatment

	Prednisolone	Prednisone	20α-dihydroprednisolone	20β-dihydroprednisolone
A1. Oral growth-promoting treatment				
N° positive	12	0	8	12
C_{min} (μg L^{-1})	0.027	-	0.153	0.695
C_{max} (μg L^{-1})	1.17	-	3.41	14.10
Mean (μg L^{-1})	0.832	-	0.771	4.35
SD (μg L^{-1})	0.381	-	0.544	2.44
A2. Intramuscular growth-promoting treatment				
N° positive	12	4	8	12
C_{min} (μg L^{-1})	0.014	0.030	0.138	0.938
C_{max} (μg L^{-1})	8.44	2.17	1.79	14.2
Mean (μg L^{-1})	1.16	0.311	0.472	4.91
SD (μg L^{-1})	1.08	0.413	0.308	3.15
B1. Oral therapeutic treatment				
N° positive	12	2	8	12
C_{min} (μg L^{-1})	0.038	0.033	0.156	1.07
C_{max} (μg L^{-1})	1.36	0.306	2.85	15.15
Mean (μg L^{-1})	0.922	0.125	0.552	5.13
SD (μg L^{-1})	0.428	0.108	0.635	1.20
B2. Intramuscular therapeutic treatment				
N° positive	12	12	12	12
C_{min} (μg L^{-1})	0.528	1.08	3.32	8.97
C_{max} (μg L^{-1})	189	22.5	127	100
Mean (μg L^{-1})	31.3	8.17	14.9	37.9
SD (μg L^{-1})	40.7	5.91	26.0	25.0

For each of the treatment set-ups (A1, A2, B1, B2), 12 bovines were considered. In case that a glucocorticoid was not found in the urine samples of all animals, means ± SD were determined based on the positive urine samples only

the hypothalamic-pituitary-adrenal axis. In this study, detectable concentration levels of prednisolone, prednisone, 20β-dihydroprednisolone and 20α-dihydroprednisolone were observed under this pharmacologically-induced stress. Hereby, concentration levels for prednisolone in urine ranged from 0.120 to 6.45 μg L^{-1} (average 1.45 μg L^{-1}), 4 h after tetracosactide hexaacetate administration (Day + 1 and Day + 2). After 6 h, prednisolone concentration levels were significantly lower (p-value ≤ 0.05), although still detectable with a concentration range from 0.169 to 0.729 μg L^{-1} (average 0.318 μg L^{-1}). The metabolites prednisone, 20α-, and 20β-dihydroprednisolone were also detected, 4 h after tetracosactide hexaacetate administration (Day + 1 and Day + 2), showing concentrations that ranged from 0.697 to 14.4 μg L^{-1} (average 3.51 μg L^{-1}), 3.31 to 19.1 μg L^{-1} (average 6.31 μg L^{-1}), and 0.407 to 33.2 μg L^{-1} (average 8.12 μg L^{-1}), respectively. At 6 h after treatment (Day + 3 and Day + 4), the metabolite concentrations were 2 to 3 times lower, but still present at detectable levels in the urine from all animals. Eventually, 24 h after the last tetracosactide hexaacetate administration, no residues of prednisolone or its metabolites could be detected.

In this study, urinary 20β-dihydroprednisolone was thus detected upon growth-promoting (PO and IM) prednisolone treatment as well as in the pharmacologically-induced stress situation (Fig. 3). Hereby, no significant differences (p ≥ 0.05) were observed between the 20β-dihydroprednisolone concentrations after PO or IM prednisolone administration and those determined at 6 h post-ACTH treatment. This is not the case when the urinary concentrations are considered 4 h after administration of tetracosactide hexaacetate, showing a significant difference (p ≤ 0.05).

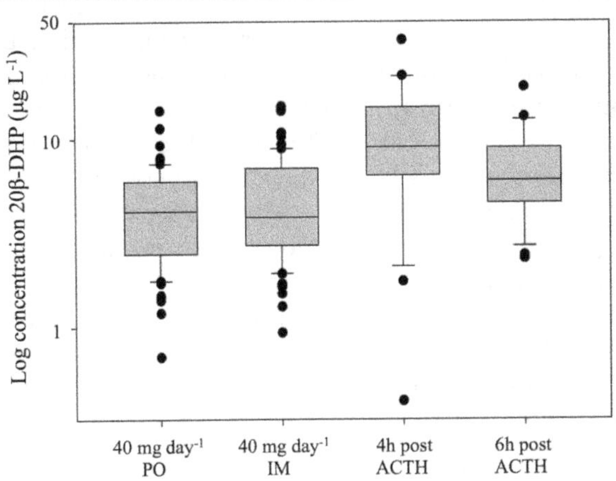

Fig. 3 Urinary concentration profile of 20β-dihydroprednisolone during growth-promoting and ACTH administration. Concentrations of 20β-dihydroprednisolone (20β-DHP) are log-transformed and presented for the oral (PO1) and intramuscular (IM1) growth-promoting treatment, as well as for the ACTH treatment (with sampling moments at 4 h and 6 h after administration)

Urinary excretion profile of natural glucocorticoids

Acclimatization

During the acclimatization period, the three most abundant steroids in urine were cortisol (ranging from 0.411 to 4.26 μg L^{-1}, average 1.79 μg L^{-1}), cortisone (ranging from 0.472 to 5.53 μg L^{-1}, average 2.68 μg L^{-1}) and dihydrocortisone (ranging from 0.222 to 9.36 μg L^{-1}, average 2.27 μg L^{-1}). Other steroids and associated metabolites were detected at significantly lower concentrations.

Growth-promoting and therapeutic treatment

The relative intensity changes of the target natural metabolites during the various treatments are visualized by a heat map (Fig. 4). It was hereby noted that the intensity of most metabolites showed a steady decrease when prednisolone dose increased.

When a growth-promoting dose of prednisolone was administered, regardless of the administration route, a significant decrease (p-value ≤ 0.05) of the urinary concentration was observed for cortisol, cortisone, dihydrocortisone, and deoxycorticosterone (i.e. compared to Blank). After ending the growth-promoting treatment, it took 5 days before cortisol and its associated metabolites reached their basal concentration levels again.

During therapeutic administration, a 2- to 5-fold intensity decrease for the urinary metabolites was noticed for the oral treatment, whereas during IM therapeutic treatment, almost no residues of the glucocorticoids dihydrocortisone, allotetrahydrocortisol, corticosterone, deoxycorticosterone, 6β-hydrocycortisol and α-cortolone remained (p-values ≤ 0.05, i.e. compared to Blank). It took 12 days after ending the therapeutic treatment, before cortisol and its metabolites reached their basal concentration levels again.

ACTH treatment

Urinary glucocorticoid profiles were evaluated during the first 2 days of ACTH treatment. It was thereby concluded that treatment with tetracosactide hexaacetate resulted in significantly (p-value ≤ 0.05) increased urinary secretion of cortisol, cortisone, dihydrocortisone, tetrahydrocortisol, 6β-hydrocycortisol and α-cortolone (Fig. 4). The most intense increases were noticed for cortisol (70-fold), cortisone (40-fold), and 6β-hydrocycortisol (35-fold). In addition, the mineralocorticoid aldosterone was evaluated as well [25], but showed only a 1.5-fold increase, which is much less than the observed 70-fold increase of cortisol.

Discussion

In this study, it was aimed to verify the validity of the prednisolone/cortisol ratio and capacity of 20β-dihydroprednisolone to discriminate between endogenous and exogenous urinary prednisolone [16, 19].

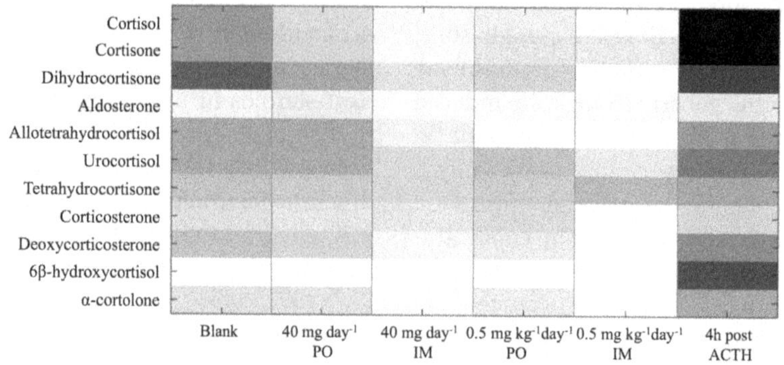

Fig. 4 Heat map with the relative abundance of urinary steroids and metabolites along in vivo treatments. Within this heat map, urinary relative abundances are presented for the acclimatization period (Blank), growth-promoting treatment (PO1 and IM1), therapeutic treatment (PO2 and IM2), and ACTH treatment. The intensities of each ion were averaged (n = 12) and then log-transformed. Shades of black and white represent, respectively, higher and lower intensities as observed for the different treatments

Indeed, there is a strong need for an adequate screening and confirmation tool that is able to unambiguously affirm the origin of detected prednisolone as the EURL suggested discriminative threshold value of 5 μg L^{-1} [12, 13] is not fully conclusive. This was also evidenced in this study as urinary prednisolone concentrations were frequently below this threshold during both growth-promoting and therapeutic treatment. In this context, the above-mentioned screening strategies were comprehensively assessed by evaluating the urinary profiles and plasma pharmacokinetics of relevant glucocorticoids, as being measured during in vivo experiments, which intended to mimic situations of endogenous prednisolone formation and dose-variant exogenous prednisolone administration.

Based on the plasma pharmacokinetics and urinary profiles, it was concluded that 20β-dihydroprednisolone is the most abundant prednisolone-derived metabolite in both matrix types, independently of administration route. These results are in line with the findings of Nebbia et al. (2014) [3], who acknowledged 20β-dihydroprednisolone as the main urinary metabolite of prednisolone in therapeutically treated bovines (n = 14). As such, based on the abundant presence of 20β-dihydroprednisolone, this metabolite was indeed considered interesting to be tested as a potential urinary discriminative marker. In the prednisolone-treated animals, this metabolite could be detected in all urine samples, independently of the prednisolone administration route or dose. However, 20β-dihydroprednisolone was also detected in all samples from the ACTH treatment, which intended to induce endogenous formation of prednisolone. Hereby, no significant differences (p-value > 0.05) could be revealed between the urinary concentrations for the growth-promoting treatment and those in the samples that were collected 6 h after tetracosactide hexaacetate administration. On the other hand, at 4 h after tetracosactide hexaacetate treatment, urinary concentrations of 20β-dihydroprednisolone were noted to be significantly higher (p-value < 0.05) than those obtained during the growth-promoting treatment. Nevertheless, it is stated that 20β-dihydroprednisolone is no adequate marker metabolite as its discriminative potential will be strongly dependent on the time of sampling, relative to the triggering (stress) moment of endogenous prednisolone formation, whereby a small shift in time may already yield a completely different decision with respect to the origin of detected prednisolone. Moreover, it would be very difficult or even impossible to set a discriminative threshold for 20β-dihydroprednisolone as a large inter-individual variation in urinary concentration was noted for this metabolite. In this regard, it can be stated that metabolic processes and their sensitivity to specific triggers are strongly depending on the individual animal, which was also concluded when considering the urinary profiles of 20α-dihydroprednisolone within the prednisolone treatments. It was hereby observed that for both the oral growth-promoting and therapeutic treatment, the same 8 out of 12 animals showed detectable concentration levels of 20α-dihydroprednisolone in their urine. As this was verified to be independent of body weight or age, individual differences in metabolism are assumed to be responsible for this.

Evaluation of the prednisolone/cortisol ratio was conducted by profiling the natural glucocorticoid metabolites during dose-variant prednisolone treatments (growth-promoting and therapeutic) as well as induced formation of endogenous prednisolone. For the prednisolone treatments, a dose-dependent decrease in relative intensities was observed for the natural urinary glucocorticoids, including cortisol. This indicates a significant effect of prednisolone administration on the regulation of the synthesis of endogenous glucocorticoids, being the result of a suppressed hypothalamic-pituitary-adrenal axis.

Hereby, prednisolone inhibits the transcription of corticotropin-releasing hormone (CRH), which also negatively affects the pro-opiomelanocortin (POMC) transcription. The associated POMC polypeptide is a precursor for ACTH, which makes that administration of prednisolone indirectly leads to the inhibition of ACTH and eventually to a decreased production of cortisol [26]. The impact of prednisolone is hereby influenced by both the dosage and administration route [27], which has been observed in this study as well. Focusing on the growth-promoting treatment, prednisolone/cortisol ratios ranged from 0.0603 to 9.55 during PO administration and from 1.57 to 36.9 during IM administration (Fig. 5). Metabolism of cortisol was also monitored during pharmacologically induced stress, triggering the hypothalamic-pituitary-adrenal axis and associated cortisol secretion. As expected, in comparison with non-stressed conditions (i.e. Blank), a significantly higher ($p < 0.05$) urinary cortisol concentration was observed upon tetracosactide hexaacetate administration. For calculation of the associated prednisolone/cortisol ratios, it was opted to also incorporate the data from a recent study of De Clercq et al. (2015) [28], considering a situation of 'natural' stress (at slaughter). As such, concentration ratios ranged from 0.00379 to 0.0763 at 4 h after ACTH treatment, from 0.0147 to 0.129 at 6 h after ACTH treatment, and from 0.00315 to 1.044 awaiting slaughter (Fig. 5). Based on the increased cortisol secretion during (induced) stress, prednisolone/cortisol ratios appeared to be significantly lower (p-value < 0.05) than during growth-promoting prednisolone treatment. However, it is here also noted that ratios tend to change rapidly with the time relative to the moment of stress. Nevertheless, this ratio shows potential to affirm the origin of detected prednisolone, and for this, a discriminative threshold was determined. To this end, a receiver operating characteristics (ROC) curve was established (Fig. 6) (SPSS Statistics 24, BMI, USA), which described the sensitivity and specificity when deciding on the origin of detected prednisolone. Hereby, the individual prednisolone/cortisol ratios associated with natural stress (at slaughter, $n = 36$), induced stress (ACTH treatment, $n = 45$), and prednisolone treatments (PO and IM, $n = 103$) were used. It should be noted that only those samples with detectable prednisolone concentrations were taken into account and that in case of cortisol concentrations below the LOD, the ratio was set as the maximum of the concerned experimental condition. The latter was the case for some samples from PO and IM, and this for both therapeutic and growth-promoting treatment. Based on the area under the curve (AUC), which is in fact a summary measure of the ROC-curve, excellent discrimination using the prednisolone/cortisol ratio was concluded as the AUC was 0.945 (p-value of 4.11 e^{-5}) and thus close to 1 [29]. Searching the balance between an optimal sensitivity and specificity, a threshold of 0.260 was decided, which was accompanied by a sensitivity of 94.2% and a specificity of 99.0%. Further studies should confirm the validity of this threshold in discriminating endogenous from exogenous prednisolone.

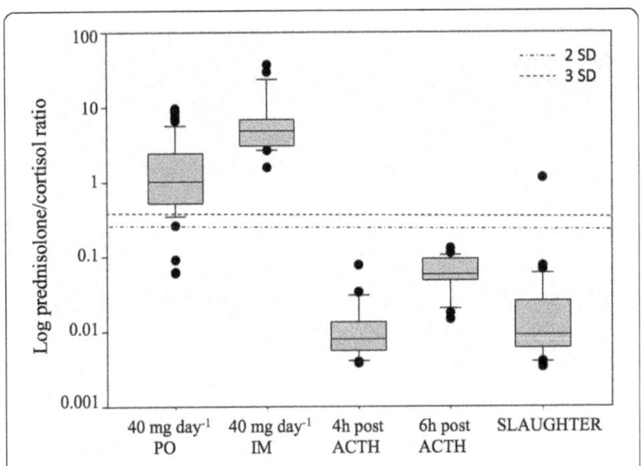

Fig. 5 Boxplot for urinary prednisolone/cortisol ratios as determined for growth-promoting, ACTH treatment and at slaughter. Urinary concentration ratios were log-transformed. Within the growth-promoting treatment, a distinction between oral (PO1) and intramuscular (IM) prednisolone treatment was made

Conclusions

This study yielded an expedient strategy to appoint the origin of detected urinary prednisolone in cattle. More

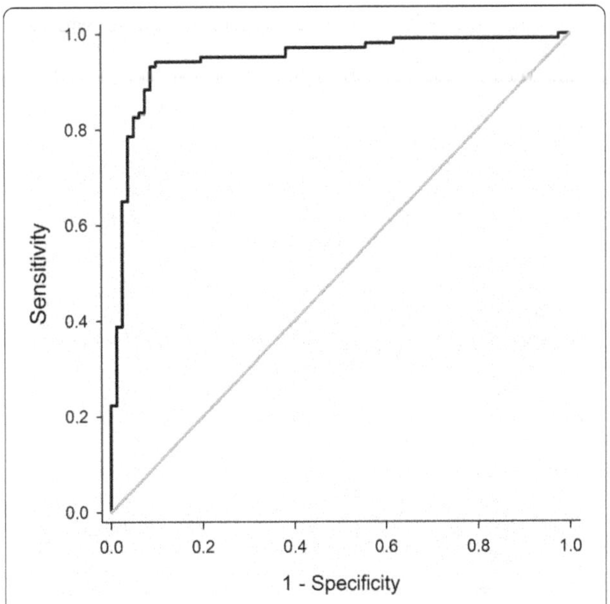

Fig. 6 ROC-curve for sensitivity and specificity in determining the origin of prednisolone using the prednisolone/cortisol ratio. Data for natural stress (slaughter, $n = 36$), pharmacologically induced stress (ACTH, $n = 45$), and exogenously administered prednisolone (PO and IM, $n = 103$) were used for establishing the ROC-curve. The diagonal line represents the class discrimination on random chance with an AUC of 0.5 whereas a perfect discrimination is represented by an AUC of 1. The AUC of this particular ROC curve was 0.945

specifically, the urinary prednisolone/cortisol ratio was found to specifically discriminate between exogenous and endogenous prednisolone, being the result of exogenous prednisolone administration and pharmacologically induced or natural stress, respectively. Hereby, a discriminative threshold value was proposed, i.e. a concentration ratio of 0.260, which rendered a sensitivity of 94.2% and specificity of 99.0%. As such, the prednisolone/cortisol ratio is believed to hold significant value to contribute towards a more righteous decision-making when monitoring for unauthorized usage of prednisolone in bovine breeding. However, it is acknowledged that the validity of the suggested threshold should be verified under varying conditions and on a larger scale before implementation of the prednisolone/cortisol ratio becomes possible. Alternatively, the discriminating potential of 20β-dihydroprednisolone was assessed as well, whereby no unambiguously significant concentration differences were noted between exogenous prednisolone administration and pharmacologically induced endogenous formation of prednisolone. Therefore, at this this point, 20β-dihydroprednisolone was not assigned any marker potential, although situations of prednisolone formation under natural stress should be considered before the marker potential of this metabolite can be disclaimed definitely. In this context and in contrast with the applied targeted approaches, an untargeted fingerprinting of the urinary metabolome may still be opportune to reveal (unknown) metabolite markers in order to transcend the sensitivity and specificity values, as currently linked with the prednisolone/cortisol ratio.

Additional files

Additional file 1: Biotransformation pathway of prednisolone into prednisone, 20α-dihydroprednisolone and 20β-dihydroprednisolone by hydroxysteroid dehydrogenases. Schematic representation of the enzymatic mechanisms, underlying the formation of the major prednisolone-related metabolites. Involved enzymes concern various hydroxysteroid dehydrogenases (HSD).

Additional file 2: MS/MS-parameters for the target glucocorticoids and internal standards. Table that contains data on the selected precursor and product ions, which were selected for each of the targeted glucocorticoids. In addition, optimal parameter settings for tandem fragmentation are presented.

Additional file 3: Performance characteristics of the method for glucocorticoid analysis in bovine plasma. Quantitative data for the performance criteria, obtained by method validation according to CD 2002/657/EC. Whereas recovery and repeatability were evaluated on the basis of 7 samples per nominal concentration, within-laboratory reproducibility was determined by considering 14 samples. RSD represent the relative standard deviation.

Abbreviations

11β-HSD2: 11β-hydroxysteroid dehydrogenase type 2; ACTH: Adrenocorticotropic hormone; $AUC_{0\text{-}inf}$: Area under the plasma concentration-time curve from time 0 to time inf; CER: Centre d'Economie Rurale; Cl/F: Apparent clearance; C_{max}: Peak plasma concentration; HESI: Heated electrospray ionization; IM: Intramuscular; k_a: Absorption rate constant; $k_{el\alpha}$: Distribution rate constant; $k_{el\beta}$: Elimination rate constant; MRL: Maximum residue limit; MRM: Multiple reaction monitoring; PO: Per os; R^2: Determination coefficient; ROC: Receiver operating characteristic; RSD: Coefficients of variation; $T_{1/2a}$: Absorption half-life; $T_{1/2el\beta}$: Elimination half-life; T_{max}: Time to reach the peak plasma concentration; UHPLC: Ultra-high performance liquid chromatography; Vd/F: Apparent volume of distribution

Acknowledgments

The authors wish to thank Mieke Naessens and Joke Goedgebuer for their technical contribution to this manuscript.

Funding

This study was funded by the Federal Public Service of Health, Food Chain Safety and Environment (RT 11/03). The members of the associated evaluation committee had an advising role, especially with regard to the design of the study and interpretation of the data.

Authors' contributions

NDC and LVM performed sample analyses, data interpretation and manuscript establishment. JVB helped with elaboration and optimization of laboratory procedures. EF and PD organized the experimental section of the in vivo study, whereby EF performed the plasma and urine sampling. MD, PD, SC, and LV participated in the study design and revised the manuscript. MD helped with the pharmacokinetics. All authors read and approved the final manuscript.

Consent for publication

Not applicable.

Competing interests

All authors declare that they have no competing interests.

Author details

[1]Faculty of Veterinary Medicine, Department of Veterinary Public Health & Food Safety, Laboratory of Chemical Analysis, Ghent University, Salisburylaan 133, 9820 Merelbeke, Belgium. [2]Faculty of Veterinary Medicine, Department of Pharmacology, Toxicology and Biochemistry, Laboratory of Pharmacology and Toxicology, Ghent University, Salisburylaan 133, 9820 Merelbeke, Belgium. [3]Département Santé, CER Groupe, Rue du Point du Jour 8, Marloie 6900, Belgium.

References

1. Geleta JN, Shimoda W, Mercer HD. Excretion of [3H]prednisolone in clinically normal and experimentally infected bovine udders. Am J Vet Res. 1984;45:1576–81.
2. Sipka A, Gurjar A, Klaessig S, Duhamel GE, Skidmore A, Swinkels J, Cox P, Schukken Y. Prednisolone and cefapirin act synergistically in resolving experimental *Escherichia coli mastitis*. J Dairy Sci. 2013;96:4406–18.
3. Nebbia C, Capra P, Leporati M, Girolami F, Barbarino G, Gatto S, Vincenti M. Profile of the urinary excretion of prednisolone and its metabolites in finishing bulls and cows treated with a therapeutic schedule. BMC Vet Res. 2014;10:237–46.

4. Courtheyn D, Le Bizec B, Brambilla G, De Brabander HF, Cobbaert E, Van de Wiele M, Vercammen J, De Wasch K. Recent developments in the use and abuse of growth promoters. Anal Chim Acta. 2002;473:71–82.
5. Cannizzo FT, Capra P, Divari S, Ciccotelli V, Biolatti B, Vincenti M. Effects of low-dose dexamethasone and prednisolone long term administration in beef calf: chemical and morphological investigation. Anal Chim Acta. 2011;700:95–104.
6. European Commission. Council directive 96/23/EC of 29 April 1996 on measures to monitor certain substances and residues thereof in live animals and animal products. Off J Eur Commun. 1996;L125:10–32.
7. European Commission. Commission Regulation 37/2010 of 22 December 2009 on pharmacologically active substances and their classification regarding maximum residue limits in foodstuffs of animal origin. Off J Eur Union. 2010;L15:1,11,26,47,56.
8. Commission staff working document on the implementation of national residue monitoring plans in the member states in 2009. Brussels, Belgium. https://ec.europa.eu/food/safety/chemical_safety/vet_med_residues_en . Accessed 12 Feb 2015.
9. Commission staff working document on the implementation of national residue monitoring plans in the member states in 2010. Brussels, Belgium. https://ec.europa.eu/food/safety/chemical_safety/vet_med_residues_en. Accessed 12 Feb 2015.
10. Commission staff working document on the implementation of national residue monitoring plans in the member states in 2011. Brussels, Belgium. https://ec.europa.eu/food/safety/chemical_safety/vet_med_residues_en . Accessed 12 Feb 2015.
11. Commission staff working document on the implementation of national residue monitoring plans in the member states in 2012. Brussels, Belgium. https://ec.europa.eu/food/safety/chemical_safety/vet_med_residues_en . Accessed 12 Feb 2015.
12. de Rijke E, Zoontjes PW, Samson D, Oostra S, Sterk SS, van Ginkel LA. Investigation of the presence of prednisolone in bovine urine. Food Addit Contam Part A-Chem. 2014;31:605–13.
13. Wetenschappelijk Comité van het Federaal Agentschap voor de veiligheid van de voedselketen. Betreft: Aanwezigheid van anabole en/of verboden stoffen van endogene oorsprong bij voedselproducerende dieren, 2013 (Amendement Advies 07). http://www.afsca.be/wetenschappelijkcomite/adviezen/2013/. Accessed 12 Feb 2015.
14. Dusi G, Vago G, Ghidelli V, Pellegrino RM, Galarini R. Analytical investigations about the presence of prednisolone in cow urine. J Mass Spectrom. 2012;47:1221–31.
15. Vincenti M, Leporati M, Capra P, Gatto S, Attucci A, Barbarino G, Nebbia C. A field survey on the presence of prednisolone and prednisone in urine samples from untreated cows. Food Addit Contam Part A-Chem. 2012;29:1893–900.
16. Delahaut P, Demoulin L, Gillard N, Fichant E, Courtheyn D. Preliminary study on the presence of prednisolone in porcine urine and liver – how to distinguish endogenous from therapeutically administered prednisolone. Drug Test Anal. 2014;6:325–35.
17. Leporati M, Capra P, Cannizzo FT, Biolatti B, Nebbia C, Vincenti M. Determination of prednisolone metabolites in beef cattle. Food Addit Contam Part A-Chem. 2013;30:1044–54.
18. Pariante CM, Papadopoulos AS, Poon L, Checkley SA, English J, Kerwin RW, Lightman S. A novel prednisolone suppression test for the hypothalamic-pituitary-adrenal axis. Biol Psychiatry. 2002;51:922–30.
19. Jerjes WK, Cleare AJ, Wood PJ, Taylor NF. Assessment of subtle changes in glucocorticoid negative feedback using prednisolone: comparison of salivary free cortisol and urinary cortisol metabolites as endpoints. Clin Chim Acta. 2006;364:279–86.
20. Fidani M, Gamberini MC, Pompa G, Mungiguerra F, Casati A, Arioli F. Presence of endogenous prednisolone in human urine. Steroids. 2002;78:121–6.
21. De Clercq N, Vanden Bussche J, Croubels S, Delahaut P, Vanhaecke L. A validated analytical method to study the long-term stability of natural and synthetic glucocorticoids in livestock urine using ultra-high performance liquid chromatography coupled to Orbitrap-high resolution mass spectrometry. J Chromatogr A. 2013;1301:111–21.
22. European Commission. 2002/657/EC: Commission Decision of 12 August 2002 implementing Council Directive 96/23/EC concerning the performance of analytical methods and the interpretation of results. Off J Eur Commun. 2002;L221:8.
23. Levine L, Fahy JP. Evaluation of urinary lead determinations. J Ind Hyg Toxicol. 1945;27:217–23.
24. Diederich S, Eigendorff E, Burkhardt P, Quinkler M, Bumke-Vogt C, Rochel M, Seidelmann D, Esperling P, Oelkers W, Bähr V. 11beta-hydroxysteroid dehydrogenase types 1 and 2: an important pharmacokinetic determinant for the activity of synthetic mineralo- and glucocorticoids. J Clin Endocrinol Metab. 2002;87:5695–701.
25. Kubzansky LD, Adler GK. Aldosterone: a forgotten mediator of the relationship between psychological stress and heart disease. Neurosci Biobehav Rev. 2010;34:80–6.
26. Tasker JG, Herman JP. Mechanisms of rapid glucocorticoid feedback inhibition of the hypothalamic-pituitary-adrenal axis. Stress. 2011;14:398–406.
27. Czock D, Keller F, Rasche FM, Häussler U. Pharmacokinetics and pharmacodynamics of systemically administered glucocorticoids. Clin Pharmacokinet. 2005;44:61–98.
28. De Clercq N, Van Meulebroek L, Vanden Bussche J, Croubels S, Delahaut P, Vanhaecke L. The impact of stress on the prevalence of prednisolone in bovine urine: a metabolic fingerprinting approach. J Steroid Biochem Mol Biol. 2015;154:206–16.
29. Parikh CR, Thiessen-Philbrook H. Key concepts and limitations of statistical methods for evaluating biomarkers of kidney disease. J Am Soc Nephrol. 2014;25:1621–9.

23

Comparison of the fecal microbiota of domestic commercial meat, laboratory, companion, and shelter rabbits (*Oryctolagus cuniculi*)

Jennifer Kylie, J. Scott Weese and Patricia V. Turner*

Abstract

Background: Rabbits are cecotrophic, hindgut-fermenters that rely heavily on their gastrointestinal microbiota for optimal digestion of plant-based diets. Dysbiosis, caused by disruption of the gastrointestinal microbiota, is known to predispose rabbits to rabbit enteritis complex (REC), a major cause of morbidity and mortality. The objectives of this study were to describe the fecal microbiota of domestic rabbits from a variety of settings (commercial meat, companion, laboratory, and shelter) and to identify how factors such as age, season, and routine antimicrobial use affect the fecal microbiota composition.

Results: A total of 86 pooled commercial meat, 54 companion, 14 pooled laboratory, and 14 shelter rabbit fecal samples were evaluated using 16S rRNA gene sequencing of the V4 region. In all sample types, the predominant bacterial phylum was Firmicutes. Other commonly identified phyla (composing ≥ 1% of the total microbiota composition) were Verrucomicrobia, Proteobacteria, and Bacteroidetes. Significant differences in composition were noted between commercial, companion, laboratory, and shelter rabbit samples for proportions of Verrucomicrobia ($P < 0.01$), Proteobacteria ($P < 0.01$), and Lentisphaerae ($P = 0.01$) within the total microbiota. Within the commercial meat rabbit samples, significant differences between the microbiota composition of growers ($n = 42$) and does ($n = 44$) were limited to one unclassified Firmicutes ($P = 0.03$) and no differences were identified at the phylum level. Significant differences were present between fecal samples taken from rabbits during the summer ($n = 44$) compared to the winter ($n = 42$), with Firmicutes ($P = 0.04$), Verrucomicrobia ($P = 0.03$), Proteobacteria ($P = 0.02$), Deinococcus-Thermus (P = 0.04), Armatimonadates ($P = 0.003$), and Actinobacteria (P = 0.03) forming significantly different proportions of the microbiota. The only significant difference in composition between those farms that routinely reported antimicrobial use and those that did not was in one unclassified Bacteroidetes ($P < 0.05$) and no differences were identified at the phylum level.

Conclusions: Rabbit husbandry and diet, in addition to season, significantly influence the fecal microbiota composition of domestic rabbits, while age of the rabbit post-weaning has minimal impact.

Keywords: Gastrointestinal microbiota, Rabbit, Rabbit enteritis complex

* Correspondence: pvturner@uoguelph.ca
Department of Pathobiology, University of Guelph, Guelph, ON N1G 2W1, Canada

Background

Rabbits are herbivorous, monogastric, hindgut-fermenting mammals that rely on cecotrophy to ensure maximum nutrient absorption from their diet. Management of this unique gastrointestinal (GI) physiology can be challenging, and, as a result, enteric disease is common in domestic rabbits. One of the most difficult aspects of managing rabbit digestion is maintaining the normal commensal gastrointestinal microbiota. In rabbits, disruption of the normal microbiota, termed dysbiosis, is commonly implicated as a cause of enteritis, with ensuing diarrhea, subsequent dehydration, inadequate nutrition, and, potentially, death as a result.

The etiopathogenesis of enteritis in rabbits is complex and generally multifactorial. Enteric pathogens such as *Escherichia coli, Clostridium spiriforme, Lawsonia intracellularis*, rotavirus, and coronavirus are commonly associated with diarrhea outbreaks in rabbits, as are other agents such as *Clostridium piliforme, Salmonella* spp., parvovirus, and astrovirus [1–6]. However, much is still unknown about initiating factors as infection with these organisms is not synonymous with disease and subclinical infection may occur with no overt clinical signs [7]. Most cases of enteritis in rabbits are caused by a combination of factors, including feeding of a low fiber diet, debility and overall health status, management-related stress, and age, along with the presence of one or more potentially pathogenic organisms [7–9].

Because of its critical importance in rabbit health, several studies have focused on understanding the composition of the rabbit enteric microbiota. Historically, researchers used culture-based techniques; however, the development of culture-independent techniques has permitted much greater in-depth analysis [10, 11]. Culture-based studies concluded that Bacteroidetes was the predominant bacterial phylum within the rabbit gastrointestinal tract, regardless of age [12]. With culture-independent sequencing Bacteroidetes are still reported as predominant in the intestinal tract of very young rabbits, but the predominant phylum in post-weaned and adult rabbits is Firmicutes, with Bacteroidetes accounting for only a small fraction [13–16]. Other predominant phyla routinely identified using culture-independent sequencing include Verrucomicrobia and Proteobacteria [14, 16].

Previous studies examining the fecal microbiota of rabbits have used small numbers of laboratory rabbits kept in well-controlled environments exposed to minimal environmental or husbandry variations, making broad applicability to other domestic rabbit conditions less likely. Factors such as diet, husbandry, and seasonal effects have been demonstrated to have effects on the fecal microbiota in both humans and other animal species [17–19], but have not been explored in rabbits. The objectives of this study were to characterize the microbiota of domestic rabbits kept in a variety of environments and to identify factors contributing to enteric microbiota variations using a culture-independent, high-throughput sequencing method. We hypothesized that significant fecal microbiota differences would be seen between commercial meat rabbits and domestic rabbits kept in other settings, largely because of differences in husbandry, including dietary composition, routine use of antimicrobials, and environmental management. Additionally, we hypothesized that these differences would be least significant between commercial meat rabbits and rabbits housed in a shelter environment (i.e., a facility where previously-owned animals have been surrendered for re-homing) due to the likely inconsistencies in the environment of both of these types of rabbits and diet (in the case of shelter rabbits), while differences would be most significant between commercial meat rabbits and both companion and laboratory rabbits due to more consistent environmental conditions, diet, care, and reduced infectious disease within these latter two groups of rabbits.

Results

A total of 168 rabbit fecal samples from various sources were included in the final analysis: 86 pooled commercial meat, 54 companion, 14 pooled laboratory, and 14 shelter animals. Twenty-three samples (14 commercial meat, 8 companion, and 1 shelter) were not included in the final analysis either due to an inability to produce bands following DNA extraction, amplification, and purification, an insufficient quantity of DNA within the sample (< 12.5 nM) at the time of normalization prior to sequencing or an insufficient number of sequences (< 5000) present following the completion of all quality control filters. A total of 10,897,154 V4 16S rRNA gene sequences passed all quality control filters. Sequence numbers per sample ranged from 6359 to 325,029, with a mean of 64,864, median of 53,721, and a standard deviation of 46,279.

The domestic rabbit fecal microbiota

The analysis was based on 168 samples, with a subsample of 4577 sequences per sample for normalization. A total of 31 bacterial phyla were identified; however, only five were present at a relative abundance of ≥ 1%. Of these five phyla, Firmicutes composed 66.4% of the total microbiota, Verrucomicrobia composed 14.1%, Proteobacteria composed 9.5%, and Bacteroidetes composed 1.54% while 6.9% of the sequences could not be identified at the phylum level (see Additional file 1: Table S1 for further information).

Comparison of the rabbit fecal microbiota based on animal source

There were several statistically significant differences in relative abundance of bacteria within all taxonomic levels based on animal source. These differences remained consistent regardless of whether the specific source from which the sample came was included as a random effect in the analysis; therefore, all relative abundance analyses that are reported below exclude specific source as a random effect. Significant differences were identified between commercial rabbits, and companion and laboratory rabbits in relative abundances of Proteobacteria ($P < 0.01$), between commercial rabbits, companion rabbits, and laboratory and shelter rabbits in relative abundances of Verrucomicrobia ($P < 0.01$), and between commercial rabbits, and companion and shelter rabbits in relative abundances of Lentisphaera ($P < 0.01$) when the p-value was corrected for false discovery rates (Fig. 1). These differences were also reflected at all levels of taxonomic classification (see Additional file 2: Table S2).

Commercial meat and companion rabbits had distinctly different fecal microbiota community structures, while those of laboratory and shelter rabbits tended to overlap with those from companion rabbits (Fig. 2). The dendrogram of community structure (Yue and Clayton index of dissimilarity) is presented in Fig. 3.

In both cases, clustering of ≥ 10 samples can be seen within large numbers of commercial and pet samples, with the laboratory and shelter rabbit fecal samples scattered intermittently between, and primarily amongst, the companion samples. Using the Jaccard tree, significant differences were noted between all possible group pairings using a parsimony test ($P < 0.02$ for all comparisons), something that was also noted with unweighted UniFrac tests ($P \leq 0.04$ for all comparisons), indicating that the fecal microbiota community membership differed significantly between all sources. Using the parsimony test with the Yue and Clayton tree, significant differences were identified between commercial meat and laboratory samples ($P = 0.03$), commercial meat and companion animal samples ($P < 0.01$), and commercial meat and shelter samples ($P < 0.01$). These differences were also detected using unweighted UniFrac (all $P < 0.01$), indicating that fecal microbiota community structure was significantly different between commercial meat rabbits and rabbits from all other sources, but the other sources did not differ amongst one another. Thirty-seven OTUs were identified to be differentially abundant via LEfSe ($P \leq 0.05$) with LDA scores ≥ 3.0 (Table 1).

Comparison of the rabbit fecal microbiota based on animal age

Forty-four samples, each consistently of pooled feces from 3 does per commercial meat farm, and 42 samples composed of pooled feces from 3 growers per commercial meat farm, were compared, with a subsample of 4577 sequences per sample. No significant differences were observed in relative abundance between the two age groups at the bacterial phylum, order, family, and genus levels (all adjusted $P > 0.05$). At the class level, there was a significant difference between does and growers for an unclassified Firmicutes, where the relative abundance in does was 5.8% and in growers was 7.7% ($P = 0.03$).

Community structure differences are visualised in the PCoA (Fig. 2b). There is significant overlap between the community structures of the two different age groups with no obvious grouping based on age. A significant

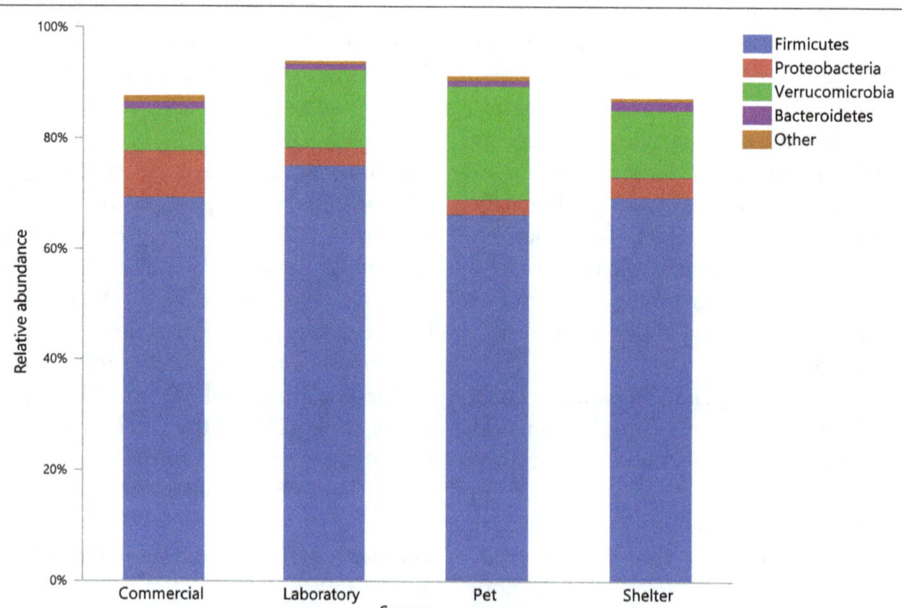

Fig. 1 Median relative abundances of predominant bacterial phyla of the rabbit fecal microbiota separated by animal source. Significant differences ($p \leq 0.05$) are present between sources for Proteobacteria, Verrucomicrobia, and Lentisphaera (included in 'Other' and composed < 1% of the total composition)

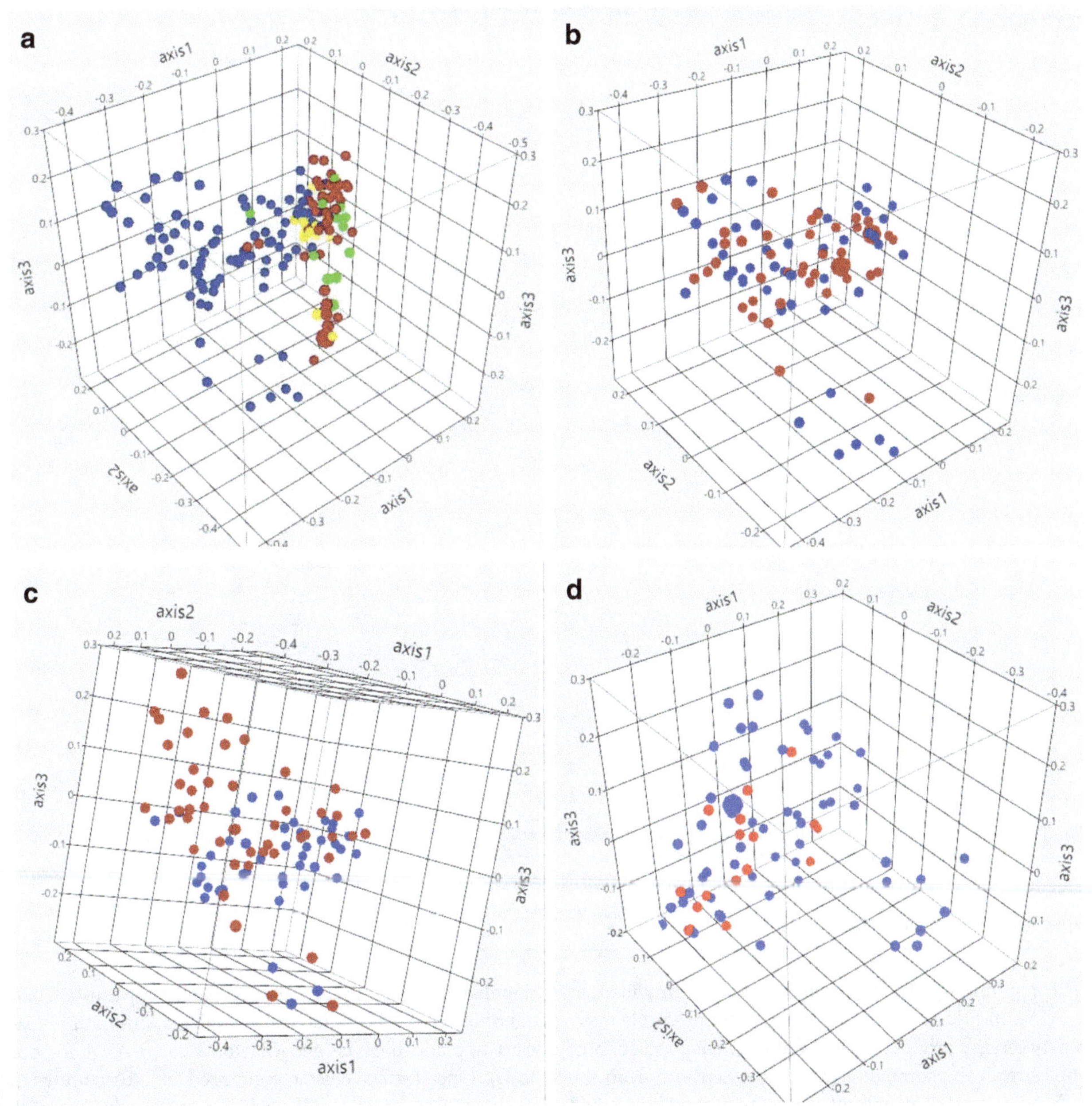

Fig. 2 Principle co-ordinates analysis (PCoA) of the rabbit fecal microbiota based on the Jaccard Index. **a** blue circles = commercial meat rabbits, red circles = companion rabbits, yellow circles = laboratory rabbits, green circles = shelter rabbits; **b**) blue circles = does, red circles = fryers; **c**) blue circles = winter, red circles = summer; **d**) blue circles = routine antimicrobial use, red circles = no routine use of antimicrobials. Clustering of markers within a plot indicates similarity in microbiota community membership. Significant differences are present between rabbit sources and between seasons, but not between ages and antimicrobial use statuses

difference between the fecal microbiota community structure of does and fryers was only noted using the Yue and Clayton tree with the parsimony test ($P = 0.04$); however, no more than five samples were noted to be clustered by age within commercial meat samples in the Yue and Clayton tree analysis (Fig. 3). Six OTUs were identified to be significantly different between ages ($P \leq 0.05$) with LEfSe LDA scores ≥ 3.0 (Fig. 4a).

Comparison of the rabbit fecal microbiota based on season

A comparison was conducted of 44 pooled fecal samples collected from meat rabbits during winter months and 42 pooled fecal samples collected during summer months, with a subsample of 4577 sequences per sample. Significant differences at all taxonomic levels of classification were identified (Table 2).

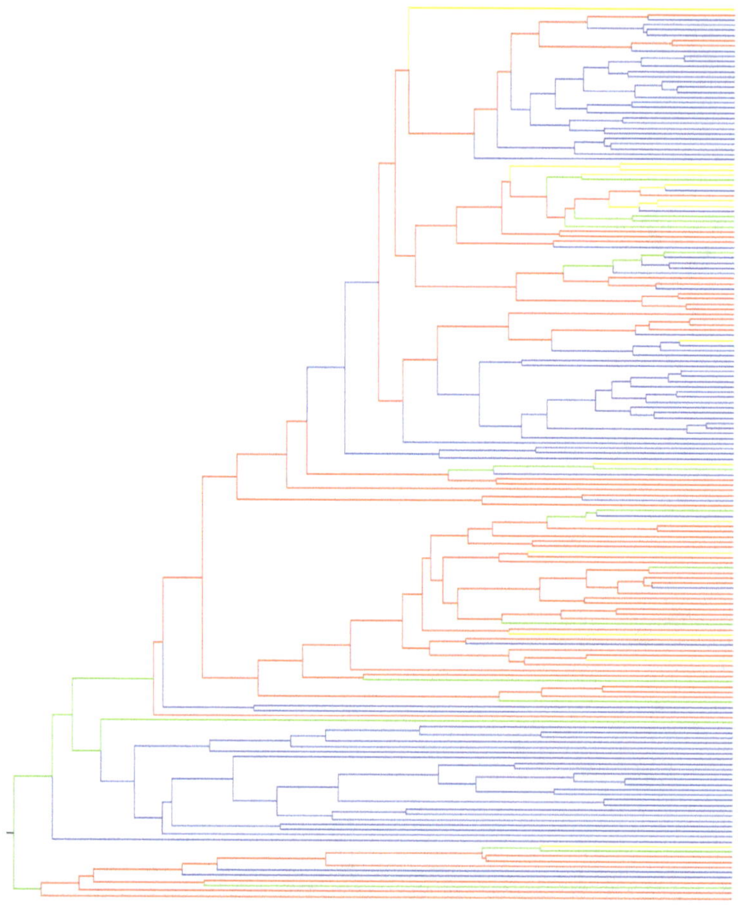

Fig. 3 Dendrogram of the rabbit fecal microbiota community structure based on the Yue and Clayton Index of Dissimilarity. Blue = commercial rabbits, red = companion rabbits, yellow = laboratory rabbits, green = shelter rabbits. Clustering of lines indicates similarity in microbiota community structure. Significant differences are present between commercial meat rabbits and all other sources. The top cluster delineated by the vertical black line indicates clustering of samples collected from commercial meat rabbits during the winter months while the clusters indicated by the lower vertical black lines indicate clustering of samples collected from commercial meat rabbits during the summer months

The community structure differences are presented in the PCoA in Fig. 2c. While there is significant visible overlap between the groups, there is a distinct subpopulation of samples from the summer group that is separate from the overlying samples. Significant differences were identified between summer and winter fecal microbiota community membership and structure using a parsimony test ($P < 0.01$) , and unweighted UniFrac tests ($P < 0.01$) with both the Jaccard tree and the Yue and Clayton tree ($P < 0.01$ for both tests). One distinct cluster comprised of ≥ 10 commercial meat rabbits samples collected during the winter months was present, as was one distinct cluster of ≥ 10 samples

Table 1 OTUs identified as significantly differentially abundant ($p \leq 0.05$) from all other rabbit sources with LDA scores ≥ 3.0

Commercial meat	Companion	Laboratory	Shelter
Unclassified Ruminococcaceae	Unclassified Bacteroidetes	Unclassified Firmicutes	*Corynebacterium*
Tissierella	Unclassified Lachnospiraceae	Unclassified Clostridia	Unclassified Bacteroides
Unclassified Aerococcaceae	Unclassified Bacillaceae_2	*Flavonifractor*	*Barnesiella*
Erysipelothrix	*Campylobacter*	*Pseudoflavonifractor*	*Acetitomaculum*
Facklamia	Unclassified Desulfovibrionaceae	*Anaerostipes*	Unclassified Erysipelotrichaceae
Unclassified Pseudomonadaceae	*TM7_genus_incertae_sedis*	*Lutispora*	*Bacillus*
Paenalcaligenes	*Persicirhabdus*	*Lachnospira*	*Pseudomonas*
Ignatzschineria	Unclassified Verrucomicrobiaceae	*Acetivibrio*	
Oligella		Unclassified Alphaproteobacteria	
Escherichia_Shigella		Unclassified Betaproteobacteria	
Oceanisphaera			
Stenotrophomonas			

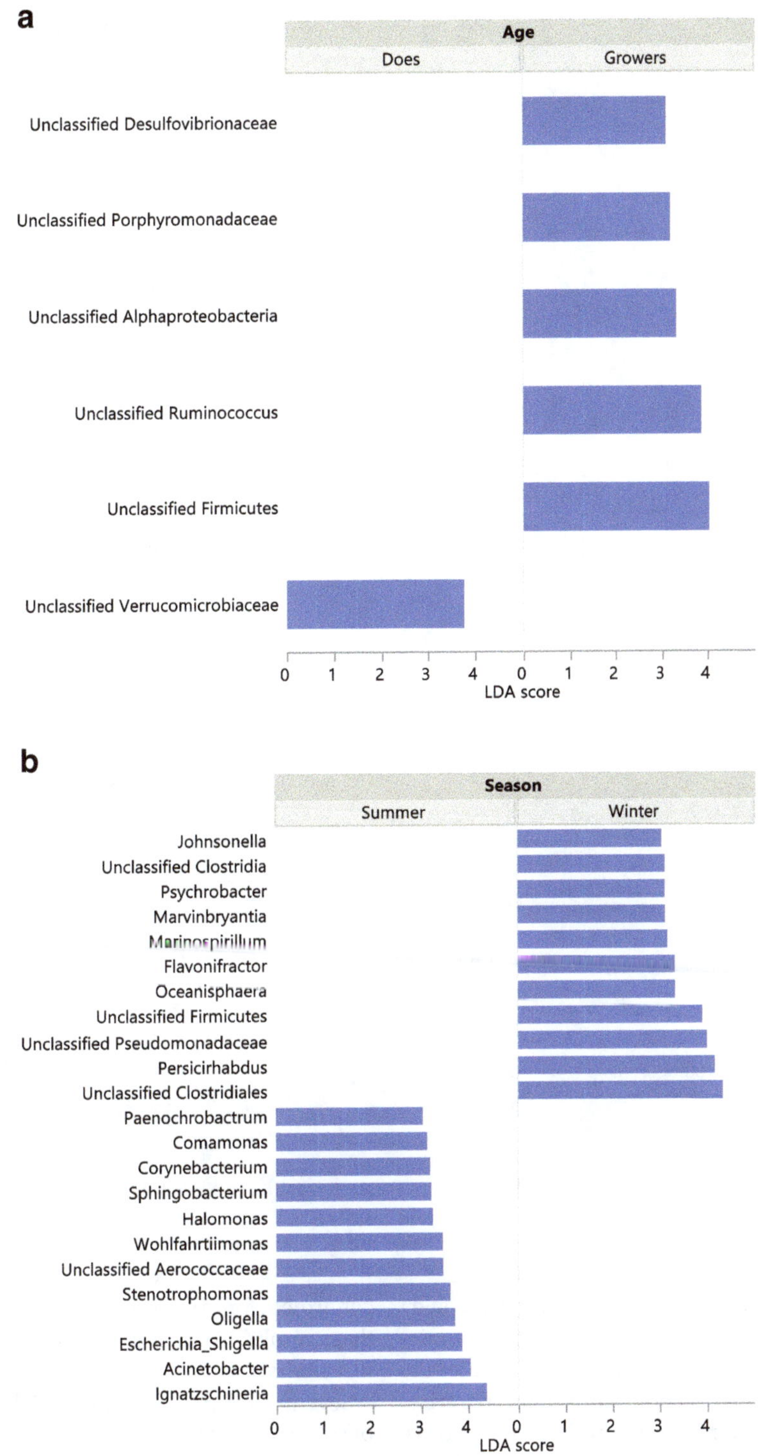

Fig. 4 OTUs noted to be significantly different between **a**) ages and **b**) seasons with LEfSe scores > 3.0

collected during the summer months within the Yue and Clayton Tree calculated based on animal source (Fig. 3). Twenty-three OTUs were identified to be significantly different between season ($P \leq 0.05$) with LDA scores ≥ 3.0 (Fig. 4b).

Comparison of the rabbit fecal microbiota based on routine antimicrobial use

Routine use of antimicrobials in feed or water was reported in 17 of 23 (73.9%) farms, while 3 farms did not respond and one farm had closed at the time of follow-

Table 2 Relative abundance and FDR *p*-values for significantly different ($P \leq 0.05$) samples from summer ($n = 44$) and winter ($n = 42$)

	Relative Abundance - Summer	Relative Abundance – Winter	FDR *P*-value
Phylum			
Actinobacteria	1.14%	0.57%	0.03
Bacteroidetes	1.90%	1.22%	0.03
Deinococcus-Thermus	0.06%	0.01%	0.04
Proteobacteria	18.57%	9.09%	0.02
Verrucomicrobia	7.29%	10.64%	0.03
Firmicutes	62.94%	69.51%	0.04
Order			
Actinomycetales	0.82%	0.17%	0.04
Flavobacteriales	0.33%	0.09%	0.04
Rhodobacterales	0.20%	0.04%	0.04
Xanthomonadales	5.86%	0.95%	0.04
Family			
Microbacteriaceae	0.06%	0.01%	0.03
Flavobacteriaceae	0.30%	0.06%	0.03
Rhodobacteraceae	0.20%	0.04%	0.05
Burkholderiaceae	0.01%	< 0.01%	0.01
Moraxellaceae	2.20%	0.55%	0.03
Xanthomonadaceae	5.86%	0.95%	0.03
Aerococcaceae	1.19%	0.38%	0.03
Unclassified Clostridiales (Firmicutes)	17.7%	22.2%	0.05
Genus			
Leucobacter	0.04%	0.01%	0.05
Flavobacterium	0.07%	< 0.01%	0.03
Myroides	0.11%	0.01%	0.05
Burkholderia	0.01%	< 0.01%	0.02
Delftia	< 0.01%	< 0.01%	0.03
Unclassified Enterobacteriaceae (Proteobacteria)	0.11%	0.01%	0.05
Acinetobacter	2.16%	0.38%	0.02
Serpens	0.04%	< 0.01%	0.04
Wohlfahrtiimonas	0.41%	0.02%	0.05
Marvinbryantia	0.19%	0.34%	0.02

up questioning. Farms for which antimicrobial use could not be confirmed were excluded from the analysis. Antimicrobials reported to be used routinely included, in order of descending frequency of use, salinomycin sodium 6%, virginiamycin, tylosin, chlortetracycline, bacitracine methylene disalicylate, sulfamethazine, sulfadimethoxine, and one anti-coccidial agent that was not further specified. Twelve of the 17 (70.6%) farms reporting routine antimicrobial use reported using ≥ 2 antimicrobials in combination, making statistical analysis of the data beyond the general category of "routine antimicrobial use" not feasible. Antimicrobials were not reported to be routinely used in any of the laboratory rabbits sampled, and antimicrobial use could not be confirmed for the companion or shelter rabbit samples; thus, results from these groups were also excluded from this analysis.

Seventy-five pooled commercial meat rabbit fecal samples were compared on the basis of routine antimicrobial use following sequence filtering and the removal of non-responders, 58/75 (77.3%) with routine antimicrobial use, with a subsample of 4577 sequences per sample. The only significant difference observed at all levels of taxonomic classification, aside from the phylum level where no significant differences were observed, was in one Bacteroidetes unclassified at the class level ($P < 0.01$ at all taxonomic levels), which was significantly higher in samples from farms where no routine antimicrobial use occurred (0.85, 0.75, 0.75, 0.57% at class, order, family, and genus levels, respectively) compared to when routine use did occur (0.29, 0.31, 0.30, 0.32%, respectively).

No significant differences in community membership or structure were identified using Jaccard or Yue and Clayton trees with both the parsimony and unweighted UniFrac tests ($p \geq 0.29$ for all tests); samples from farms that did not report routine use of antimicrobials can be seen as well-distributed amongst samples from farms that did in the PCoA in Fig. 2d. Thirteen OTUs were identified to be significantly different between use status ($P \leq 0.05$) with LDA scores ≥ 2.0; single OTUs with an LDA score ≥ 3.0 that were more frequently identified with routine antimicrobial use were from each of the following genera: *Ignatzschineria, Erysipelothrix*, and *Wohlfahrtiimonas*. One OTU with an LDA score ≥ 3 was significantly more prevalent when antimicrobials were not being routinely used was present from each of the following genera: *Acetitomaculum, Clostridium* cluster III, and *Parasporobacterium*, in addition to one unclassified Ruminococcaceae, one unclassified Desulfovibrionaceae, and one unclassified Bacteroidetes.

Discussion

Our study provides significant insight into the composition of fecal microbiota of domestic rabbits, as well as factors that may promote changes in its composition. The large number of animals sampled, combined with the variety of factors incorporated into the study, suggests that the results are applicable to rabbits in a variety of domestic settings. Consistent with previous culture independent sequencing studies, such as those conducted by Eshar and Weese [14] and Zhu et al. [16], the predominant phylum identified in the rabbit fecal microbiota, regardless of source, age, season or reported antimicrobial use was Firmicutes. Within this phylum, the Clostridia were the most abundant class identified, of which the Ruminococcaceae and the Lachnospiraceae were the most abundant families present. While the prevalence of Firmicutes in our study is lower than that reported by Eshar and Weese (66% vs. 82%, respectively) , other studies report levels of Firmicutes varying between 61 and 82% with significant individual variation, suggesting that the relative abundance of Firmicutes in the rabbit enteric microbiota falls somewhere within this range [16, 20]. In addition to being identified as the predominant phylum present in the rabbit gut, Firmicutes has been described as the most abundant phylum in the gastrointestinal microbiota of most healthy adult mammals, including humans [21–24], emphasizing its likely importance as a commensal in GI health.

Other predominant phyla identified include Verrucomicrobia, Proteobacteria, and Bacteroidetes. The relative levels identified for these phyla are consistent with previous reports, although proportions of Verrucomicrobia appear to vary considerably with the method of analysis [14, 16, 20, 25]. While Verrucomicrobia is still a relatively newly-defined group of organisms, *Akkermansia* (within this phylum) has been suggested to have a key role in hydrolysis of diverse ingested polysaccharides, contributing to more complete digestion of dietary cellulose as well as methane metabolism [26–28]. Thus, its presence as an important constituent of the rabbit fecal microbiota is unsurprising. The most well-known species in this genus is *Akkermansia muciniphila*, a mucin-degrading bacterium that has been demonstrated to be beneficial in both human and animal health [29, 30]. For example, increases in the proportion of fecal *Akkermansia mucinophila* have been associated with a healthier metabolic status in both humans and mice [29, 30]. While the impact of *Akkermansia muciniphila* on rabbit health is still unknown, it is known that the ability to breakdown mucin is especially important during cecotrophy for optimal nutrient extraction [8]. In vitro studies have also identified a positive correlation between the proportion of Verrucomicrobiaceae and concentrations of proprionate and acetate, volatile fatty acids that are found in high concentrations within rabbit ceca following the breakdown of fiber-rich carbohydrates, and significant energy sources [20, 31]. *Akkermansia mucinophila* levels have also been inversely correlated with several inflammatory markers in mice [32], indicating that a decrease in *Akkermansia mucinophila* levels may result in a more pro-inflammatory gut environment. A decreased proportion of Verrucomicrobia within the fecal microbiota of commercial meat rabbits overall, and particularly during the summer months, as found in this study, suggests less optimal gut health and nutrient extraction in this group of rabbits, as well as a pro-inflammatory state. This most likely reflects the lack of hay in the diet of commercial meat rabbits, compared to rabbits from other sources, as well as metabolic distress potentially due to heat stress, discussed in further detail below.

While small proportions of Proteobacteria are routinely observed within the enteric microbiota of all mammals, it has been suggested that increased relative abundance of Proteobacteria should be considered as a diagnostic indicator of underlying dysbiosis, predisposing individuals to enteric disease or indicating the presence of disease [33]. Relative increases in Proteobacteria with or without a concurrent reduction in Firmicutes have been observed in several species in cases of metabolic gastrointestinal disorders, such as genetically-related and diet-induced obesity [34, 35], as well as in chronic intestinal inflammation, such as inflammatory bowel disease and ulcerative colitis [36, 37]. It is hypothesized that the resultant bacterial population shift caused by increasing relative proportions of Proteobacteria stimulates the host gastrointestinal immune system, resulting in a pro-inflammatory response [38]. Therefore, the increased relative proportion of Proteobacteria observed within commercial meat rabbits overall, and specifically during the summer, suggests a shift away from the normal gut microbiota in these animals, increasing their risk for disease development. This idea is supported by the higher proportion of potentially pathogenic bacteria associated with REC identified in commercial meat rabbit fecal samples overall as well as in the summer at the OTU level. In both cases, elevations in *Escherichia/Shigella* accounted for significant differences in fecal microbiota composition when compared to feces from rabbits from other sources.

No significant differences were observed between does and growers in this study. This is consistent with previous reports suggesting that the rabbit fecal microbial community rapidly reaches a steady state at, or just after, weaning [20]. This stabilization has been observed in several other species, including mice [39] and pigs [40]. Additionally, no significant differences were observed between samples from farms in which antimicrobials were routinely used compared to farms where they were not. In 2007, Abecia et al. examined the effects of bacitracin and tiamulin on the cecal microbiota of lactating rabbit does. The study demonstrated that significant microbiota compositional changes were highly dependent on the specific antimicrobial used, with bacitracin having minimal effects on the cecal microbiota composition and tiamulin causing significant changes [41]. In the current study, a variety of antimicrobials with different pharmacologic mechanisms were reported in use alone or in combination, including those with anticoccidial activity and those used to treat respiratory disease. Effects of specific agents on the gut microbiota may have been masked by the concurrent use of other antimicrobial agents; additional studies into the effects of specific antimicrobial agents on the microbiota composition will help to differentiate those antimicrobials likely to have a significant effect versus those that have minimal effect.

Several factors that may contribute to gut microbiota composition are thought to differ significantly between domestic rabbit sources – in particular, the diet. Once animals are weaned, commercial meat rabbits are almost exclusively fed extruded pellet diets relatively low in fiber (15–20%) and high in carbohydrates to encourage rapid growth prior to slaughter [42]. This contrasts with recommended feeding practices for companion rabbits, which suggest a high fiber hay-based diet (e.g., timothy hay) that is supplemented (< 5%) by lower fiber pellets to ensure that all nutritional requirements are met while optimizing gastrointestinal function [9, 43]. Companion rabbit owners also frequently supplement this recommended dietary regimen with other fiber-rich fruits and vegetables. While the diet of laboratory rabbits is also primarily that of high carbohydrate pellets, the fiber content of many of the commercially available laboratory diets tends to be closer to 25%. Laboratory rabbits are also frequently given hay and vegetables as enrichment, although generally at more restricted levels than companion rabbits, while the dietary history of domestic rabbits in shelters is largely unknown. There is also significant variation in how long these animals may have been in a shelter receiving a balanced diet. Dietary fiber source, content, and digestibility are critical components of the rabbit diet, in which changes are directly and significantly correlated with enteritis and mortality in growing meat rabbits [44, 45]. It was beyond the scope of this study to evaluate specific changes in dietary fiber source, content, and type in relation to the rabbit fecal microbiota; however, this likely contributes to the majority of differences noted in microbiota between commercial meat and other sources of rabbits and is an area of further investigation.

Studies in other species examining the influence of season on the gut microbiota have identified decreases in the relative abundance of Verrucomicrobia during the summer as observed in the current study, but not relative increases in Bacteroidetes and Proteobacteria as were seen in this study [19]. The seasonal changes in the microbiota of Arctic ground squirrels observed in the Stevenson et al. 2014 study were attributed to diet availability and variation between seasons. In the current study, seasonality was only examined in commercial meat rabbits, in which the diet remains relatively consistent with fixed content proportions year-round (although changes in plant source and feed quality may vary from batch to batch). Thus, it is unlikely that the seasonal changes in relative abundance of different phyla were related to diet. Rabbits are much more tolerant of colder temperatures and low humidity and they are especially prone to heat stress [9, 46]. In general, Canadian rabbit barns do not have environmental controls for temperature or relative humidity and rabbits are exposed to hot and humid ambient conditions in July and August. The relative reduction in levels of the two beneficial phyla (Firmicutes and Verrucomicrobia), and the relative increase in less beneficial phyla (Proteobacteria) could relate to seasonal-related climate changes and directly impact rabbit health, susceptibility to enteritis, and possibly feed conversion efficiency. Additional studies are needed to explore these possibilities. Studies of potential seasonal differences in gut microbiota of rabbits from other sources are also needed.

A potential limitation of this study is whether the fecal microbiota is reflective of the gastrointestinal microbiota of rabbits in general. Michelland et al. [47] demonstrated no significant differences in bacterial community diversity between soft and hard feces or cecal content in rabbits. In addition, Schoster et al. [48] demonstrated that while significant differences existed between the microbiota of the stomach, duodenum, ileum, large colon, and feces in healthy horses, another hindgut-fermenting species, the microbiota profile remained stable from the cecum to the feces. These studies suggest that, at least in the case of hindgut-fermenting species, the fecal microbiota is representative of the distal gastrointestinal tract. For rabbits, in which the cecal microbiota is of primary consideration for overall animal health, the fecal microbiota provides an accurate and non-invasive method for studying their gastrointestinal health.

This study exclusively characterized the bacterial fecal microbiota of rabbits. It is well known that other prokaryotic and eukaryotic microorganisms, such as viruses, bacteriophages, protozoa, archaea and fungi, are essential components of the gastrointestinal microbiota, and can play significant roles in human and animal health [23, 49]. As pathogenic viruses, in addition to pathogenic bacteria, are significant contributors to rabbit dysbiosis and REC, a greater understanding of the rabbit gut virome would provide further insight into understanding rabbit health.

Lastly, it is unknown whether the organisms identified using next generation sequencing methods are functionally or metabolically active. Future computational studies are needed to specifically examine the metabolomics of the bacteria identified.

Conclusions

This study characterized the composition of the domestic rabbit fecal microbiota, as well as potential factors influencing its composition, such as rabbit source, age, and season, and the routine use of antimicrobials. By gaining an increased understanding of the rabbit enteric microbiota and factors that influence its composition, rabbit health and welfare can be better managed.

Methods

Animals and study approval

Commercial meat rabbit producers were contacted through Ontario Rabbit, a rabbit producer group, and asked to voluntarily participate in the study. Feces from domestic rabbits from 27 commercial farms (representing approximately 25% of large rabbit farms in Ontario, Canada) were collected for this study. Rabbit feces were sampled based on age (does and growers, aka fryers) and fecal samples were collected during summer and winter months. Feces from an additional 62 clinically healthy adult companion rabbits of varying ages and breeds were included. Rabbit fecal samples from one commercial laboratory rabbit vendor and seven laboratory research facilities in Ontario were also included, as were rabbit feces from four shelters in southwestern Ontario. All known history for samples collected is listed in Table 3. In all cases, participation in the study was voluntary, with companion, laboratory, and shelter organizations contacted directly by the researchers of the study.

Fecal sample collection

Hard feces of commercial meat rabbits ($n = 100$ samples) and laboratory rabbits ($n = 14$ samples) were collected from pans beneath rabbit home cages. In all cases, attempts were made to collect the freshest samples from the top layer of feces in the collecting pan (i.e., the most recently voided samples) or by placing a clean pan within 48 h prior to collection. Pooled fecal samples were collected from 3 separate cages per age group that were well-dispersed throughout each barn or facility and mixed thoroughly in sterile plastic bags. For commercial rabbits, one sample bag was submitted for each of two age groups, growers (aged 5–12 weeks) and does (reproductively active, adult, females) per farm. Samples from commercial rabbits were collected during summer (July-Aug) and winter (Feb-Mar) months, when possible. Producers were also asked to verbally report any antimicrobial use, both routine and sporadic, at the time of collection; this information was later confirmed by email or telephone follow-up. At research facilities, when possible, multiple samples (up to 3) were collected from the same facility if there were enough number of rabbits kept in the same room to allow for multiple collections (1 facility), rabbits were kept in multiple rooms or multiple sites throughout the facility (1 facility), significantly different age groups were present within the facility (1 facility), an opportunity was provided to collect samples in repeated years (1 facility), and an opportunity occurred to collect samples immediately following rabbit shipping/arrival to the facility and then following a period of acclimation (1 facility). Fecal samples from companion rabbits were collected from clinically normal rabbits whose owners attended a regional rabbit exposition ($n = 55$) and from healthy patients visiting the Ontario Veterinary College's Avian and Exotic Service for dental procedures ($n = 7$). Samples were chilled or placed on ice and transported for coding and processing to a central laboratory where 0.2 g of feces from each sample were isolated for DNA extraction while the remaining sample was frozen at -80 °C.

DNA extraction and quality control

DNA extraction was performed using the E.N.Z.A. Stool DNA Kit (Omega Bio-Tek Inc., Doraville, Georgia, USA) following the manufacturer's protocol for pathogen detection. Quantity and quality of extracted nucleic acids were assessed by spectrophotometry (NanoDrop, Roche, Mississauga, ON, Canada).

Table 3 History of samples collected by source

Facility number	Sample number	Age group	Sample submission date	Sample type
Commercial				
1	1	Does	Summer 2012	Pooled
	2	Growers	Summer 2012	Pooled
	3	Does	Winter 2013	Pooled
	4	Growers	Winter 2013	Pooled
2	1	Does	Summer 2012	Pooled
	2	Growers	Summer 2012	Pooled
	3	Does	Winter 2014	Pooled
	4	Growers	Winter 2014	Pooled
3	1	Does	Summer 2012	Pooled
	2	Growers	Summer 2012	Pooled
	3	Does	Winter 2013	Pooled
	4	Growers	Winter 2013	Pooled
	5	Does	Winter 2013	Pooled
4	1	Does	Summer 2012	Pooled
	2	Growers	Summer 2012	Pooled
	3	Does	Winter 2013	Pooled
	4	Growers	Winter 2013	Pooled
5	1	Does	Summer 2012	Pooled
	2	Growers	Summer 2012	Pooled
	3	Does	Winter 2013	Pooled
	4	Growers	Winter 2013	Pooled
6	1	Does	Summer 2012	Pooled
	2	Growers	Summer 2012	Pooled
	3	Does	Winter 2014	Pooled
	4	Growers	Winter 2014	Pooled
7	1	Does	Summer 2012	Pooled
	2	Growers	Summer 2012	Pooled
	3	Does	Winter 2014	Pooled
	4	Growers	Winter 2014	Pooled
8	1	Growers	Summer 2013	Pooled
	2	Growers	Summer 2013	Pooled
9	1	Does	Winter 2014	Pooled
	2	Growers	Winter 2014	Pooled
10	1	Does	Summer 2013	Pooled
	2	Growers	Summer 2013	Pooled
	3	Does	Winter 2014	Pooled
	4	Growers	Winter 2014	Pooled
11	1	Does	Winter 2014	Pooled
	2	Growers	Winter 2014	Pooled
	3	Does	Summer 2014	Pooled
	4	Growers	Summer 2014	Pooled

Table 3 History of samples collected by source *(Continued)*

Facility number	Sample number	Age group	Sample submission date	Sample type
	5	Diarrheic animal	Summer 2014	Individual
12	1	Does	Summer 2013	Pooled
	2	Growers	Summer 2013	Pooled
	3	Does	Winter 2014	Pooled
	4	Growers	Winter 2014	Pooled
13	1	Does	Summer 2013	Pooled
	2	Growers	Summer 2013	Pooled
	3	Does	Winter 2014	Pooled
	4	Growers	Winter 2014	Pooled
14	1	Does	Summer 2013	Pooled
	2	Growers	Summer 2013	Pooled
	3	Does	Winter 2014	Pooled
	4	Growers	Winter 2014	Pooled
15	1	Does	Summer 2013	Pooled
	2	Growers	Summer 2013	Pooled
	3	Does	Winter 2014	Pooled
	4	Growers	Winter 2014	Pooled
16	1	Does	Winter 2014	Pooled
	2	Growers	Winter 2014	Pooled
17	1	Does	Summer 2013	Pooled
	2	Growers	Summer 2013	Pooled
	3	Does	Summer 2014	Pooled
	4	Growers	Summer 2014	Pooled
18	1	Does	Summer 2013	Pooled
	2	Growers	Summer 2013	Pooled
	3	Does	Winter 2014	Pooled
	4	Growers	Winter 2014	Pooled
19	1	Does	Summer 2013	Pooled
	2	Growers	Summer 2013	Pooled
	3	Does	Winter 2014	Pooled
	4	Growers	Winter 2014	Pooled
20	1	Does	Summer 2013	Pooled
	2	Growers	Summer 2013	Pooled
	3	Does	Winter 2014	Pooled
	4	Growers	Winter 2014	Pooled
21	1	Does	Summer 2013	Pooled
	2	Growers	Summer 2013	Pooled
	3	Does	Winter 2014	Pooled
	4	Growers	Winter 2014	Pooled
22	1	Does	Summer 2013	Pooled
	2	Growers	Summer 2013	Pooled
	3	Does	Winter 2014	Pooled

Table 3 History of samples collected by source *(Continued)*

Facility number	Sample number	Age group	Sample submission date	Sample type
	4	Growers	Winter 2014	Pooled
23	1	Does	Summer 2013	Pooled
	2	Growers	Summer 2013	Pooled
	3	Does	Winter 2014	Pooled
	4	Growers	Winter 2014	Pooled
24	1	Does	Summer 2013	Pooled
	2	Growers	Summer 2013	Pooled
	3	Does	Winter 2014	Pooled
	4	Growers	Winter 2014	Pooled
25	1	Does	Summer 2013	Pooled
	2	Growers	Summer 2013	Pooled
26	1	Does	Winter 2014	Pooled
	2	Growers	Winter 2014	Pooled
	3	Does	Summer 2014	Pooled
	4	Growers	Summer 2014	Pooled
27	1	Does	Winter 2014	Pooled
	2	Growers	Winter 2014	Pooled
Laboratory				
1	1 (2014)	Adults	Winter 2014	Pooled
	2 (2015)	Adults	Spring 2015	Pooled
2	1	Adults	Winter 2014	Pooled
3	1	Fryers	Winter 2014	Pooled
	2	Adults	Winter 2014	Pooled
	3	Adults	Winter 2014	Pooled
4	1	Adults	Spring 2015	Pooled
5	1	Adults	Spring 2015	Pooled
	2	Adults	Spring 2015	Pooled
6	1 (Site 1)	Adults	Spring 2015 (Site 1)	Pooled
	2 (Site 2)	Adults	Spring 2015 (Site 2)	Pooled
7	1 (New arrivals)	Adults	Spring 2015	Pooled
	2 (8 weeks following arrival)	Adults	Spring 2015	Pooled
8	1	Adults	Spring 2015	Pooled
Shelter				
1	1	Adult	Fall 2013	Individual
	2	Adult	Fall 2013	Individual
	3	Adult	Fall 2013	Individual
2	1	Adult	Spring 2015	Individual
3	1	Adult	Spring 2015	Individual
	2	Adult	Spring 2015	Individual
	3	Adult	Spring 2015	Individual
	4	Adult	Spring 2015	Individual

Table 3 History of samples collected by source *(Continued)*

Facility number	Sample number	Age group	Sample submission date	Sample type
	5	Adult	Spring 2015	Individual
4	1	Adult	Spring 2015	Individual
	2	Adult	Spring 2015	Individual
	3	Adult	Spring 2015	Individual
	4	Adult	Spring 2015	Individual
	5	Adult	Spring 2015	Individual
	6	Adult	Spring 2015	Individual
Companion				
1				Individual
2				Individual
3				Individual
4				Individual
5				Individual
6				Individual
7				Individual
8				Individual
9				Individual
10				Individual
11				Individual
12				Individual
13				Individual
14				Individual
15				Individual
16				Individual
17				Individual
18				Individual
19				Individual
20				Individual
21				Individual
22				Individual
23				Individual
24				Individual
25				Individual
26				Individual
27				Individual
28				Individual
29				Individual
30				Individual
31				Individual
32				Individual
33				Individual
34				Individual
35				Individual

Table 3 History of samples collected by source *(Continued)*

Facility number	Sample number	Age group	Sample submission date	Sample type
36				Individual
37				Individual
38				Individual
39				Individual
40				Individual
41				Individual
42				Individual
43				Individual
44				Individual
45				Individual
46				Individual
47				Individual
48				Individual
49				Individual
50				Individual
51				Individual
52				Individual
53				Individual
54				Individual
55				Individual
56	1	Adult	Spring 2015	Individual
	2	Adult	Spring 2015	Individual
57	1	Adult	Spring 2015	Individual
	2	Adult	Spring 2015	Individual
	3	Adult	Spring 2015	Individual
58	1	Adult	Spring 2015	Individual
59	1	Adult	Spring 2015	Individual

16S rRNA gene amplification, purification, and sequencing

Using the protocol described by Caporaso et al. [50] and the primers recommended by Klindworth et al. [51], the V4 region of the 16S rRNA gene was amplified by PCR using the forward primer S-D-Bact-0564-a-S-15 (5'-AYTGGGYDTAAGNG-3′) and the reverse primer S-D-Bact-0785-b-A-18 (5'-TACNVGGGTATCTAATCC-3′), with an expected product size of 240 bp. These forward and reverse primers contained a region that overlapped the Illumina forward and reverse sequencing primers (TCGTCGGCAGCGTCAGATGTGTATAAGAGACAG and GTCTCGTGGGCTCGGAGATGTGTATAAGAGA CAG, respectively), allowing them to anneal to the primers containing the Illumina adaptors plus the 8 bp identifier indices (forward: AATGATACGGCGACCACC GAGATCTACAC-index-TCGTCGGCAGCGTC; reverse: CAGCAGAAGACGGCATACGAGAT-index-GTCTCGT GGGCTCGG). For each extracted sample, a 25uL reaction was performed using 12.5uL KAPA Ready Mix, 9.0uL sterile water, 0.5uL each forward and reverse primers (10pM/uL), and 2.5uL DNA template (5 ng/uL). The PCR conditions were as follows: 1) 3 min at 94 °C for denaturation, 2) 45 s at 94 °C for denaturation, 3) 60 s at 53 °C for denaturation, 4) 1.5 min at 72 °C for elongation, and 5) 10 min at 72 °C. Steps 2–4 were repeated for a total of 27 cycles. PCR products were stored at 4 °C until purification was completed. Electrophoresis of PCR products was conducted in 2% agarose gel to evaluate the products for the presence of bands of the appropriate length (~ 240 bp). Purification of PCR products was conducted using Agencourt AMPure XP (Beckman Coulter Inc., Mississauga, ON, Canada); 20uL of AMPure XP was mixed with the PCR product on a 96 well plate. Following 2 min at room temperature, the mixture was transferred to a magnetic plate, left for 2 min, and then the supernatant was discarded. Beads were then washed with 200uL freshly made 80% ethanol twice, air dried for 10 min, and separated from the magnet. The beads were then rinsed with 52.5uL of 10 mM Tris pH 8.5 buffer, placed back onto the magnetic plate, and 50uL of the supernatant of each sample was transferred to a new tube.

A second reaction was performed using 2.5uL purified product, 12.5uL KAPA Ready mix, 9.0uL sterile water, and 1.0uL each Illumina Forward Index Primer (I501-I508 or S513, S15-S18, S20-S22) (10pM/uL) and Illumina Reverse Index Primer (I701–712 or N716, N718-N729) for each sample. An additional PCR was conducted with the following conditions: 1) 3 min at 94 °C, 2) 45 s at 94 °C, 3) 60 s at 50 °C, 4) 1.5 min at 72 °C, and 5) 10 min at 72 °C. Steps 2–4 were repeated for a total of 8 cycles completed. Again, the second PCR product was purified using AMPure XP using a similar procedure to that described above, with 40uL of AMPure XP and 37uL 10 mM Tris pH 8.5 Buffer. An evaluation of final products was completed using electrophoresis in 2% agarose gel, again observing for bands of the appropriate length.

When bands were not visible or of an inappropriate length, spectrophotometry was performed to identify nucleic acid quantity; adjustments to the volumes of KAPA Ready mix, DNA product, and sterile water were made based on the quantity of nucleic acids identified as needed to produce bands of the appropriate size.

Purified samples were normalized to a final concentration of 12.5 nM and submitted for sequencing to the University of Guelph's Advanced Analysis Centre. An Illumina MiSeq (San Diego, California, USA) and 2 × 250 chemistry were utilized for sequencing of the library pool.

Microbiota assessment and analyses

Analysis of the sequencing results was conducted using Mothur software (v1.35) [52]. Paired-end reads were aligned and sequences greater than 244 bp or less than 237 bp in length were removed from the data set. Any sequences containing long runs (> 8 bp) of holopolymers, as well as ambiguous base calls, sequences that did not align with the 16S rRNA gene V4 region, or that were identified as chimeras were also removed. Sequences from mitochondria, chloroplasts, Archaea, and eukaryotes were also removed. Sequences were binned into operational taxonomic units (OTUs) at the 3% dissimilarity level using nearest neighbour clustering using open OTU picking. Comparison of relative abundances of different taxa was conducted using one-way ANOVAs within the JMP 12 Response Screening Platform (SAS Institute Inc., Cary, NC, USA). Adjustment of p values to account for false discovery rate (FDR) was performed using the Benjamini-Hochberg technique. Analysis was performed both with facility (i.e., where the animal came from) named as a random effect and without. Follow-up post-hoc testing of taxa identified as significantly different between groups was conducted using the Steel-Dwass nonparametric test. Results were considered significant when adjusted P values were ≤ 0.05. Differences in microbiota composition based on age (fryers versus does) and season (summer versus winter), were calculated exclusively for commercial meat rabbits.

For subsequent analysis, subsampling was performed to normalize sequence numbers. Good's Coverage was used to assess coverage to ensure that the microbial population was adequately represented within the samples. Population richness was assessed using Chao1 to identify the number of different organisms present within each sample and the inverse Simpson's index was used to describe population diversity to determine the abundance of the different organisms present within each sample. The Jaccard index (which measures community membership by comparing the number of shared OTUs, but not their abundance) and Yue and Clayton measure of dissimilarity (which measures community structure by examining shared OTUs and their relative abundances) were used to assess population dissimilarity and to create dendrograms to compare how closely related the microbial communities of each sample were to one another. These were compared between groups for source, age and season using unweighted UniFrac (which measures the phylogenetic distance between communities based on membership), as well as parsimony tests (which examines community membership similarily). Figures were created using FigTree (v1.4.2) (http://tree.bio.ed.ac.uk) and JMP 12. Principal coordinate analysis (PCoA) was also performed to visualize data similarities and dissimilarities between microbial communities and figures were created in JMP 12. LEfse was also performed to identify OTUs that were differentially abundant between groups.

Additional files

Additional file 1: Table S1. Relative abundance of predominant (≥ 1%) taxonomic classifications of bacteria isolated from the feces of domestic rabbits ($n = 168$).

Additional file 2: Table S2. Relative abundance and FDR p-values for significantly different bacterial phyla, classes, orders, families, and genera in the rabbit fecal microbiota when compared between commercial ($n = 86$), companion ($n = 54$), laboratory ($n = 14$), and shelter ($n = 14$) rabbit samples.

Abbreviations

ANOVA: Analysis of variance; FDR: False discovery rate; GI: Gastrointestinal; LDA: Linear discriminant analysis; LEfSe: Linear discriminant analysis effect size; OTU: Operational taxonomic units; PCoA: Principal coordinate analysis; REC: Rabbit enteritis complex

Acknowledgements

We thank Joyce Rousseau, Mackenzie Slifierz, Mohammed Jalai, and Jutta Hammermeuller for technical assistance, and Patrick Boerlin and Scott McEwen for editorial assistance.

Funding

This project was funded by a grant from the Ontario Ministry of Agriculture, Food, and Rural Affairs (200494), Farm and Food Care Ontario, Floradale Feed Mill, and BW Feeds. The funding sources had no influence on the study design, outcomes or interpretation of results.

Authors' contributions

PVT and JSW conceived of the work and prepared the grant; PVT, JSW, and JK recruited samples for the study, reviewed and analyzed the results, and prepared and reviewed the manuscript; and JK conducted the work. All authors read and approved the final manuscript.

Consent for publication

All authors consent to publication of this original article.

Competing interests

The authors declare that they have no competing interests.

References

1. Greenham LW. Some preliminary observations on rabbit mucoid enteritis. Vet Rec. 1999;74:79–85.
2. Kahn CM, editor. The Merck veterinary manual. 3rd ed. Whitehouse Station: Merck; 2005.
3. Peeters JE, Pohl P, Charlier G. Infectious agents associated with diarrhoea in commercial rabbits: a field study. Ann Rech Vet. 1984;15:335–40.
4. Peeters JE, Geeroms R, Carman RJ, Wilkins TD. Significance of *Clostridium spiroforme* in the enteritis-complex of commercial rabbits. Vet Microbiol. 1986;12:25–31.
5. Percy DH, Muckle CA, Hampson RJ, Brash ML. The enteritis complex in domestic rabbits: a field study. Can Vet J. 1993;34:95–102.
6. Whitney JC. A review of non-specific enteritis in the rabbit. Lab Anim. 1976; 10:209–21.
7. Bennegadi N, Gidenne T, Licois D. Impact of fibre deficiency and sanitary status on non-specific enteropathy of the growing rabbit. Anim Res. 2001; 50:401–13.

8. Davies RR, Davies JA. Rabbit gastrointestinal physiology. Vet Clin North Am Exot Anim Pract. 2003;6:139–53.
9. Harkness JE, Turner PV, Van de Woude S, Wheler CL. Harkness and Wagner's biology and medicine of rabbits and rodents. 5th Ames: Wiley-Blackwell; 2010.
10. Karger BL, Guttman A. DNA sequencing by CE. Electrophoresis. 2009;30 Suppl 1:S196–202.
11. Patel JB. 16S rRNA gene sequencing for bacterial pathogen identification in the clinical laboratory. Mol Diagn. 2001;6:313–21.
12. Gouet P, Fonty G. Changes in the digestive microflora of holoxenic rabbits from birth until adulthood. Ann Biol Anim Biochim Biophys. 1979;19:553–66.
13. Combes S, Gidenne T, Cauquil L, Bouchez O, Fortun-Lamothe L. Coprophagous behavior of rabbit pups affects implantation of cecal microbiota and health status. J Anim Sci. 2014;92:652–65.
14. Eshar D, Weese JS. Molecular analysis of the microbiota in hard feces from healthy rabbits (*Oryctolagus cuniculus*) medicated with long term oral meloxicam. BMC Vet Res. 2014;10:62.
15. Monteils V, Cauquil L, Combes S, Godon JJ, Gidenne T. Potential core species and satellite species in the bacterial community within the rabbit caecum. FEMS Microbiol Ecol. 2008;66:620–9.
16. Zhu Y, Wang C, Li F. Impact of dietary fiber/starch ratio in shaping caecal microbiota in rabbits. Can J Microbiol. 2015;61:771–84.
17. Davenport ER, Mizrahi-Man O, Michelini K, Barreiro LB, Ober C, Gilad Y. Seasonal variation in human gut microbiome composition. PLoS One. 2014;9:e90731.
18. Rausch P, Basic M, Batra A, Bischoff SC, Blaut M, Clavel T, et al. Analysis of factors contributing to variation in the C57BL/6J fecal microbiota across German animal facilities. Int J Med Microbiol. 2016;306:343–55.
19. Stevenson TJ, Duddleston KN, Buck CL. Effects of season and host physiological state on the diversity, density, and activity of the arctic ground squirrel cecal microbiota. Appl Environ Microbiol. 2014;80:5611–22.
20. Combes S, Michelland RJ, Monteils V, Cauquil L, Soulie V, Tran NU, et al. Postnatal development of the rabbit caecal microbiota composition and activity. FEMS Microbiol Ecol. 2011;77:680–9.
21. Costa MC, Arroyo LG, Allen-Vercoe E, Stämpfli HR, Kim PT, Sturgeon A, et al. Comparison of the fecal microbiota of healthy horses and horses with colitis by high throughput sequencing of the V3-V5 region of the 16S rRNA gene. PLoS One. 2012;7:e41484.
22. Guinane CM, Cotter PD. Role of the gut microbiota in health and chronic gastrointestinal disease: understanding a hidden metabolic organ. Ther Adv Gastroenterol. 2013;6:295–308.
23. Lim ES, Zhou Y, Zhao G, Bauer IK, Droit L, Ndao IM, et al. Early life dynamics of the human gut virome and bacterial microbiome in infants. Nat Med. 2015;21:1228–34.
24. Xiao L, Feng Q, Liang S, Sonne SB, Xia Z, Qui X, et al. A catalog of the mouse gut metagenome. Nat Biotechnol. 2015;33:1103–8.
25. Zeng B, Han S, Wang P, Wen B, Jian W, Guo W, et al. The bacterial communities associated with fecal types and body weight of rex rabbits. Sci Rep. 2015;5:9342.
26. Dunfield PF, Yuryev A, Senin P, Smirnova AV, Stott MB, Hou S, et al. Methane oxidation by an extremely acidophilic bacterium of the phylum Verrucomicrobia. Nature. 2007;450:879–82.
27. Martinez-Garcia M, Brazel DM, Swan BK, Arnosti C, Chain PSG, Reitenga KG, et al. Capturing single cell genomes of active polysaccharide degraders: an unexpected contribution of verrucomicrobia. PLoS One. 2012;7:e35314.
28. Wertz JT, Kim E, Breznak JA, Schmidt TM, Rodrigues JL. Genomic and physiological characterization of the Verrucomicrobia isolate *Diplosphaera colitermitum* gen. Nov., sp. nov., reveals microaerophily and nitrogen fixation genes. Appl Environ Microbiol. 2012;78:1544–55.
29. Dao MC, Everard A, Aron-Wisnewsky J, Sokolovska N, Prifti E, Verger EO, et al. *Akkermansia muciniphila* and improved metabolic health during a dietary intervention in obesity: relationship with gut microbiome richness and ecology. Gut. 2016;65:426–36.
30. Everard A, Belzer C, Geurts L, Ouwerkerk JP, Druart C, Bindels LB, et al. Cross-talk between *Akkermansia muciniphila* and intestinal epithelium controls diet-induced obesity. Proc Natl Acad Sci U S A. 2013;110:9066–71.
31. Yang J, Martinez I, Walter J, Keshavarzian A, Rose DJ. In vitro characterization of the impact of selected dietary fibers on fecal microbiota composition and short chain fatty acid production. Anaerobe. 2013;23:74–81.
32. Schneeberger M, Everard A, Gómez-Valadés AG, Matamoros S, Ramírez S, Delzenne NM, et al. *Akkermansia muciniphila* inversely correlates with the onset of inflammation, altered adipose tissue metabolism, and metabolic disorders during obesity in mice. Sci Rep. 2015;5:166643.
33. Shin NR, Whon TW, Bae JW. Proteobacteria: microbial signature of dysbiosis in gut microbiota. Trends Biotechnol. 2015;33:496–503.
34. Geurts L, Lazarevic V, Derrien M, Everard A, Van Roye M, Knauf C, et al. Altered gut microbiota and endocannabinoid system tone in obese and diabetic leptin-resistant mice: impact on apelin regulation in adipose tissue. Front Microbiol. 2011;2:149.
35. Zhang C, Zhang M, Pang X, Zhao Y, Wang L, Zhao L. Structural resilience of the gut microbiota in adult mice under high-fat dietary perturbations. ISME J. 2012;6:1848–57.
36. Lavelle A, Lennon G, O'Sullivan O, Docherty N, Balfe A, Maguire A, et al. Spatial variation of the colonic microbiota in patients with ulcerative colitis and control volunteers. Gut. 2015;64:1553–61.
37. Morgan XC, Tickle TL, Sokol H, Gevers D, Devaney KL, Ward DV, et al. Dysfunction of the intestinal microbiome in inflammatory bowel disease and treatment. Genome Biol. 2012;13:R79.
38. Carvalho FA, Koren O, Goodrich JK, Johansson MEV, Nalbantoglu I, Aitken JD, et al. Transient inability to manage proteobacteria promotes chronic gut inflammation in TLR5-deficient mice. Cell Host Microbe. 2012;12:139–52.
39. Schloss PD, Schuber AM, Zackular JP, Iverson KD, Young VB, Petrosino JF. Stabilization of the murine gut microbiome following weaning. Gut Microbes. 2012;3:383–93.
40. Mach N, Berri M, Estellé J, Levenez F, Lemonnier G, Denis C, et al. Early-life establishment of the swine gut microbiome and impact on host phenotypes. Environ Microbiol Rep. 2015;7:554–69.
41. Abecia L, Fondevila M, Balcells J, Lobley GE, McEwan NR. The effect of medicated diets and level of feeding on caecal microbiota of lactating rabbit does. J Appl Microbiol. 2007;103:787–93.
42. Carrilho MC, Lopez M, Campo MM. Effect of the fattening diet on the development of the fatty acid profile in rabbits from weaning. Meat Sci. 2009;83:88–95.
43. Harkness JE, Turner PV, VandeWoude S, Wheler CL. Harkness and Wagner's Biology and Medicine of Rabbits and Rodents, 5th ed. Ames: IA,Wiley-Blackwell; 2010. pp 35–37.
44. De Blas JC, Pérez E, Fraga MJ, Rodriguez JM, Gálvez JF. Effect of diet on feed intake and growth of rabbits from weaning to slaughter at different ages and weights. J Anim Sci. 1981;52:1225–32.
45. Gidenne T. Fibres in rabbit feeding for digestive troubles prevention: respective role of low-digested and digestible fibre. Livest Prod Sci. 2003;81:105–17.
46. Marai IFM, Habeeb AAM, Gad AE. Rabbits' productive, reproductive and physiological performance traits as affected by heat stress: a review. Livest Prod Sci. 2002;78:71–90.
47 Michelland RJ, Combes S, Monteils V, Cauquil L, Gidenne T, Fortun-Lamothe L. Molecular analysis of the bacterial community in digestive tract of rabbit. Anaerobe. 2010;16:61–5.
48. Schoster A, Arroyo LG, Staempfli HR, Weese JS. Comparison of microbial populations in the small intestine, large intestine and feces of healthy horses using terminal restriction fragment length polymorphism. BMC Res Notes. 2013;6:1–9.
49. Cadwell K. Expanding the role of the virome: commensalism in the gut. J Virol. 2015;89:1951–3.
50. Caporaso JG, Kuczynski J, Stombaugh J, Bittinger K, Bushman FD, Costello EK, et al. QIIME allows analysis of high-throughput community sequencing data. Nat Methods. 2010;7:335–6.
51. Klindworth A, Pruesse E, Schweer T, Peplies J, Quast C, Horn M, et al. Evaluation of general 16S ribosomal RNA gene PCR primers for classical and next-generation sequencing-based diversity studies. Nucleic Acids Res. 2013;e1:41.
52. Kozich JJ, Westcott SL, Baxter NT, Highlander SK, Schloss PD. Development of a dual-index sequencing strategy and curation pipeline for analyzing amplicon sequence data on the MiSeq Illumina sequencing platform. Appl Environ Microbiol. 2013;79:5112–20.

24

Molecular cloning and characterization of the family of feline leucine-rich glioma-inactivated (LGI) genes, and mutational analysis in familial spontaneous epileptic cats

Yoshihiko Yu*, Daisuke Hasegawa*, Aki Fujiwara-Igarashi, Yuji Hamamoto, Shunta Mizoguchi, Takayuki Kuwabara and Michio Fujita

Abstract

Background: Leucine-rich glioma-inactivated (LGI) proteins play a critical role in synaptic transmission. Dysfunction of these genes and encoded proteins is associated with neurological disorders such as genetic epilepsy or autoimmune limbic encephalitis in animals and human. Familial spontaneous epileptic cats (FSECs) are the only feline strain and animal model of familial temporal lobe epilepsy. The seizure semiology of FSECs comprises recurrent limbic seizures with or without evolution into generalized epileptic seizures, while cats with antibodies against voltage-gated potassium channel complexed/LGI1 show limbic encephalitis and recurrent limbic seizures. However, it remains unclear whether the genetics underlying FSECs are associated with LGI family genes. In the present study, we cloned and characterized the feline LGI1–4 genes and examined their association with FSECs. Conventional PCR techniques were performed for cloning and mutational analysis. Characterization was predicted using bioinformatics software.

Results: The cDNAs of feline *LGI1–4* contained 1674-bp, 1650-bp, 1647-bp, and 1617-bp open reading frames, respectively, and encoded proteins comprising 557, 549, 548, and 538 amino acid residues, respectively. The feline LGI1–4 putative protein sequences showed high homology with *Homo sapiens*, *Canis familiaris*, *Bos taurus*, *Sus scrofa*, and *Equus caballus* (92%–100%). Mutational analysis in 8 FSECs and 8 controls for LGI family genes revealed 3 non-synonymous and 14 synonymous single nucleotide polymorphisms in the coding region. Only one non-synonymous single nucleotide polymorphism in LGI4 was found in 3 out of 8 FSECs. Using three separate computational tools, this mutation was not predicted to be disease causing. No co-segregation of the disease was found with any variant.

Conclusions: We cloned the cDNAs of the four feline LGI genes, analyzed the amino acid sequences, and revealed that epilepsy in FSEC is not a monogenic disorder associated with LGI genes.

Keywords: Feline, Epilepsy, Lgi, Cloning and sequence analysis, Molecular characterization

* Correspondence: yoshy@shinkei.com; disk-hsgw@nvlu.ac.jp
Department of Clinical Veterinary Medicine, Nippon Veterinary and Life Science University, 1-7-1 Kyonan-cho, Musashino-shi, Tokyo 180-8602, Japan

Background

Epilepsy is a chronic functional neurological disorder characterized by recurrent, unprovoked epileptic seizures and a range of loss of consciousness, salivation, muscle spasms, and severe and prolonged convulsion. Epilepsy affects over 50 million people worldwide, and is one of the most common neurological diseases [1]. Although the causes of epilepsy are variable, approximately 70% is believed to be associated with genetic factors [2]. Thus, understanding the genetic causes is important for developing effective therapeutic strategies for epilepsy [3–5]. Recently, it was also reported that treatment with a chemical corrector, 4-phenylbutyrate ameliorated the increased seizure susceptibility of the LGI1E383A model mouse, a mouse model of familial epilepsy [6].

In 2009, we identified a feline family line with spontaneous recurrent epileptic seizures, and established a colony strain of spontaneous epileptic cats (familial spontaneous epileptic cats [FSECs]) [7]. The FSEC colony consists of large multigenerational pedigrees with multiple cases. FSECs are healthy except for the presence of recurrent epileptic seizures, which have a variable frequency between FSECs. FSECs have two types of clinical seizures, with some FSECs showing both or one seizure pattern(s), while others are asymptomatic. Spontaneous focal limbic seizures with or without evolving into generalized epileptic seizures is one type of seizure observed in FSECs. This seizure type is similar to the historical limbic kindling and/or kainate model of epilepsy [8], as also represents the common seizure type in cats [9–11]. Vestibular stimulation-induced generalized epileptic seizures is the other seizure type in FSECs, and is similar to the widely used EL mouse model, which shows genetic epilepsy [12]. As both the kindling/kainate model and the EL mouse are used to model human mesial temporal lobe epilepsy (MTLE), we consider that FSECs are a natural genetic model of human and feline TLE. We previously reported their clinical, electrophysiological and magnetic resonance imaging findings, which resembled those of human MTLE [13–16]. Further, a familial form of MTLE (FMTLE) was reported in humans [17–20]. Thus, our studies provide support that the FSEC is an animal model of human FMTLE. As such, understanding the genetic causes of FSECs may be useful in exploring the genetics of familial epilepsy.

The leucine-rich glioma-inactivated (LGI) protein family (LGI1–4) play important roles in the development and function of the vertebrate nervous system, including synaptic transmission and myelination. Indeed, dysfunction of these genes and encoded proteins are associated with neurological disorders including genetic epilepsy or autoimmune limbic encephalitis in animals and human [21, 22]. LGI1 has been shown to be causative in the lateral form of familial TLE (also termed autosomal dominant lateral TLE) [23–25]. In veterinary medicine, feline complex partial seizures with orofacial involvement (FEPSO; also termed feline TLE), characterized by recurrent limbic seizures (e.g., episodic orofacial automatism) with salivation, chewing, licking, and facial twitching, was previously reported [26–28]. Some of those cats have increased antibodies against the voltage-gated potassium channel (VGKC)/LGI1 complex [27]. Thus, FEPSO is considered to involve, at least in part, VGKC/LGI1 complex antibody-mediated limbic encephalitis (LE), resembling LE in humans.

Interestingly, while FSEC was associated with loss of neurons in the CA3 subarea of the hippocampus [13, 29], the VGKC/LGI1 complex antibody LE in humans is associated with focal CA3 atrophy [30]. A protein-truncating nonsense mutation in the LGI2 gene was identified as a cause of benign familial juvenile epilepsy in the Lagotto Romagnolo dog [31]. Further, LGI4 may contribute to susceptibility to benign familial infantile convulsions and childhood absence epilepsy in humans [32, 33]. Despite these overall findings, there has been no known association of the LGI3 gene with human or veterinary diseases, although LGI3 is highly expressed in the mouse brain in a developmentally- and transcriptionally-regulated manner [34]. As LGI gene family members are highly conserved and have the same overall structure, they may also have similar functions [21], including a predisposition to epilepsy.

In the present study, we examined the hypothesis that the etiology of FSECs is associated with LGI protein family dysfunction [22]. As the cDNA sequences of the feline LGI (fLGI) genes were not previously reported, we first cloned the cDNA of LGI family genes in the *Felis catus*, predicted the corresponding protein sequence, obtained their basic physical and chemical properties, and then performed phylogenetic and structural analysis. Next, we performed fLGI mutational analysis in FSECs and healthy cats to determine their roles in epilepsy.

Results

Characterization of full-length feline LGI cDNAs

We cloned and sequenced the fLGI1, fLGI2, fLGI3, and fLGI4 cDNAs, and sequences were submitted to the DNA Databank of Japan under accession numbers LC309277, LC309278, LC309279, and LC309280, respectively. Nucleotide sequence analysis showed that fLGI1 cDNA contained a 1674-base pair (bp) open reading frame (ORF) encoding a 557-amino acid peptide, fLGI2 cDNA contained a 1650-bp ORF encoding a 549-amino acid peptide, fLGI3 cDNA contained a 1647-bp ORF encoding a 548-amino acid peptide, and fLGI4 cDNA contained a 1617-bp ORF encoding a 538-amino acid peptide.

Amino acid sequence analysis of the feline LGI proteins

The physicochemical properties of the four LGI proteins were predicted using ProtParam software (Table 1). The

Table 1 Physiochemical characteristics of the feline leucine-rich glioma-inactivated (LGI) proteins

Physiochemical characteristics	LGI1	LGI2	LGI3	LGI4
Amino acid	557	549	548	538
Total number of atoms	8959	8728	8683	8323
Molecular weight (Da)	63,817.99	62,249.12	61,887.77	58,979.10
Isoelectric point	8.39	6.21	8.46	7.60
Asp + Glu	56	63	51	49
Arg + Lys	61	58	56	50
Extinction coefficients	84520[a]/83770[b]	80955[a]/80330[b]	91050[a]/90300[b]	71805[a]/70930[b]
Aliphatic index	85.75	88.23	88.47	97.25
Instability index	42.89	53.34	44.27	47.50
Grand average of hydropathicity	−0.227	−0.119	−0.143	0.064

[a]Computed value based on the assumption that all cysteine residues appear as half cysteine's; [b]Assuming that no cysteine appears as a half cysteine

fLGI1, fLGI2, fLGI3, and fLGI4 proteins were predicted to have a signal peptide located at 1–34, 1–34, 1–30, and 1–20 amino acids, respectively; three, four, ten, and four O-glycosylation sites, respectively; three, four, three, and one N-glycosylation sites, respectively; 66, 57, 50, and 44 phosphorylation sites, respectively; and five, four, five, and five disulfide bonds, respectively (Fig. 1). The subcellular distribution of the fLGI protein was predicted and summarized in Additional file 1.

Prediction of the structures and features of feline LGI proteins

Secondary structural analysis predicted the proportion of alpha helix, beta sheet, and random coils of the putative fLGI proteins as: fLGI1: 2.15%, 30.70%, and 7.15%, respectively; fLGI2: 5.65%, 24.95%, and 69.40%, respectively; fLGI3: 3.65%, 25.73%, and 70.62%, respectively; and fLGI4: 3.90%, 24.90%, and 71.20%, respectively (Fig. 2). Analysis of each deduced amino acid sequence using SMART (Simple Modular Architecture Research Tool) revealed that the leucine-rich repeat domain flanked by the cysteine-rich region (C-terminal) at the N-terminal followed by epitempin (EPTP) domain(s) was common to all fLGI proteins (Fig. 3, Additional file 2). While SMART showed two or three EPTP domains within the LGI4 protein in other mammals, with the exception of *Felis catus* and *Canis familiaris* (see Fig. 3), two EPTP domains of fLGI4 positioned in the corresponding regions to other mammals were excluded from the diagram because of E-value thresholds of 0.00075 and 0.0039. Further, the fLGI family proteins were predicted not to have an interaction in their respective pathways (Additional file 3).

Exonic structure analysis, multiple alignments, and phylogenetic analysis

The fLGI1–3 genes included eight exons and seven introns, while the fLGI4 gene included nine exons and eight introns. All four genes shared a similar exon structure with those of other mammals (Additional file 4) based on the amino acid and genomic sequences listed in Additional file 5. Homology analysis indicated that the amino acid sequences of the predicted fLGI1–4 proteins were 94.7, 92.7, 88.5, and 86.3% identical, respectively, to the other species listed in Table 2. However, when compared with most typical mammalians including *Homo sapiens*, *Canis familiaris*, *Bos taurus*, *Sus scrofa* and *Equus caballus*, the identities were over 92%.

The amino acid sequences of the LGI proteins were aligned with sequences from other species using DNAMAN version 9.122 (Trial version; Lynnon Biosoft, San Ramon, CA, USA) (Additional files 6, 7, 8 and 9). Phylogenetic trees were constructed using MEGA 7.0 (Molecular Evolutionary Genetics Analysis Version 7.0) based on the amino acid sequences of the LGI family listed in Additional file 10 (Fig. 4), and included the proteins identified as homologous to LGI 1–4. The evolutionary history was inferred using the neighbor-joining method. The optimal trees with branch length sums of 0.27374760, 0.40249836, 0.38710421, and 0.76533180 are shown. The trees are drawn to scale, with branch lengths in the same units as those of the evolutionary distances used to infer the phylogenetic tree. While phylogenetic tree analysis based on the available amino acid sequences revealed that fLGI1, fLGI3, and fLGI4 shared the closest evolutionary relationship with *Canis familiaris*, fLGI2 showed the closest evolutionary relationship with *Sus scrofa* and *Bos taurus*.

Mutational analysis and allele frequency

Except for exon1 of fLGI2, all exons that contained coding sequences were amplified from the genomic DNA from eight FSECs and eight control cats. It was impossible to design primers for exon 1 of fLGI2 because of its GC rich content. PCR products were compared

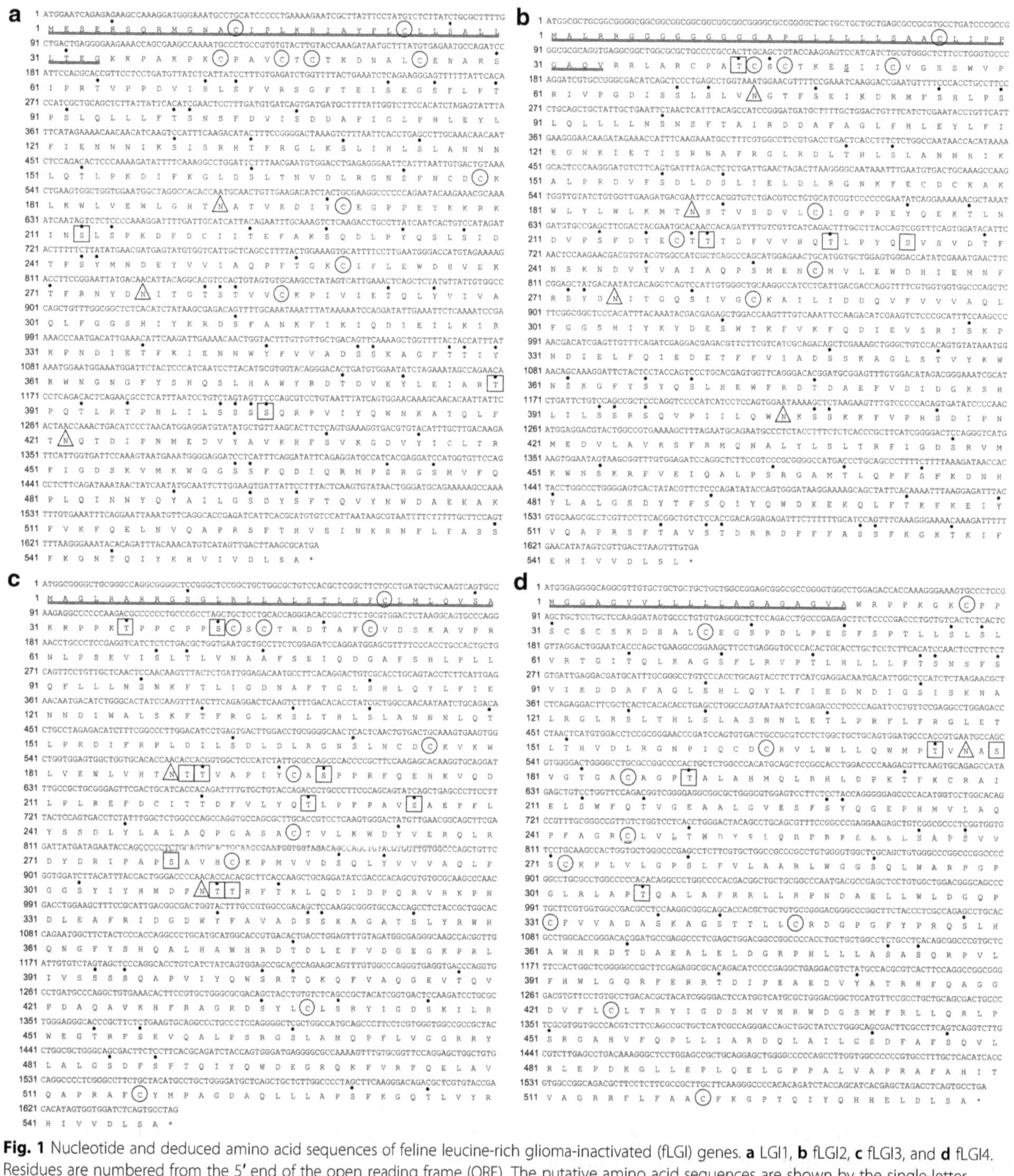

Fig. 1 Nucleotide and deduced amino acid sequences of feline leucine-rich glioma-inactivated (fLGI) genes. **a** LGI1, **b** fLGI2, **c** fLGI3, and **d** fLGI4. Residues are numbered from the 5′ end of the open reading frame (ORF). The putative amino acid sequences are shown by the single-letter amino acid codes. Asterisk indicates the stop codon. The signal peptide sequence is double-underlined. The cysteine residues required for formation of disulfide bonds are indicated with circles. The putative N-linked or O-linked glycosylation sites are indicated with triangles or squares, respectively. The predicted phosphorylation sites are indicated by a dot above the single-letter amino acid code. The sequences reported in this paper have been deposited in the DNA Data Bank of Japan (DDBJ) (LC309277, LC309278, LC309279, and LC309280)

with feline reference genomic sequences (NC_018733.2, NC_018726.2, NC_018726.2, and NC_018737.2). Sequence analysis of the fLGI gene family revealed 41 variants, the majority of which were not in the National Center for Biotechnology Information single nucleotide polymorphism (SNP) database (https://www.ncbi.nlm.nih.gov/projects/SNP/). Among them, three non-synonymous and 14 synonymous SNPs in the coding region were found. The

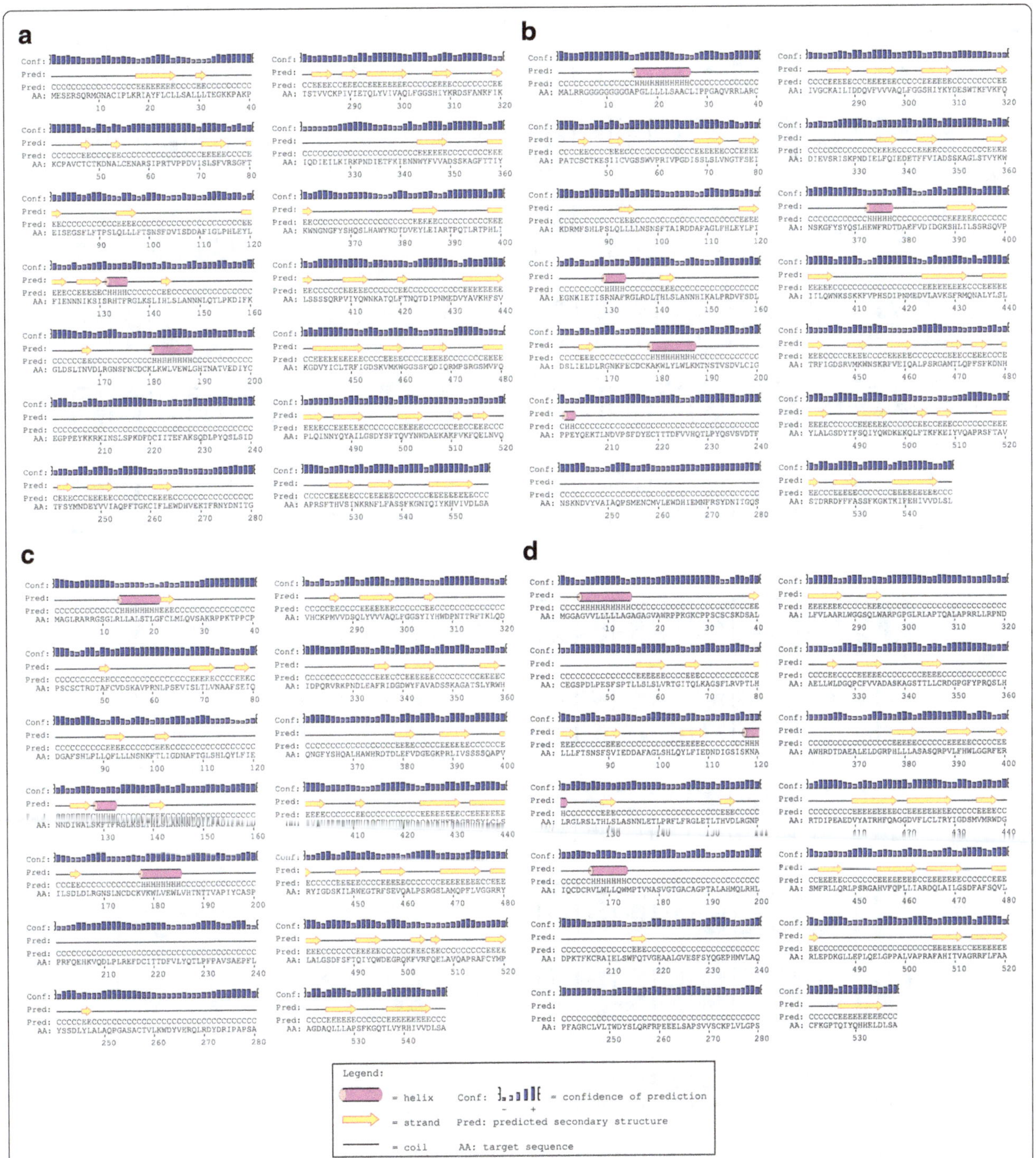

Fig. 2 The predicted secondary structure of the fLGI proteins. Secondary structure of (**a**) fLGI1, (**b**) fLGI2, (**c**) fLGI3, and (**d**) fLGI4

three SNPs were found in *fLGI1*, which included one synonymous SNPs in the coding region and two SNPs in the intron region. Six synonymous SNPs in the coding region and 11 SNPs in the intron and non-coding regions were found in *fLGI2*. As for *fLGI3*, one non-synonymous SNP, four synonymous SNPs, and four intronic SNPs were detected. In fLGI4, two non-synonymous SNPs, three synonymous SNPs, and seven intronic SNPs were found. For the three non-synonymous SNPs found in the *fLGI* genes, P33A in *fLGI3* was heterozygous in a control cat, A17T in *fLGI4* was also heterozygous in a control cat, while E49K in *fLGI4* was heterozygous in three FSECs. No co-segregation of the disease was found with any

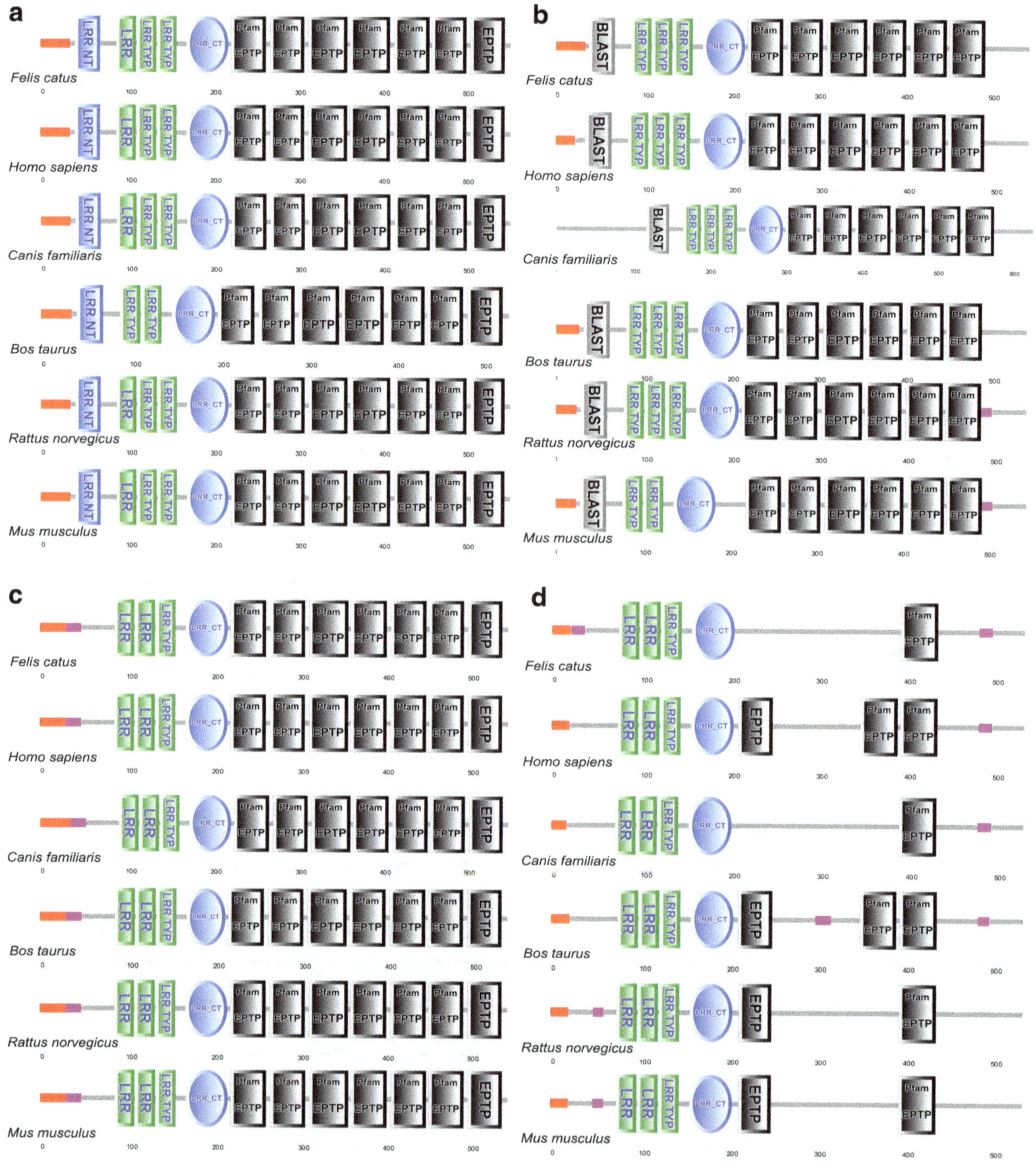

Fig. 3 Confidently predicted domains, repeats, motifs, and features using SMART (Simple Modular Architecture Research Tool). This analysis included *Felis catus*, *Homo sapiens*, *Canis familiaris*, *Bos taurus*, *Rattus norvegicus*, and *Mus musculus*. LRR NT: Leucine rich repeat N-terminal domain; LRR: Leucine-rich repeats; LRR TYP: Leucine-rich repeats, typical subfamily; LRR_CT: Leucine rich repeat C-terminal domain; EPTP: Epitempin repeat. Note that BLAST also shows LRR NT. **a** LGI1, **b** LGI2, **c** LGI3, and **d** LGI4

variant. These results are summarized in Table 3 and Additional file 11.

In silico functional analysis for one non-synonymous SNP (P33A) in *fLGI3* and two non-synonymous SNPs (A17T, E49K) in *fLGI4* were performed using SIFT (Sorting Intolerant From Tolerant), PolyPhen-2 (Polymorphism Phenotyping v2), and PROVEAN (Protein Variation Effect Analyzer). SIFT predicted P33A in *fLGI3* as deleterious, and A17T and E49K in *fLGI4* as tolerated (SIFT scores were 0.02, 0.26, and 0.27, respectively). PP2

Table 2 Identity of amino acid sequences of the LGI family in other species

Species	LGI1 (%)	LGI2 (%)	LGI3 (%)	LGI4 (%)
Homo sapiens	99.3	96.2	97.6	93.5
Rattus norvegicus	97.1	95.1	96.5	88.1
Mus musculus	97.1	85.7	97.1	89.0
Canis familiaris	100.0	96.8	96.9	96.1
Bos taurus	95.0	96.2	96.7	92.9
Sus scrofa	99.1	96.6	98.4	92.8
Equus caballus	99.5	97.5	98.0	92.9
Gallus gallus	84.5	87.0	73.9	N/A
Xenopus tropicalis	80.7	81.6	N/A	43.7
All of the above species	94.7	92.7	88.5	86.3

N/A Not available

predicted P33A in *fLGI3* as benign, A17T in *fLGI4* as unknown, and E49K in *fLGI4* as benign (PP2 scores were 0.002, not available, and 0.185, respectively). PROVEAN predicted all SNPs as neutral (PROVEAN scores were −0.528, −0.346, and 0.948, respectively). These results are also summarized in Table 3.

Discussion

LGI proteins are known to play an important role in synaptic transmission, and their dysfunction may cause neuronal hyperexcitability [22]. Although LGI1 gene mutations can cause autosomal dominant lateral TLE in humans (but not FMTLE), *LGI1* conditional knockout mice were reported to have epileptic discharges that started in the hippocampus [35]. Similarly, we previously reported that epileptic seizures in FSECs originated from the hippocampus and/or amygdala [13]. Thus, these data suggest that *LGI1* dysfunction may cause seizure onset in the mesial temporal lobe. Mutations of the LGI gene family are also associated with genetic epilepsy in both humans and animals [23–25, 31–33], although the association of *LGI3* with disease occurrence remains unclear. Nevertheless, LGI3 was reported to be broadly expressed in the adult mouse brain [34], and to play a regulatory role in neuronal exocytosis [36]. In the present study, we cloned cDNA of the fLGI gene family from feline brain tissue, analyzed their potential functions, and assessed their associations with feline familial epilepsy.

All fLGI family members cloned in this study showed a predicted molecular mass of approximately 60 kDa, similar to those in humans [37]. All fLGI family genes were predicted to have a signal peptide followed by a leucine-rich repeat domain flanked by cysteine-rich sequences, consistent with the reported previously features in humans [38]. Exonic structural analysis indicated conserved exonic numbers and bps, especially between mammalian species. Further, multiple alignments, homology analysis, and phylogenic tree analysis revealed that the LGI amino acid sequences were conserved with sequences of their analogous in other species, particularly in *Homo sapiens, Canis familiaris, Bos taurus, Sus scrofa*, and *Equus caballus* (>90% homology). LGI1 showed the highest conserved amino acid sequence, suggesting that it may have similar functions to those in other species. Domain analysis also showed conservative structures between mammalian species. Although there were occasional mismatched structures in some mammalian sequences, those sequences were considered not completely accurate. Interaction analysis suggested that the LGI1, 3, and 4 proteins interacted with the a disintegrin and metalloprotease (ADAM) family proteins. ADAM22 and ADAM23 genes were reported to be associated with progressive encephalopathy with epilepsy in human, and with genetic epilepsy in canine, respectively [39–41]. Thus, LGI-ADAM interactions are an area of important focus for future epilepsy research.

In our mutational analysis, we only evaluated exons and exon-intron boundaries, except for exon1 of *fLGI2* (we were unable to design the primers because of the high GC content). Thus, we cannot exclude the possibility that haplotypes within genomic regions of fLGI family genes may be associated with FSEC. Additionally, we cannot exclude other types of intronic mutations that could also cause splicing disruptions. Therefore, there is still a possibility that fLGI genes may be causative of epilepsy in FSECs. Furthermore, c.145G > A in *fLGI4* which caused E49K was seen in the three affected cats, suggesting this mutation could potentially cause increased risk for epilepsy. We found that FSECs did not have any coding mutations concordant for causing epilepsy in these genes. In veterinary medicine, VGKC/LGI1 complex antibody-mediated LE in feline TLE [27], and the *LGI2* mutation in benign familial juvenile epilepsy in Lagotto Romagnolo dogs [31], are the only two known diseases associated with LGI genes/proteins. Thus, further studies are required to determine the association of LGI proteins and genes with animal disease. It was reported that rats with a *LGI1* missense mutation (L385R) has sound-induced generalized tonic-clonic seizures [42].

Several forms of human familial TLE have been reported, including autosomal dominant and complex inheritance [17–20]. The initial pedigree analysis at the time we identified FSEC, presumed that FSEC might have an autosomal recessive inheritance pattern [7], however, the current extended pedigree also implied the possibilities for other inheritance patterns, such as low-penetrance autosomal dominant or complex inheritance as well. Genetic studies have been performed on multiple human families with FMTLE, and several loci have been mapped in large pedigrees by linkage analysis [43–47]. Most of these loci have not been replicated in other families,

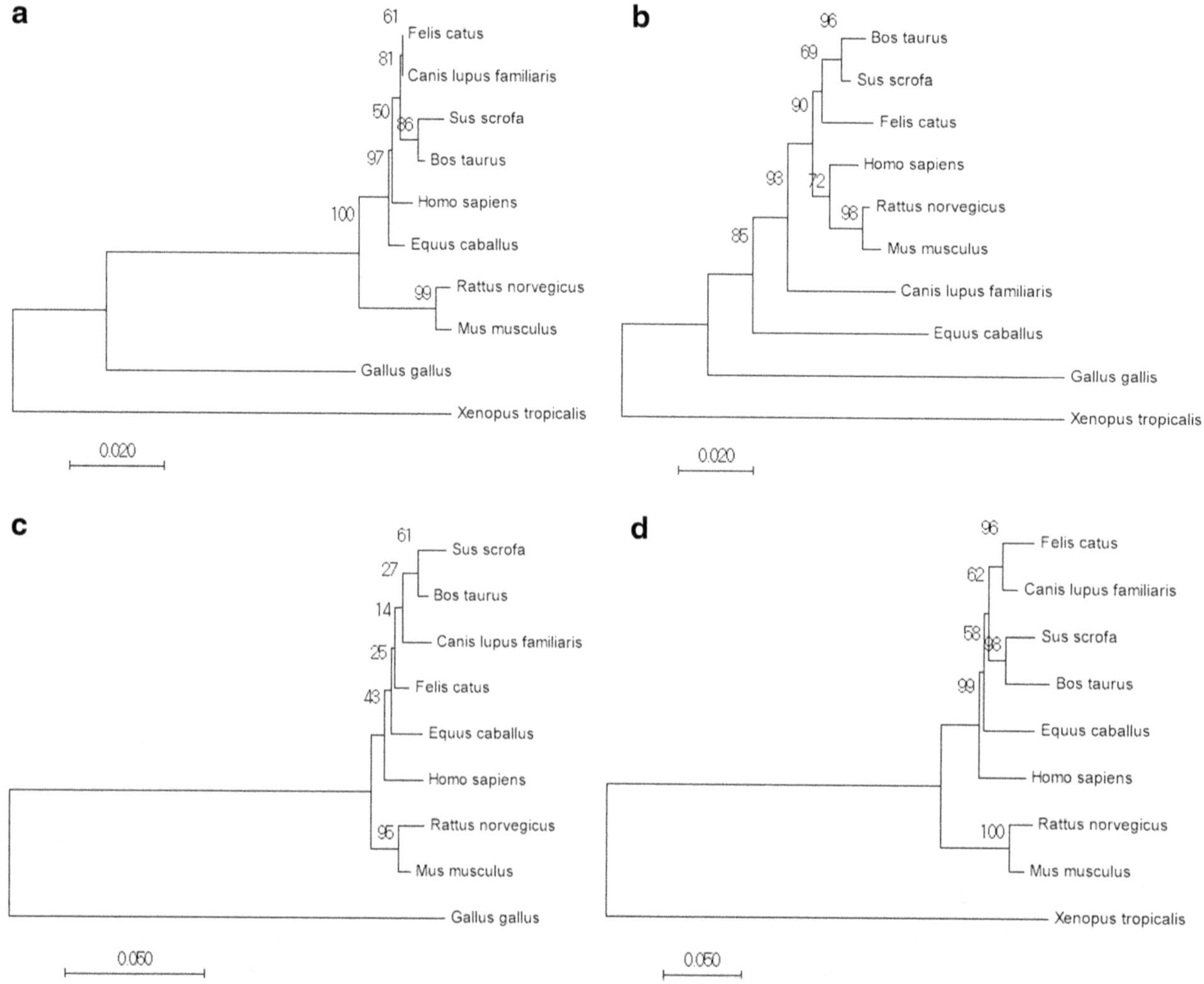

Fig. 4 Phylogenetic trees of the LGI family. The phylogenetic trees of the LGI family proteins were constructed to investigate the evolutionary relationships using the neighbor-joining method with Molecular Evolutionary Genetics Analysis Version (MEGA) 7.0 to calculate the p-distance, 1000 bootstrap replication, and pairwise deletion for the gaps/missing data treatment. Amino acid sequences of the LGI family used for this construction were obtained from GenBank, and their accession numbers are shown in Additional file 10. **a** LGI1 protein, **b** LGI2 protein, **c** LGI3 protein, and **d** LGI4 protein. The numbers at the nodes indicate bootstrap majority consensus values from 1000 replicates

Table 3 Allelic and genotypic distribution of non-synonymous mutation found in LGI1–4 in familial spontaneous epileptic cats (FSECs) and controls

	Nucleotide	Amino Acid	SIFT prediction	PP2 prediction	PROVEAN prediction	Group (n)	Genotype frequencies			Allele frequencies	
LGI3							C/C	C/G	G/G	f(C)	f(G)
	c.97C > G	p.P33A	Deleteriouss	Benign	Neutral	FSECs(8)	8	0	0	1	0
						Controls(8)	7	1	0	0.9375	0.0625
LGI4							G/G	G/A	A/A	f(G)	f(A)
	c.49G > A	p.A17T	Tolerated	Unknown	Neutral	FSECs(8)	8	0	0	1	0
						Controls(8)	7	1	0	0.9375	0.0625
							G/G	G/A	A/A	f(G)	f(A)
	c.145G > A	p.E49K	Tolerated	Benign	Neutral	FSECs(8)	5	3	0	0.8125	0.1875
						Controls(8)	8	0	0	1	0

potentially because of their genetic heterogeneity. Only one of these studies performed whole exome sequencing in addition to linkage analysis, although no putative pathogenic variants were found in the region suggested by linkage analysis [47]. It is possible that whole genome sequencing combined with linkage analysis may reveal the genetic cause of human FMTLE, such as regulatory variants or risk haplotype outside of the coding regions, or genomic rearrangement. Recently, genome-wide analyses including linkage analysis, the transmission disequilibrium test, genome-wide association analysis using the feline SNP array, and whole genome sequencing have become available for feline genetic disorders [48, 49], providing new possibilities for genetic analysis of FSECs.

Conclusion

In the present study, we cloned, sequenced, and characterized the cDNA sequences of the feline LGI1–4 genes. Using deduced amino acid sequences, we also predicted their physical and chemical properties, performed structural analyses, evaluated the evolutionary association between species, and examined their association with disease in FSECs. We found that the fLGI1–4 amino acid sequences were highly conserved with those of other mammals. However, mutational analysis revealed that the non-synonymous substitutions found in the fLGI family genes were not involved in disease occurrence in FSECs. Further studies using genome-wide strategies, including combinations of linkage analysis, the transmission disequilibrium test, or next generation sequencing, are required to identify the genes involved in epilepsy in FSECs. Nevertheless, our findings provide a further understanding of the functions of the fLGI genes and proteins, and emphasize the presence of FMTLE unrelated to only single mutations within coding regions of LGI family genes.

Methods

Experimental animals and sample collection

This study was approved by the Animal Care and Use Committee and the Bioethics Committee of Nippon Veterinary and Life Science University (accession #26 K-29, 27 K-10, 28 K-4; representative researcher was D.H.). FSECs and control cats were housed in the facility for rearing animal at Nippon Veterinary and Life Science University. Founder cats for the FSEC colony were originally purchased from a commercial laboratory (Narc, Inc., Chiba, Japan; already closed down.) in 2009 and have since been maintained as a colony at Nippon Veterinary and Life Science University [7]. All control cats were obtained from two other commercial laboratories (Shiraishi Laboratory Animals Co., Ltd., Saitama, Japan; already closed down, and Liberty Research, Inc., Waverly, NY, USA). For cDNA cloning, brain tissues were obtained from a normal cat unrelated to the FSEC strain and euthanized previously for another study [29]. After euthanasia, brain tissues (cerebral cortex) were collected within 30 min and snap frozen in liquid nitrogen. For mutation analysis, eight FSECs (male:female = 6:2; median age: 95.5 months [range: 82–180 months]; median body weight: 3.9 kg [range: 3.0–5.6 kg]) and eight healthy cats without history of seizures, abnormal findings on magnetic resonance imaging or scalp electroencephalography, or relationship with FSECs (male:female = 5:3; median age: 73 months [range: 33–74 months]; median body weight: 3.8 kg [range: 3.0–6.0 kg]) were included.

A 0.5 ml peripheral blood sample was collected by jugular or inner thigh venipuncture without sedation to extract genomic DNA. The median age of the seizure onset in FSECs was 8 months (range: 3–35 months). Six out of eight FSECs showed both seizure forms, one cat showed only spontaneous limbic seizures evolving into generalized epileptic seizures, and the other showed only vestibular stimulation-induced generalized epileptic seizures. All FSECs used in this study had interictal spikes on scalp electroencephalography, which predominantly arose from the temporal region. All cats were monitored by a 24-h video monitoring system for more than 1 year. Spontaneous seizure frequencies were variable among FSECs (range: 0–36/year). Clinical data of FSECs included in this study are summarized in Table 4.

RNA extraction and first strand cDNA synthesis

Total RNA was extracted from a normal cat brain using Illustra RNA spin columns (GE Healthcare UK Ltd., Little Chalfont, England), according to the manufacturer's instructions. Total RNA was reverse transcribed into first-strand cDNA using ReverTra Ace reverse transcriptase (Toyobo, Osaka, Japan). The cDNA was used as the template to amplify the fLGI1, 2, 3, and 4 genes.

Cloning of full-length fLGI cDNAs

To amplify overlapping fragments including ORFs of the fLGI1–4 genes, oligonucleotide primers were designed based on the predicted mRNA sequences of the *Felis catus* LGI1–4 genes (GenBank accession numbers: XM_003994222.3, XM_011281979.1, XM_003984713.3, and XM_003997904.3, respectively) using Primer3.0 online software (http://www.bioinformatics.nl/cgi-bin/primer3plus/primer3plus.cgi/). PCR was performed with AmpliTaq Gold 360 Master Mix (Thermo Fisher Scientific, Waltham, MA, USA) using brain cDNA as a template. PCR cycle conditions were follows: 95 °C for 10 min, followed by 38 cycles of denaturation (95 °C for 30 s), annealing (30 s), and extension (72 °C for 60 s), followed by a final extension (72 °C for 7 min). The set of primers used and each annealing temperature are summarized in Additional file 12. PCR products were detected by 2% agarose gel electrophoresis, isolated from the agarose,

Table 4 Clinical summary of FSECs included in this study

FSECs	Age (months)	Sex	Seizure phenotype	Seizure dominant form	Spontaneous seizure frequency (/year)	Age at Onset (months)	Father	Mother
#1	84	M	SS	SS	About 36	8	Asymptomatic*	Asymptomatic
#2	74	M	SS&VSS	SS	About 24	8	Asymptomatic†	Asymptomatic
#3	61	F	SS&VSS	SS	0–2	10	Asymptomatic†	Asymptomatic
#4	67	M	SS&VSS	VSS	About 2	17	Symptomatic (#1)	Symptomatic (#6)
#5	129	M	SS&VSS	SS	0–4	36	Asymptomatic	Asymptomatic
#6	87	F	SS&VSS	VSS	0–2	8	Asymptomatic*	Asymptomatic
#7	74	M	SS&VSS	VSS	0–1	35	Symptomatic¶	Symptomatic‡¶
#8	79	M	VSS	VSS	N/A	4	Asymptomatic	Symptomatic‡¶

*, †, ‡Cats with the same symbol are the same individual. ¶Cats showed spontaneous seizures (SS) only. Vestibular-stimulated seizures (VSS) were rare in all cats used in this study. *M* Male. *F* Female

and purified using the Wizard SV Gel and PCR Clean-Up System (Promega, Fitchburg, WI, USA).

For TA cloning, purified cDNA were ligated with T4 DNA ligase and cloned into the pGEM-T Easy Vector System (Promega). The vector containing purified PCR product was transformed into competent high DH5α cells (Toyobo). Plasmids were isolated from DH5α cells using the NucleoSpin Plasmid QuickPure Kit (Takara Bio, Shiga, Japan). As the 5′-region of the coding sequence of fLGI2 was not represented in the predicted sequences (GenBank accession numbers: XM_011281979.1), 3′- and 5′-rapid amplification of cDNA ends PCR was performed. The sequences at the 5′-end of LGI2 were amplified using the SMARTer RACE 5′/3' Kit (Takara Bio), following the manufacturer's instructions.

DNA extraction from peripheral blood, PCR for mutation detection, and product purification

Genomic DNA from eight FSECs and eight control cats was extracted from peripheral blood collected in tubes containing ethylenediaminetetraacetic acid using the QIAamp DNA Mini Kit (Qiagen, Hilden, Germany), according to the manufacturer's instructions. PCR was performed as described above for cloning. Primers (flanking the intron/exon boundaries) were designed based on the predicted genomic sequences for each of the fLGI1–4 genes (NC_018733.2, NC_018726.2, NC_018726.2, and NC_018737.2, respectively) using Primer 3.0 online software. Detection and purification of PCR products was performed as described above for LGI gene cloning, except that the concentration of agarose gel used was 1.8%.

Table 5 List of bioinformatics analysis software used in this study

Bioinformatics analysis software	URL	Prediction purpose
ORF finder	https://www.ncbi.nlm.nih.gov/orffinder/	Predict ORF
ProtParam	http://web.expasy.org/protparam/	Basic properties
PsiPred	http://bioinf.cs.ucl.ac.uk/psipred/	Secondary structures
NetOGlyc 4.0	http://www.cbs.dtu.dk/services/NetOGlyc/	O-glycosylation sites
NetNGlyc 1.0	http://www.cbs.dtu.dk/services/NetNGlyc/	N-glycosylation sites
NetPhos 3.1	http://www.cbs.dtu.dk/services/NetPhos/	Phosphorylation sites
TMHMM Server v. 2.0	http://www.cbs.dtu.dk/services/TMHMM/	Transmembrane domains
SignalP 4.1	http://www.cbs.dtu.dk/services/SignalP/	Signal peptides
SCRATCH	http://scratch.proteomics.ics.uci.edu/	Disulfide bonds
PSORT II	https://psort.hgc.jp/form2.html	Sub cellular distribution
LALIGN	http://www.ch.embnet.org/software/LALIGN_form.html	Pairwise alignments
SMART	http://smart.embl.de/	Structural domains
STRING 10.0	http://string-db.org/	Proteins interaction
SIFT	http://sift.bii.a-star.edu.sg/	Predicting pathogenicity
PP2	http://genetics.bwh.harvard.edu/pph2/	Predicting pathogenicity
PROVEAN	http://provean.jcvi.org	Predicting pathogenicity

Primer sequences and annealing temperatures are shown in Additional file 13.

Sequencing

Purified DNA and purified PCR products were sequenced using an Applied Biosystems 3130xl Genetic Analyzer (Applied Biosystems, Foster City, CA, USA) or 3730xl DNA Analyzer (Applied Biosystems) using BigDye Terminator v3.1 (Applied Biosystems). Sequencing results were analyzed using the CLC sequence viewer (Version 7.0; CLC Bio, Waltham, MA, USA). For mutation analysis, direct sequencing of the PCR products was performed twice.

Bioinformatics analyses of fLGI genes

The full-length cDNA sequences of the fLGI genes were assembled using CLC Sequence Viewer. The basic bioinformatics analysis software used in this study are shown in Table 5. The amino acid sequences were deduced from our cDNA sequences. The genomic sequences of LGI1–4 genes from other species (accession numbers shown in Additional file 5) were used to perform exonic sequence structure analysis. All amino acid sequences used for multiple sequence alignment and homology analysis are summarized in Additional file 10. Pairwise alignments between the *Felis catus* and other species were performed with LALIGN, using the following parameters: scoring matrix (BLOSUM50), gap open/extension penalty (−12/−2). Multiple sequence alignments were constructed using DNAMAN version 9.122 (Trial version; Lynnon Biosoft, San Ramon, CA, USA). A phylogenetic analysis was performed using the neighbor-joining methods (bootstrap phylogeny test, 1000 replicates) with MEGA 7.0 software to calculate the p-distance. In silico functional analysis of non-synonymous mutations was performed using SIFT, PP2 and PROVEAN. In SIFT analysis, the amino acid substitution are predicted damaging if the score is ≤0.05, and tolerated if the score is >0.05. PP2 score ranges from 0.0 (tolerated) to 1.0 (deleterious). PROVEAN was used with a threshold value of −2.5.

Additional files

Additional file 1: The subcellular distribution of feline leucine-rich glioma-inactivated (fLGI) proteins. The subcellular distribution of fLGI proteins are represented in pie charts.

Additional file 2: Confidently predicted domains, repeats, and motifs of LGI proteins by SMART (Simple Modular Architecture Research Tool).

Additional file 3: The confidence views of the LGI protein interaction. Stronger associations are represented by thicker lines. (**a**) Confidence views of fLGI1 protein interactions, (**b**) fLGI2 protein interactions, (**c**) fLGI3 protein interactions, and (**d**) fLGI4 protein interactions.

Additional file 4: Exonic structures of the coding sequences of the LGI family genes from *Felis catus* and other species. (**a–d**) show comparison of exonic structures between species for the LGI1–LGI4 genes, respectively. Amino acid sequences and genomic sequences are provided in Additional file 5. Colored blocks represent exons. Gray blocks represent introns. Numbers over the colored blocks indicate base pairs that construct exons.

Additional file 5 Accession numbers of the amino acid sequences and genomic sequences used for exonic structural analysis.

Additional file 6 Multiple alignment of LGI1 amino acid sequences from *Felis catus* and other species. Multiple alignment was constructed using DNAMAN 9.122. The black, red, and light blue shading represent 100% conserved, less-conserved (≥75%), and non-conserved (≥50%) amino acids, respectively.

Additional file 7 Multiple alignment of LGI2 amino acid sequences from *Felis catus* and other species. Multiple alignment was constructed using DNAMAN 9.122. The black, red, and light blue shading represent 100% conserved, less-conserved (≥75%), and non-conserved (≥50%) amino acids, respectively.

Additional file 8 Multiple alignment of LGI3 amino acid sequences from *Felis catus* and other species. Multiple alignment was constructed using DNAMAN 9.122. The black, red, and light blue shading represent 100% conserved, less-conserved (≥75%), and non-conserved (≥50%) amino acids, respectively.

Additional file 9 Multiple alignment of LGI4 amino acid sequences from *Felis catus* and other species. Multiple alignment was constructed using DNAMAN 9.122. The black, red, and light blue shading represent 100% conserved, less-conserved (≥75%), and non-conserved (≥50%) amino acids, respectively.

Additional file 10 List of amino acid sequences of LGI proteins used in the analysis.

Additional file 11 Allelic and genotypic distribution of synonymous and intronic polymorphisms other than non-synonymous mutation found in LGI1–4 genes in familial spontaneous epileptic cats (FPSCs) and controls.

Additional file 12 List of oligonucleotide primers used for molecular cloning of ORFs of fLGI genes. In rapid-amplification of cDNA ends (RACE), touchdown PCR was performed, with annealing temperatures of 70 °C for five cycles and 68 °C for 20 cycles.

Additional file 13 List of oligonucleotide primers used in sequencing and mutation analysis of the fLGI1–4 genes.

Abbreviations

ADAM: A disintegrin and metalloprotease; ADLTE: Autosomal dominant lateral temporal lobe epilepsy; Bp: Base pair(s); cDNA: DNA complementary to RNA; EPTP: Epitempin; FEPSO: Feline complex partial seizure with orofacial involvement; fLGI: Feline leucine-rich glioma inactivated; FMTLE: Familial mesial temporal lobe epilepsy; FSEC: Familial spontaneous epileptic cats; LE: Limbic encephalitis; LGI: Leucine-rich glioma inactivated; LRR: Leucine rich repeat; ORF: Open reading frame; RACE: Rapid-amplification of cDNA ends; RT-PCR: Reverse transcription-polymerase chain reaction; SNPs: Single nucleotide polymorphisms; TLE: Temporal lobe epilepsy; VGKC: Voltage-gated K Channel

Acknowledgements

We thank Dr. Hirotaka Igarashi for critical review of this manuscript.

Funding

This study was partially supported by a Grant of the Science Research Promotion Fund from the Promotion and Mutual Corporation for Private School of Japan (2015–2017 [representative researcher: DH]). The funders had no role in the design of the study and experiments, analysis, and the interpretation of data and in writing the manuscript.

Authors' contributions

DH and YY conceived and designed the study. YY and AFI performed the experiments and analyzed the data. DH, YY, YH, SM, and TK coordinated the clinical evaluation of the studied animals and the collection of samples. YY drafted the manuscript. YY, DH, AFI, and MF finalized the manuscript. All authors read and approved the final manuscript.

Consent for publication
Not applicable.

Competing interests
The authors declare that they have no competing interests.

References

1. Hauser WA. Incidence and prevalence. In: Engel J, Pedley TA, editors. Epilepsy: a comprehensive textbook. Philadelphia: Lippincott-Raven; 1997. p. 47–59.
2. Hardies K, Weckhuysen S, De Jonghe P, Suls A. Lessons learned from gene identification studies in Mendelian epilepsy disorders. Eur J Hum Genet. 2016;24:961–7.
3. EpiPM Consortium. A roadmap for precision medicine in the epilepsies. Lancet Neurol. 2015;14:1219–28.
4. Walker LE, Mirza N, Yip VL, Marson AG, Pirmohamed M. Personalized medicine approaches in epilepsy. J Intern Med. 2015;277:218–34.
5. Reif PS, Tsai MH, Helbig I, Rosenow F, Klein KM. Precision medicine in genetic epilepsies: break of dawn? Expert Rev Neurother. 2017;17:381–92.
6. Yokoi N, Fukata Y, Kase D, Miyazaki T, Jaegle M, Ohkawa T, Takahashi N, Iwanari H, Mochizuki Y, Hamakubo T, Imoto K, Meijer D, Watanabe M, Fukata M. Chemical corrector treatment ameliorates increased seizure susceptibility in a mouse model of familial epilepsy. Nat Med. 2015;21:19–26.
7. Kuwabara T, Hasegawa D, Ogawa F, Kobayashi M, Fujita M, Suzuki H, Matsuki N, Orima H. A familial spontaneous epileptic feline strain: a novel model of idiopathic/genetic epilepsy. Epilepsy Res. 2010;92:85–8.
8. Kitz S, Thalhammer JG, Glantschnigg U, Wrzosek M, Klang A, Halasz P, Shouse MN, Pakozdy A. Feline temporal lobe epilepsy: review of the experimental literature. J Vet Intern Med. 2017;31:633–40.
9. Cizinauskas S, Fatzer R, Schenkel M, et al. Can idiopathic epilepsy be confirmed in cats? J Vet Intern Med. 2003, 246;17 abstract
10. Pakozdy A, Sarchahi AA, Leschnik M, Tichy AG, Halasz P, Thalhammer JG. Treatment and long-term follow-up of cats with suspected primary epilepsy. J Feline Med Surg. 2013;15:267–73.
11. Wahle AM, Brühschwein A, Matiasek K, Putschbach K, Wagner E, Mueller RS, Fischer A. Clinical characterization of epilepsy of unknown cause in cats. J Vet Intern Med. 2014;28:182–8.
12. King JT Jr, LaMotte CC. El mouse as a model of focal epilepsy: a review. Epilepsia 1989;30:257-265.
13. Hasegawa D, Mizoguchi S, Kuwabara T, Hamamoto Y, Ogawa F, Matsuki N, Uchida K, Fujita M. Electroencephalographic features of familial spontaneous epileptic cats. Epilepsy Res. 2014;108:1018–25.
14. Mizoguchi S, Hasegawa D, Kuwabara T, Hamamoto Y, Ogawa F, Fujiwara A, Matsuki N, Fujita M. Magnetic resonance volumetry of the hippocampus in familial spontaneous epileptic cats. Epilepsy Res. 2014;108:1940–4.
15. Mizoguchi S, Hasegawa D, Hamamoto Y, Yu Y, Kuwabara T, Fujiwara-Igarashi A, Fujita M. Interictal diffusion and perfusion magnetic resonance imaging features of cats with familial spontaneous epilepsy. Am J Vet Res. 2017;78:305–10.
16. Hamamoto Y, Hasegawa D, Mizoguchi S, Yu Y, Wada M, Kuwabara T, Fujiwara-Igarashi A, Fujita M. Changes in the interictal and early postictal diffusion and perfusion magnetic resonance parameters in familial spontaneous epileptic cats. Epilepsy Res. 2017;133:76–82.
17. Berkovic SF, McIntosh A, Howell RA, Mitchell A, Sheffield LJ, Hopper JL. Familial temporal lobe epilepsy: a common disorder identified in twins. Ann Neurol. 1996;40:227–35.
18. Baulac S, Gourfinkel-An I, Nabbout R, Huberfeld G, Serratosa J, Leguern E, Baulac M. Fever, genes, and epilepsy. Lancet Neurol. 2004;3:421–30.
19. Striano P, Gambardella A, Coppola A, Di Bonaventura C, Bovo G, Diani E, Boaretto F, Egeo G, Ciampa C, Labate A, Testoni S, Passarelli D, Manna I, Sferro C, Aguglia U, Caranci F, Giallonardo AT, Striano S, Nobile C, Michelucci R. Familial mesial temporal lobe epilepsy (FMTLE) : a clinical and genetic study of 15 Italian families. J Neurol. 2008;255:16–23.
20. Crompton DE, Scheffer IE, Taylor I, Cook MJ, McKelvie PA, Vears DF, Lawrence KM, McMahon JM, Grinton BE, McIntosh AM, Berkovic SF. Familial mesial temporal lobe epilepsy: a benign epilepsy syndrome showing complex inheritance. Brain. 2010;133:3221–31.
21. Kegel L, Aunin E, Meijer D, Bermingham JR. LGI proteins in the nervous system. ASN Neuro. 2013;5:167–81.
22. Pakozdy A, Patzl M, Zimmermann L, Jokinen TS, Glantschnigg U, Kelemen A, Hasegawa D. LGI Proteins and epilepsy in human and animals. J Vet Intern Med. 2015;29:997–1005.
23. Gu W, Wevers A, Schröder H, Grzeschik KH, Derst C, Brodtkorb E, de Vos R, Steinlein OK. The LGI1 gene involved in lateral temporal lobe epilepsy belongs to a new subfamily of leucine-rich repeat proteins. FEBS Lett. 2002;519:71–6.
24. Kalachikov S, Evgrafov O, Ross B, Winawer M, Barker-Cummings C, Martinelli Boneschi F, Choi C, Morozov P, Das K, Teplitskaya E, Yu A, Cayanis E, Penchaszadeh G, Kottmann AH, Pedley TA, Hauser WA, Ottman R, Gilliam TC. Mutations in LGI1 cause autosomal-dominant partial epilepsy with auditory features. Nat Genet. 2002;30:335–41.
25. Morante-Redolat JM, Gorostidi-Pagola A, Piquer-Sirerol S, Sáenz A, Poza JJ, Galán J, Gesk S, Sarafidou T, Mautner VF, Binelli S, Staub E, Hinzmann B, French L, Prud'homme JF, Passarelli D, Scannapieco P, Tassinari CA, Avanzini G, Martí-Massó JF, Kluwe L, Deloukas P, Moschonas NK, Michelucci R, Siebert R, Nobile C, Pérez-Tur J, López de Munain A. Mutations in the LGI1/ Epitempin gene on 10q24 cause autosomal dominant lateral temporal epilepsy. Hum Mol Genet. 2002;11:1119–28.
26. Pakozdy A, Gruber A, Kneissl S, Leschnik M, Halasz P, Thalhammer JG. Complex partial cluster seizures in cats with orofacial involvement. J Feline Med Surg. 2011;13:687–93.
27. Pakozdy A, Halasz P, Klang A, Bauer J, Leschnik M, Tichy A, Thalhammer JG, Lang B, Vincent A. Suspected limbic encephalitis and seizure in cats associated with voltage-gated potassium channel (VGKC) complex antibody. J Vet Intern Med. 2013;27:212–4.
28. Pakozdy A, Glantschnigg U, Leschnik M, Hechinger H, Moloney T, Lang B, Halasz P, Vincent A. EEG-confirmed epileptic activity in a cat with VGKC-complex/LGI1 antibody-associated limbic encephalitis. Epileptic Disord. 2014;16:116–20.
29. Yu Y, Hasegawa D, Hamamoto Y, Mizoguchi S, Kuwabara T, Fujiwara-Igarashi A, Tsuboi M, Chambers JK, Fujita M, Uchida K. Neuropathological features of the hippocampus and amygdala in familial spontaneous epileptic cats. Am J Vet Res. In Press
30. Miller TD, Chong TT, Aimola Davies AM, Ng TW, Johnson MR, Irani SR, Vincent A, Husain M, Jacob S, Maddison P, Kennard C, Gowland PA, Rosenthal CR. Focal CA3 hippocampal subfield atrophy following LGI1 VGKC-complex antibody limbic encephalitis. Brain. 2017;140:1212–9.
31. Seppälä EH, Jokinen TS, Fukata M, Fukata Y, Webster MT, Karlsson EK, Kilpinen SK, Steffen F, Dietschi E, Leeb T, Eklund R, Zhao X, Rilstone JJ, Lindblad-Toh K, Minassian BA, Lohi H. LGI2 truncation causes a remitting focal epilepsy in dogs. PLoS Genet. 2011;7:e1002194.
32. Gu W, Sander T, Becker T, Steinlein OK. Genotypic association of exonic LGI4 polymorphisms and childhood absence epilepsy. Neurogenetics. 2004;5:41–4.
33. Ishii A, Zhang B, Kaneko S, Hirose S. Positive association between benign familial infantile convulsions and LGI4. Brain Dev. 2010;32:538–43.
34. Lee SE, Lee AY, Park WJ, Jun DH, Kwon NS, Baek KJ, Kim YG, Yun HY. Mouse LGI3 gene: expression in brain and promoter analysis. Gene. 2006;372:8–17.
35. Boillot M, Huneau C, Marsan E, Lehongre K, Navarro V, Ishida S, Dufresnois B, Ozkaynak E, Garrigue J, Miles R, Martin B, Leguern E, Anderson MP, Baulac S. Glutamatergic neuron-targeted loss of LGI1 epilepsy gene results in seizures. Brain. 2014;137:2984–96.
36. Park WJ, Lee SE, Kwon NS, Baek KJ, Kim DS, Yun HY. Leucine-rich glioma inactivated 3 associates with syntaxin 1. Neurosci Lett. 2008;444:240–4.
37. Chernova OB, Somerville RP, Cowell JK. A novel gene, LGI1, from 10q24 is rearranged and downregulated in malignant brain tumors. Oncogene. 1998; 17:2873–81.
38. Kobe B, Kajava AV. The leucine-rich repeat as a protein recognition motif. Curr Opin Struct Biol. 2001;11:725–32.
39. Koskinen LL, Seppälä EH, Belanger JM, Arumilli M, Hakosalo O, Jokinen P, Nevalainen EM, Viitmaa R, Jokinen TS, Oberbauer AM, Lohi H. Identification of a common risk haplotype for canine idiopathic epilepsy in the ADAM23 gene. BMC Genomics. 2015;16:465.
40. Muona M, Fukata Y, Anttonen AK, Laari A, Palotie A, Pihko H, Lönnqvist T, Valanne L, Somer M, Fukata M, Lehesjoki AE. Dysfunctional ADAM22 implicated in progressive encephalopathy with cortical atrophy and epilepsy. Neurol Genet. 2016;2:e46.
41. Koskinen LL, Seppälä EH, Weissl J, Jokinen TS, Viitmaa R, Hänninen RL, Quignon P, Fischer A, André C, Lohi H. ADAM23 is a common risk gene for canine idiopathic epilepsy. BMC Genet. 2017;18:8.
42. Baulac S, Ishida S, Mashimo T, Boillot M, Fumoto N, Kuwamura M, Ohno Y, Takizawa A, Aoto T, Ueda M, Ikeda A, LeGuern E, Takahashi R, Serikawa T. A rat model for LGI1-related epilepsies. Hum Mol Genet. 2012;21:3546–57.
43. Baulac S, Picard F, Herman A, Feingold J, Genin E, Hirsch E, Prud'homme JF, Baulac M, Brice A, LeGuern E. Evidence for digenic inheritance in a family

with both febrile convulsions and temporal lobe epilepsy implicating chromosomes 18qter and 1q25-q31. Ann Neurol. 2001;49:786–92.
44. Claes L, Audenaert D, Deprez L, Van Paesschen W, Depondt C, Goossens D, Del-Favero J, Van Broeckhoven C, De Jonghe P. Novel locus on chromosome 12q22-q23.3 responsible for familial temporal lobe epilepsy associated with febrile seizures. J Med Genet. 2004;41:710–4.
45. Hedera P, Blair MA, Andermann E, Andermann F, D'Agostino D, Taylor KA, Chahine L, Pandolfo M, Bradford Y, Haines JL, Abou-Khalil B. Familial mesial temporal lobe epilepsy maps to chromosome 4q13.2-q21.3. Neurology. 2007;68:2107–12.
46. Chahine L, Abou-Khalil B, Siren A, Andermann F, Hedera P, Ge Q, Andermann E, Pandolfo M. A new locus for familial temporal lobe epilepsy on chromosome 3q. Epilepsy Res. 2013;106:338–44.
47. Fanciulli M, Di Bonaventura C, Egeo G, Fattouch J, Dazzo E, Radovic S, Spadotto A, Giallonardo AT, Nobile C. Suggestive linkage of familial mesial temporal lobe epilepsy to chromosome 3q26. Epilepsy Res. 2014;108:232–40.
48. Alhaddad H, Gandolfi B, Grahn RA, Rah HC, Peterson CB, Maggs DJ, Good KL, Pedersen NC, Lyons LA. Genome-wide association and linkage analyses localize a progressive retinal atrophy locus in Persian cats. Mamm Genome. 2014;25:354–62.
49. Lyons LA, Creighton EK, Alhaddad H, Beale HC, Grahn RA, Rah H, Maggs DJ, Helps CR, Gandolfi B. Whole genome sequencing in cats, identifies new models for blindness in AIPL1 and somite segmentation in HES7. BMC Genomics. 2016;17:265.

Metagenomic analysis of captive Amur tiger faecal microbiome

Fengping He[1], Dan Liu[2], Le Zhang[1], Jiancheng Zhai[1], Yue Ma[1,3], Yanchun Xu[1,3], Guangshun Jiang[1,4], Ke Rong[1,4*†] and Jianzhang Ma[1,4*†]

Abstract

Background: The gastrointestinal tracts of animals are home to large, complex communities of microbes. The compositions of these communities ultimately reflect the coevolution of microorganisms with their animal host and are influenced by the living environment, diet and immune status of the host. Gut microbes have been shown to be important for human disease and health, but little research exists in the gut microbiome of the Amur tiger, which is one of the most endangered species in the world.

Results: In this study, we present the use of whole-metagenome shotgun sequencing to analyze the composition and functional structures of the gut microbiota in captive Amur tigers. Our results showed a high abundance of four major phyla in captive Amur tigers, including Proteobacteria, Firmicutes, Actinobacteria and Fusobacteria. Moreover, at the genus level, *Escherichia*, *Collinsella* and *Fusobacterium* were most abundant in the captive Amur tiger fecal metagenome. At the species level, *Escherichia coli*, *Fusobacterium ulcerans* and *Fusobacterium varium* were the species with highest abundances in the captive Amur tiger gut microbiota. The primary functional categories of the Amur tiger faecal metagenome were associated mainly with Carbohydrate metabolism, Membrane transport and Amino acid metabolism based on the KEGG pathway database. The comparative metagenomic analyses showed that the captive Amur tiger fecal metagenome had a lower abundance of Spirochaetes, Cyanobacteria and Ascomycota than other animals, and the primary functional categories were primarily associated with carbohydrate metabolism subsystems, clustering-based subsystems and protein metabolism.

Conclusions: We presented here for the first time the use of the shotgun metagenomic sequencing approach to study the composition and functional structures of the gut microbiota in captive Amur tiger.

Keywords: Gastrointestinal microbiota, Amur tiger, *Panthera tigris altaica*, Metagenomics, Pyrosequencing

Background

The Amur tiger (*Panthera tigris altaica*), also called the Siberian tiger, is the largest extant tiger subspecies in the genus *Panthera* (Mammalia, Carnivora, Felidae) [1]. Amur tigers, which are found in the Russian Far East [2] and Northeast China [3], are listed as Endangered on the IUCN Red List of Threatened Species™ and are included in CITES Appendix I. The population of wild Amur tiger continues to decline due to habitat loss and degradation, poaching and prey depletion [4].

Fortunately, the Amur tiger has been successfully bred in China, and the population of the Amur tiger has increased from 27 to approximately 1000 after more than 30 years of hard work. However, with the growing population of the Amur tiger, veterinary antibiotics and antiparasitics have been widely used to maintain the healthy development of the population in the Heilongjiang Siberian Tiger Park.

Many studies have shown that the gastrointestinal tracts of humans and animals contain large, complex microbial communities [5–7]. The gut microbiota is now recognized as a coevolutionary partner that facilitates host nutritional acquisition, immune modulation, and homeostasis in response to profound lifestyle changes [8–12]. The diversity and function of the gut microbiota may indicate host

* Correspondence: rongke@nefu.edu.cn; jianzhangma@163.com
†Ke Rong and Jianzhang Ma contributed equally to this work.
[1]College of Wildlife Resources, Northeast Forestry University, Harbin 150040, China
Full list of author information is available at the end of the article

genotypic characteristics and reflect an adaptive ecosystem response to the host diet and living habits.

In recent years, metagenomic sequencing based on next-generation sequencing technologies [13] has been used to describe the microbial diversity and functional capacity of microbial communities in the gastrointestinal tracts of humans [14, 15] as well as some animal species [16–22]. In this study, for the first time, we used whole metagenome shotgun sequencing to profile the microbial flora inhabiting the digestive system of captive Amur tiger and identify the functional attributes encoded in the gut microbiome.

Results

We sequenced the faecal metagenomes of 3 captive Amur tigers using the Illumina platform and obtained 32.39 GB of high-quality bases that were free of adaptor and tiger DNA contaminants (Additional file 1). The unique sequence reads that passed the quality control filtering step were then subjected to further analyses focused on biodiversity and functional annotation. The metagenomic sequence data from this study have been submitted to the National Center for Biotechnology Information (NCBI) Sequence Read Archive (SRA) under accession numbers SRP119699.

Phylogenetic analysis of Amur tiger faecal bacteria, eukaryotes, archaea, and viruses

The phylogenetic computation revealed a profile comprising 98.10% bacteria, 1.89% viruses, 0.01% eukaryotes and 0.003% archaea. In the Amur tiger intestinal metagenome, Proteobacteria was the most predominant phylum (44.39%), followed by Firmicutes (31.38%), Actinobacteria (9.92%), and Fusobacteria (8.20%) (Fig. 1).

Of the Proteobacteria, most belonged to Enterobacteriaceae, and a very small amount were Betaproteobacteria or Pseudomonadales (Additional file 2). The dominant family of intestinal microbes in the Amur tiger is Enterobacteriaceae, and most of the Enterobacteriaceae were *Escherichia coli*. Firmicutes was the second most predominant phylum in captive Amur tiger gastrointestinal tract, with Clostridiales as the primary contributor to the Firmicutes population, followed by Erysipelotrichales and Selenomonadales (Additional file 2). Among Clostridiales, Lachnospiraceae, Peptostreptococcaceae and Clostridiaceae were the families with the highest abundance. A relatively high proportion of the Clostridiales content was attributable to *Ruminococcus gnavus*, *Clostridium hiranonis* and *Clostridium perfringens*. Erysipelotrichales contains a single family, Erysipelotrichaceae, and this family was represented mainly of *Erysipelotrichaceae bacterium nk3d112*, *Solobacterium moorei* and *Holdemanella biformis*. Selenomonadales was mostly represented by Veillonellaceae, including *Megamonas funiformis*, *M. rupellensis* and *M. hypermegale*.

Similarly, Coriobacteriia was the primary contributor to the population belonging to the phylum Actinobacteria, followed by the class Actinobacteria. The major genus in the Actinobacteria phylum was *Collinsella*. *Collinsella stercoris* and *C. intestinalis* were the predominant species

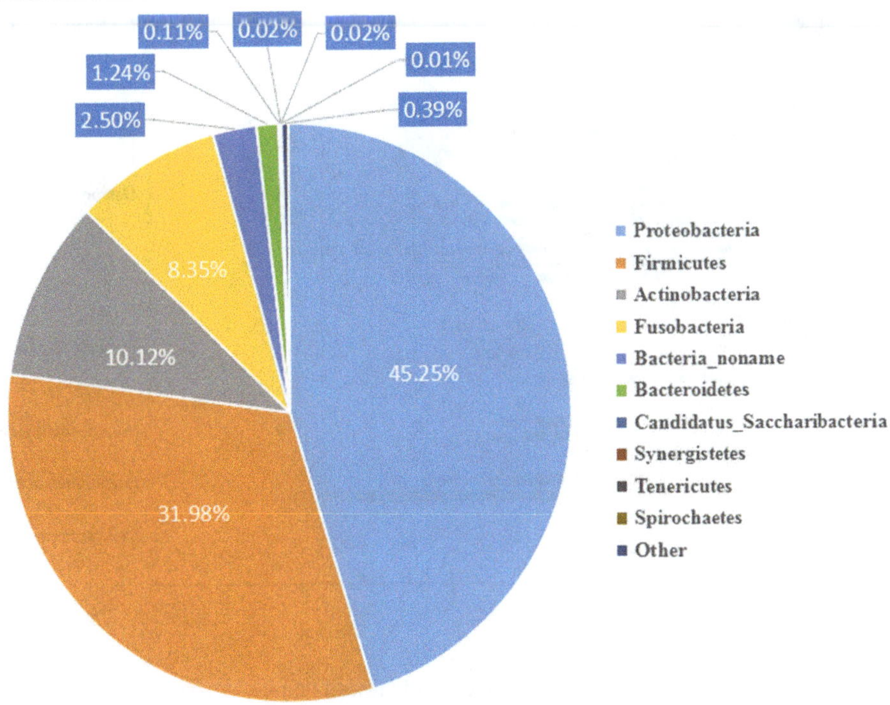

Fig. 1 Bacterial phylum profiles of the Amur tiger microbiome

among *Collinsella* in the Amur tiger metagenome. Actinobacteria was also represented by *Bifidobacterium*, *Actinomycetes* and *Corynebacterium*, with each genus represented by a variety of microbial species, such as *Actinomyces cardiffensis*, *Actinomyces turicensis*, *Corynebacterium diphtheriae* and *Bifidobacterium breve*. The major genus in the Fusobacteria phylum was *Fusobacterium*. *Fusobacterium ulcerans*, *F. varium*, *F. mortiferum* and *F. perfoetens* were the main species among the Fusobacteria in the Amur tiger metagenome. Fusobacteria are a phylum of bacteria that were significantly more abundant in Carnivora (e.g., Felidae and Canidae) [23]. A high proportion of Fusobacteria were also discovered in the gut microbiomes of some carnivorous vertebrates, such as vultures and alligators [24, 25].

Eukaryota was a minor constituent (0.01%) of the Amur tiger metagenome. Most of the Eukaryota were Ascomycota, with a small fraction of Basidiomycota (Additional file 3). Ascomycota is the largest Eukaryota phylum. *Trichophyton tonsurans* was the primary contributor to the Ascomycota population, followed by *Pseudogymnoascus pannorum*. Archaea sequences had very low abundance (0.003%) in the Amur tiger metagenome, with Euryarchaeota the primary contributor (Additional file 4). In the Amur tiger faecal metagenome, Methanosarcinaceae was the major Archaea component and included *Methanosarcina sp. WH1* and *Methanomethylovorans hollandica*. Only 1.89% of the Amur tiger metagenome sequences were viruses, of which Caudovirales was the only order identified (Additional file 5). The major family in Caudovirales was Podoviridae, followed by Siphoviridae and Myoviridae.

Metabolic profiles of the Amur tiger metagenome

In addition to providing novel insights on the taxonomic diversity of the characteristic microbial consortium, our metagenomic research enabled the identification of the gene functions involved in the symbiotic functions with the host. Based on the KEGG PATHWAY database, hits were classified into 6 groups comprising 42 functional categories (Fig. 2).

Metabolism was the largest group, with higher proportions of Carbohydrate metabolism, Amino acid metabolism, Nucleotide metabolism, Metabolism of cofactors and vitamins and Energy metabolism. Collectively, the 12 functional categories in the metabolism group accounted for 86.62% of the hits. Carbohydrate metabolism and Amino acid metabolism were the most abundant functional categories, representing 16.75 and 11.96% of the Amur tiger faecal metagenome, respectively. Environmental information processing was the

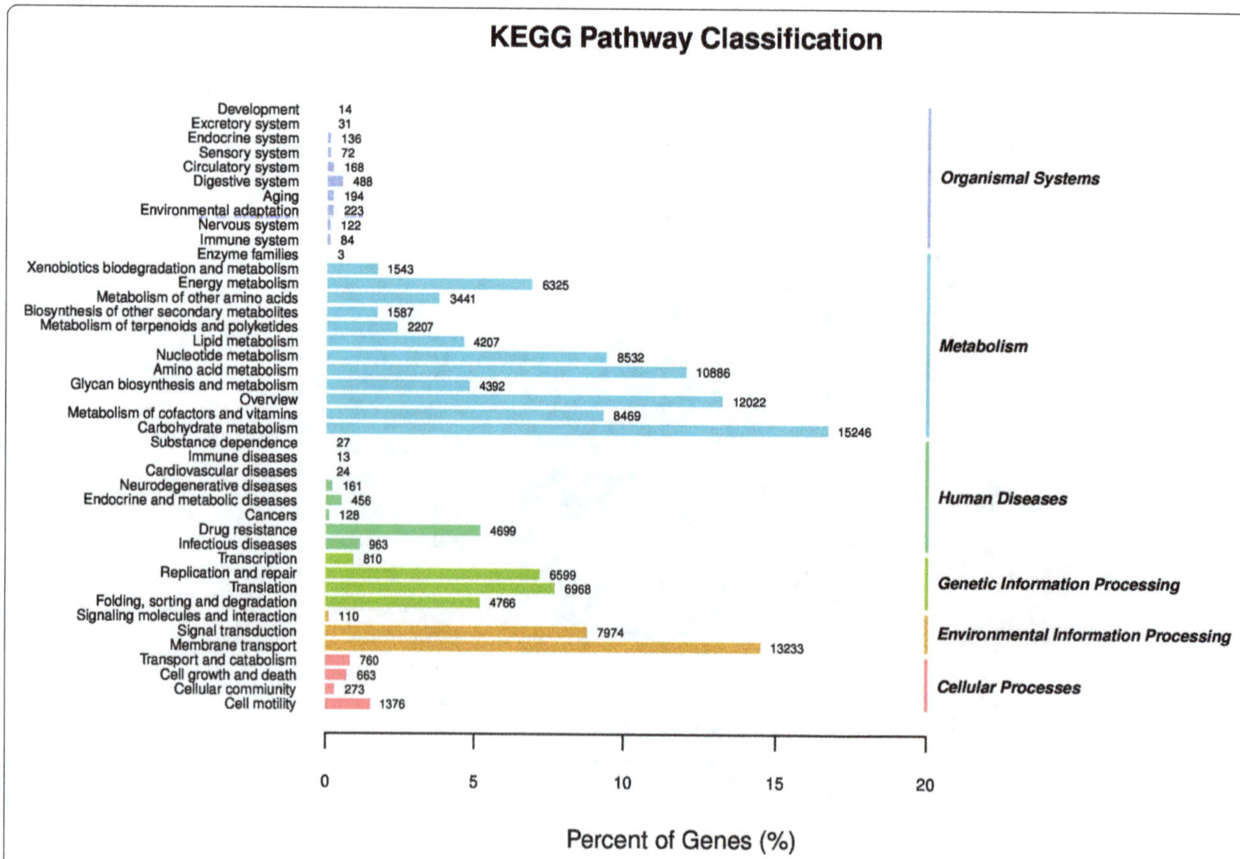

Fig. 2 Functional composition of the Amur tiger microbiome

second most prominent functional group, Membrane transport was the most abundant functional categories, followed by Signal transduction and Signalling molecules and interaction. Approximately 14.54% of the annotated reads from the Amur tiger faecal metagenomes were categorized within Membrane transport.

The third most prominent functional group was Genetic information processing, which included the categories of Translation, Replication and repair, Folding, sorting and degradation. The fourth most prominent group, Human diseases, was dominated by the categories Drug resistance, Endocrine and metabolic diseases and Neurodegenerative diseases. The remaining two groups of captive Amur tiger faecal metagenomes were Cellular processes and Organismal systems. Cell motility, Transport and catabolism and Cell growth and death were important categories within Cellular processes. Most hits of the Organismal system group were distributed among the Digestive system, Environmental adaptation and Aging.

To fully describe the attributes of the genes and gene products identified by faecal metagenome sequencing of the Amur tiger, we performed GO annotations of the unigenes obtained from sequencing. A total of 401,606 unigenes were annotated with 7961 GO functions belonging to molecular function, biological process and cellular components (Additional file 6). The biological processes group contained 157,188 (39.14%) unigenes that were annotated with 4506 GO functions. The most abundant in the biological process group was biological processes, followed by transport and regulation of transcription, DNA templated (Additional file 7). In the cellular components group, a total of 76,428 (19.03%) unigenes were annotated with 851 GO functions, mostly belonging to the cytosol, plasma membrane and cellular components. A total of 167,942 (41.82%) unigenes were annotated with 3051 GO functions in the molecular function group, in which molecular function was the largest category, followed by protein binding and ATP binding.

To further understand the carbohydrate enzymes present in the Amur tiger gut microbiome, we submitted the samples to the Carbohydrate-Active enZYmes database (CAZy). A total of 21,404 annotation results were obtained for the faeces metagenome sequences of the Amur tiger (Additional file 8). Among the 6 large functional CAZy classes, glycosyl transferase (GT) families were the most abundant, followed by glycoside hydrolase (GH) families (Additional file 9). In the further functional subclasses, GT4 and GT2 belonging to the GT family were the most abundant, followed by CBM50 of the CBM family and GH23 and GH13 of the GH family.

Discussion

In this study, whole-metagenome shotgun sequencing was performed to assess the composition and functional structure of the gut microbiota of the captive Amur tiger. In our study, we observed a high abundance of four major phyla, Proteobacteria, Firmicutes, Actinobacteria and Fusobacteria. Moreover, at the genus level, *Escherichia*, *Collinsella* and *Fusobacterium* were most abundant in the captive Amur tiger fecal metagenome. Importantly, at the species level, *Escherichia coli*, *Fusobacterium ulcerans* and *Fusobacterium varium* were the species with the highest abundances in the captive Amur tiger gut microbiota.

Despite extensive variation among individuals, the gut microbiota of members of the same species are often more similar to one another compared with those of other species. Thus, it is important to provide a comparison between the gut microbiota of the Amur tiger and those of other animals. The results of this study were compared with data sets from different animals, including humans, in the MG-RAST database. Paired data from other studies were chosen, including three wild Amur tigers (WT1, WT2, and WT3), two cats (cat 1 and cat 2), two chickens (chicken 1 and chicken 2), two humans (human 1 and human 2), two mice (mouse 1 and mouse 2), two pandas (panda 1 and panda 2), two pigs (pig 1 and pig 2) and two wolves (wolf 1 and wolf 2), which were compared with Amur tigers in captivity (ptg_z1, ptg_z2, and ptg_z3).

The comparisons were performed at the phylogenetic (Fig. 3) and the metabolic levels (Fig. 4). In the phylogenetic comparison, Actinobacteria, Bacteroidetes, Firmicutes and Proteobacteria were the most abundant in all the samples, and the captive Amur tiger samples clustered with the wild Amur tiger samples. Interestingly, the abundance of Apicomplexa and Euryarchaeota were lower in the captive Amur tiger samples than in those from the wild Amur tigers. In addition, the heat map shows that the captive Amur tiger fecal metagenome had a lower abundance of Spirochaetes, Cyanobacteria and Ascomycota than other animals. These findings suggest that the characteristics of gut microbial diversity may adapt to the habits and diet of the Amur tiger in captivity. The metabolic comparison showed that the captive Amur tiger, wild Amur tiger, cat, panda, wolf and human samples clustered together and separated from those of pigs. As expected, all the gut metagenomes were dominated by carbohydrate metabolism subsystems, and the Protein Metabolism and Clustering-based subsystems were represented in relatively high abundance as well.

Intestinal microbial community structure is the result of the coevolution of the microbes and host animal and its environment, and intestinal microorganisms influence physiological function. The intestinal microbial community is also affected by the survival environment and feeding habit of the host animal [26]. Wild felids are susceptible to changes in metabolism and behaviour when

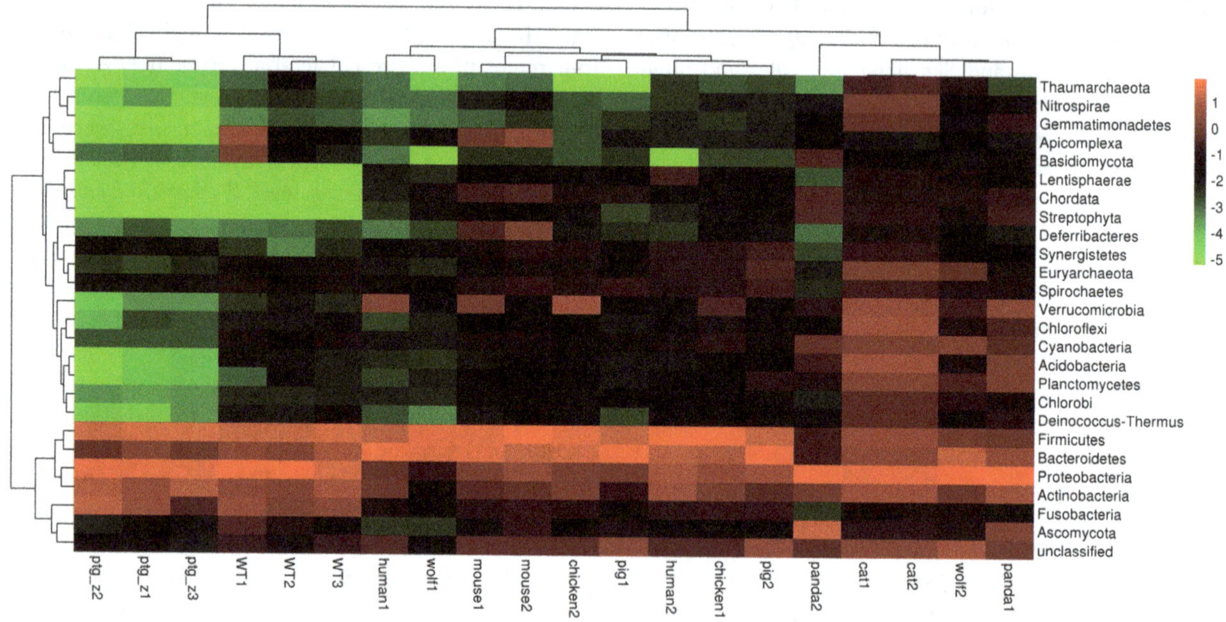

Fig. 3 Heat map of phylogenetic clustering of the wild Amur tiger gut metagenome compared to those of other animals

kept in captivity; these changes are linked to differences from their natural habitat and feeding patterns [27–31].

Conclusions

In this study, we present the use of whole-metagenome shotgun sequencing to analyze the composition and functional structures of the gut microbiota in captive Amur tigers. Our results showed a high abundance of four major phyla in captive Amur tigers, including Proteobacteria, Firmicutes, Actinobacteria and Fusobacteria. Moreover, at the genus level, *Escherichia*, *Collinsella* and *Fusobacterium* were most abundant in the captive Amur tiger fecal metagenome. At the species level, *Escherichia coli*, *Fusobacterium ulcerans* and *Fusobacterium varium* were the species with highest abundances in the captive Amur tiger gut microbiota. The primary functional categories of the Amur tiger faecal metagenome were associated mainly with Carbohydrate metabolism, Membrane transport and Amino acid metabolism based on the KEGG pathway database. The comparative metagenomic analyses showed

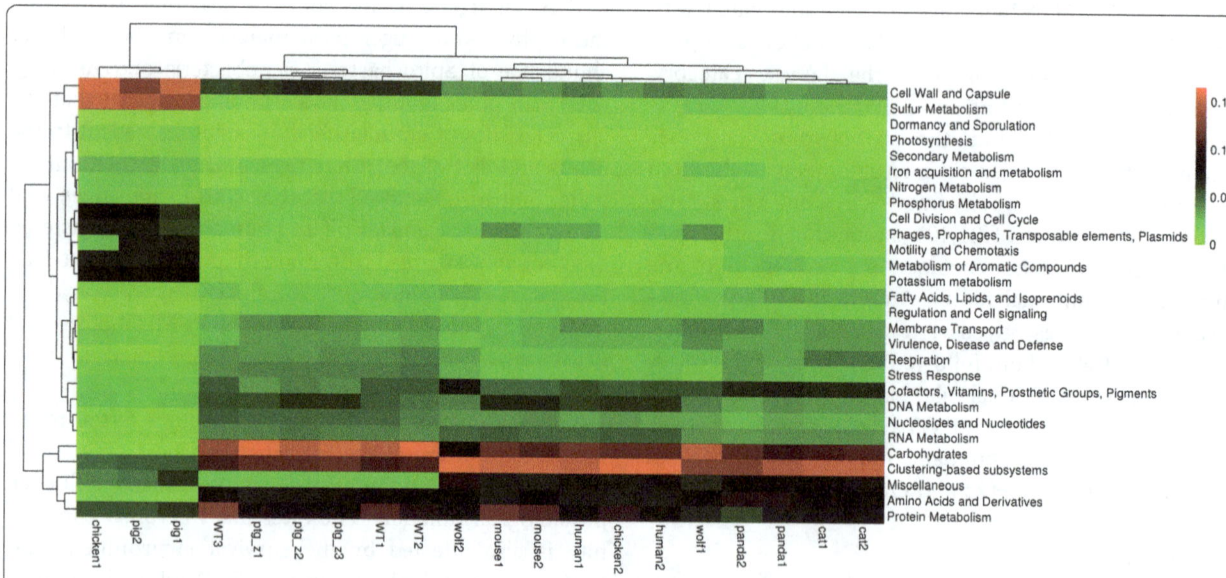

Fig. 4 Heat map of metabolic clustering of the wild Amur tiger gut metagenome compared to those of other animals

that the captive Amur tiger fecal metagenome had a lower abundance of Spirochaetes, Cyanobacteria and Ascomycota than other animals, and the primary functional categories were primarily associated with carbohydrate metabolism subsystems, clustering-based subsystems and protein metabolism. Taken together, these findings reveal the composition and functional structures of the gut microbiota in captive Amur tiger.

Methods

Faecal sample collection

Fresh faecal samples from 3 Amur tigers were collected at a single time point from the Heilongjiang Siberian Tiger Park in Heilongjiang Province, China, with permission form the authorities of the Heilongjiang Siberian Tiger Park. The age, sex and diet fed in the 10 days prior to fecal sampling are shown in Table 1 and 2. We randomly selected healthy Amur tigers in the Siberian Tiger Park, and faecal samples were collected aseptically immediately after defecation. The fresh faecal samples were transported to the laboratory on dry ice within 24 h of collection and stored at − 80 °C until DNA extraction. We brought no toxic substance that would interfere with the animal habitats. The research complied with the protocols established by the China Wildlife Conservation Association and the legal requirements of China.

DNA extraction

DNA was extracted from the faecal samples using the E.Z.N.A.® Stool DNA Kit (D4015–02, Omega, Inc., USA) according to the manufacturer's instructions. This reagent, which is designed to recover DNA from trace amounts of sample, has been shown to be effective for the preparation of DNA from most bacteria. Sample blanks consisted of unused swabs processed by DNA extraction and verified to contain no DNA amplicons. The total DNA was eluted in 50 μl of Elution buffer by modification of the procedure described by the manufacturer (QIAGEN) and stored at − 80 °C until measurement by PCR by LC-BIO TECHNOLOGIES (HANGZHOU) CO., LTD., Hang Zhou, Zhejiang Province, China.

DNA library construction

The DNA library was constructed using a TruSeq Nano DNA LT Library Preparation Kit (FC-121-4001). DNA was fragmented by dsDNA Fragmentase (NEB, M0348S) with incubation at 37 °C for 30 min. Library construction began with fragmented cDNA. Blunt-end DNA fragments were generated using a combination of fill-in reactions and exonuclease activity, and size selection was performed with the provided sample purification beads. An A-base was then added to the blunt ends of each strand to prepare them for ligation to the indexed adapters. Each adapter contained a T-base overhang to ligate the adapter to the A-tailed fragmented DNA. These adapters contained the full complement of the sequencing primer hybridization sites for the single, paired-end, indexed reads. Single- or dual-index adapters were ligated to the fragments, and the ligated products were amplified by PCR under the following conditions: initial denaturation at 95 °C for 3 min; 8 cycles of denaturation at 98 °C for 15 s, annealing at 60 °C for 15 s, and extension at 72 °C for 30 s; and final extension at 37 °C for 5 min.

Table 1 Sex, Age and Physical condition of captive Amur tiger in Siberian Tiger Park

Sample	Sex	Age (year)	Physical condition
ptg_z1	Male	7	Healthy
ptg_z2	Male	7	Healthy
ptg_z3	Female	12	Healthy

Data analysis

Raw sequencing reads were processed to obtain valid reads for further analysis. First, sequencing adapters were removed from the sequencing reads using cutadapt v1.9. Second, low-quality reads were trimmed by fqtrim v0.94 using a sliding-window algorithm. Third, the reads were aligned to the host genome using bowtie2 v2.2.0 to remove host contamination. The quality-filtered reads were then de novo assembled to construct the metagenome for each sample by SPAdes v3.10.0. All coding regions (CDS) of the metagenomic contigs were predicted by MetaGeneMark v3.26.

The CDS sequences of all samples were clustered by CD-HIT v4.6.1 to obtain unigenes. The unigene abundance for a certain sample was estimated by TPM based on the number of aligned reads by bowtie2 v2.2.0. The lowest common ancestor taxonomy of the unigenes was obtained by aligning them against the NCBI NR database using DIAMOND v 0.7.12. Similarly, the functional annotation (GO, KEGG, CAZy) of the unigenes was obtained. Based on the taxonomic and functional annotations and abundance profiles of the unigenes, differential analysis was performed at the taxonomic, functional or gene level using Fisher's exact test (non-replicated groups) or the Kruskal-Wallis test (replicated groups).

Comparative metagenomic analysis

Comparative metagenomic analysis was performed using the MG-RAST pipelines. The metagenomic runs from the captive Amur tiger data were compared with the current publicly available gut metagenomes. In the MG-RAST metagenomic annotation pipeline, the captive Amur tiger fecal metagenomic datasets were compared with those of wild Amur tigers (WT1, WT2, and WT3) and fourteen public datasets from other animals, including cat 1 (mgm

Table 2 The diet of captive Amur tiger in the 10 days before the sampling in Siberian Tiger Park

Date	ptg_z1		ptg_z2		ptg_z3	
	Diet	Quantity (kg)	Diet	Quantity (kg)	Diet	Quantity (kg)
2017-6-10	Fasting	–	Fasting	–	Fasting	–
2017-6-11	Duck	3.5	Duck	3.5	Duck	3.5
2017-6-12	Duck	3.5	Duck	3.5	Duck	3.5
2017-6-13	Duck	3.5	Duck	3.5	Duck	3.5
2017-6-14	Fasting	–	Fasting	–	Fasting	–
2017-6-15	Duck	3.5	Duck	3.5	Duck	3.5
2017-6-16	Duck	3.5	Duck	3.5	Duck	3.5
2017-6-17	Fasting	–	Fasting	–	Fasting	–
2017-6-18	Duck	3.5	Duck	3.5	Duck	3.5
2017-6-19	Duck	3.5	Duck	3.5	Duck	3.5

4,626,753.3), cat 2 (mgm4626754.3), chicken 1 (mgm4743765.3), chicken 2 (mgm4440284.3), human 1 (mgm4472483.3), human 2 (mgm4440941.3), mouse 1 (mgm4537490.3), mouse 2 (mgm4540251.3), panda 1 (mgm4694746.3), panda 2 (mgm4683980.3), pig 1 (mgm 4745745.3), pig 2 (mgm4745743.3), wolf 1 (mgm45356 26.3) and wolf 2 (mgm4441601.3).

Integrate phylum level abundance information of captive Amur tiger and other species, standardize as a percentage, take the 25 phylum with the highest percentage, others are unclassified, take the log10 for heat map drawing (the value with a percentage of 0 is replaced by 1/2 of the minimum value in all data), heat map drawing using the pheatmap package. Download the subsystems database on the SEED website (http://www.theseed.org) and comparison to unigenes of captive Amur tiger. Next, calculate the abundance of each category of subsystems, integrate abundance information of Amur tigers and other species subsystems, standardized as a percentage, using the pheatmap package to draw the heat map.

Additional files

Additional file 1: Information regarding the sequence data.

Additional file 2: Phylogenetic classification of the bacteria in the Amur tiger metagenome.

Additional file 3: Phylogenetic classification of Eukaryota in the Amur tiger metagenome.

Additional file 4: Phylogenetic classification of Archaea in the Amur tiger metagenome.

Additional file 5: Phylogenetic classification of the viruses in the Amur tiger metagenome.

Additional file 6: GO annotations of the Amur tiger faecal metagenome.

Additional file 7: GO annotations of the Amur tiger faecal metagenome.

Additional file 8: CAZy annotations of the Amur tiger metagenome.

Additional file 9: CAZy classification of the Amur tiger faecal metagenome.

Abbreviations

CAZy: Carbohydrate-active enzymes; CBM: Carbohydratebinding modules; CITES: Convention on International Trade in Endangered Species of Wild Fauna and Flora; DNA: Deoxyribonucleic acid; GH: Glycoside hydrolase; GO: Gene ontology; GT: Glycosyl transferase; IUCN: International union for conservation of nature; KEGG: Kyoto encyclopedia of genes and genomes; NCBI: National center for biotechnology information; SRA: Short read archive

Acknowledgements

We thank Haitao Xu, Yurong Guo and Xuanmin Kong for sample collection.

Funding

This work was funded by the National Natural Science Foundation of China (31372209). This study also supported by "The Fundamental Research Funds for the Central Universities" (2572017AA20).

Authors' contributions

FH participated with the study design, bioinformatic analyses and manuscript preparation. LZ carried out sample collection and sample processing. JZ participated with statistical analyses. YM participated with bioinformatic analyses. DL provided faecal materials and back ground information of tigers for the study, and monitored the diet of the captive tigers before sample collection. YX contributed with bioinformatic and statistical analyses. GJ contributed analysis tools for the study and participated with bioinformatic analyses. KR and JM collaborated in the design and coordination and helped to draft the manuscript. All authors read and approved the final manuscript.

Consent for publication

Not applicable.

Competing interests

The authors declare that they have no competing interests.

Author details

[1]College of Wildlife Resources, Northeast Forestry University, Harbin 150040, China. [2]Heilongjiang Siberian Tiger Park, Harbin 150040, China. [3]State Forestry Administration Detecting Center of Wildlife, Harbin 150040, China. [4]China Feline Research Center of Chinese State Forestry Administration, Harbin 150040, China.

References

1. Mazak J. Panthera tigris. Mamm Species. 1981;152:1–8.
2. Miquelle DG, Pikunov DG, Dunishenko YM, Aramilev VV, Nikolaev IG, Abramov VK, Smirnov EN, Salkina GP, Seryodkin IV, Gaponov VV. 2005 Amur Tiger Census. Cat News. 2007;46:14–5.
3. Zhang C, Zhang M, Stott P. Does prey density limit Amur tiger Panthera tigris altaica recovery in northeastern China? Wildlife Biol. 2013;19(4):452–61.
4. Ripple WJ, Estes JA, Beschta RL, Wilmers CC, Ritchie EG, Hebblewhite M, Berger J, Elmhagen B, Letnic M, Nelson MP. Status and ecological effects of the World's largest carnivores. Science. 2014;343(6167):1241484.
5. Ley RE, Hamady M, Lozupone C, Turnbaugh PJ, Ramey RR, Bircher JS, Schlegel ML, Tucker TA, Schrenzel MD, Knight R. Evolution of mammals and their gut microbes. Science. 2008;320(5883):1647–51.

6. Clemente JC, Ursell LK, Parfrey LW, Knight R. The impact of the gut microbiota on human health: an integrative view. Cell. 2012;148(6):1258–70.
7. Kau AL, Ahern PP, Griffin NW, Goodman AL, Gordon JI. Human nutrition, the gut microbiome and the immune system. Nature. 2011;474(7351):327–36.
8. Ley R. Microbial ecology: human gut microbes associated with obesity. Nature. 2006;444(7122):1022.
9. Qin J, Li R, Raes J, Arumugam M, Burgdorf KS, Manichanh C, Nielsen T, Pons N, Levenez F, Yamada T. A human gut microbial gene catalogue established by metagenomic sequencing. Nature. 2010; 464(7285):59–65.
10. David LA, Maurice CF, Carmody RN, Gootenberg DB, Button JE, Wolfe BE, Ling AV, Devlin AS, Varma Y, Fischbach MA. Diet rapidly and reproducibly alters the human gut microbiome. Nature. 2014;505(7484):559.
11. Vital M, Gao J, Rizzo M, Harrison T, Tiedje JM. Diet is a major factor governing the fecal butyrate-producing community structure across Mammalia, Aves and Reptilia. Isme J. 2015;9(4):832.
12. Wang J, Tang H, Zhang C, Zhao Y, Derrien M, Rocher E, Vanhylckama JV, Strissel K, Zhao L, Obin M. Modulation of gut microbiota during probiotic-mediated attenuation of metabolic syndrome in high fat diet-fed mice. Isme J Multidiscipli. 2015;9(1):1.
13. Goodwin S, McPherson JD, McCombie WR. Coming of age: ten years of next-generation sequencing technologies. Nat Rev Genet. 2016;17(6):333.
14. Gill SR, Pop M, Deboy RT, Eckburg PB, Turnbaugh PJ, Samuel BS, Gordon JI, Relman DA, Fraserliggett CM, Nelson KE. Metagenomic analysis of the human distal gut microbiome. Science. 2006;312(5778):1355–9.
15. Turnbaugh PJ, Hamady M, Yatsunenko T, Cantarel BL, Duncan A, Ley RE, Sogin ML, Jones WJ, Roe BA, Affourtit JP. A core gut microbiome in obese and lean twins. Nature. 2009;457(7228):480–4.
16. Warnecke F, Luginbühl P, Ivanova N, Ghassemian M, Richardson TH, Stege JT, Cayouette M, McHardy AC, Djordjevic G, Aboushadi N. Metagenomic and functional analysis of hindgut microbiota of a wood-feeding higher termite. Nature. 2007;450(7169):560–5.
17. Hess M, Sczyrba A, Egan R, Kim TW, Chokhawala H, Schroth G, Luo S, Clark DS, Chen F, Zhang T. Metagenomic discovery of biomass-degrading genes and genomes from cow rumen. Science. 2011;331(6016):463.
18. Lamendella R, Domingo JWS, Ghosh S, Martinson J, Oerther DB. Comparative fecal metagenomics unveils unique functional capacity of the swine gut. BMC Microbiol. 2011;11(1):1–17.
19. Singh KM, Ahir VB, Tripathi AK, Ramani UV, Sajnani M, Koringa PG, Jakhesara S, Pandya PR, Rank DN, Murty DS. Metagenomic analysis of Surti buffalo (*Bubalus bubalis*) rumen: a preliminary study. Mol Biol Rep. 2012;39(4):4841.
20. Li RW, Connor EE, Li C, Baldwin Vi RL, Sparks ME. Characterization of the rumen microbiota of pre-ruminant calves using metagenomic tools. Environ Microbiol. 2012;14(1):129.
21. Lu HP, Wang YB, Huang SW, Lin CY, Wu M, Chih-Hao H, Yu HT. Metagenomic analysis reveals a functional signature for biomass degradation by cecal microbiota in the leaf-eating flying squirrel (*Petaurista alborufus lena*). BMC Genomics. 2012;13(1):466.
22. Bo X, Xu W, Li J, Dai L, Xiong C, Tang X, Yang Y, Mu Y, Zhou J, Ding J. Metagenomic analysis of the Rhinopithecus bieti fecal microbiome reveals a broad diversity of bacterial and glycoside hydrolase profiles related to lignocellulose degradation. BMC Genomics. 2015;16(1):174.
23. Zhu L, Wu Q, Deng C, Zhang M, Zhang C, Chen H, Lu G, Wei F. Adaptive evolution to a high purine and fat diet of carnivorans revealed by gut microbiomes and host genomes. Environ Microbiol. 2018;20(5):1711–22.
24. Roggenbuck M, Bærholm Schnell I, Blom N, Bælum J, Bertelsen MF, Sicheritz-Pontén T, Sørensen SJ, Gilbert MT, Graves GR, Hansen LH. The microbiome of New World vultures. Nat Commun. 2014;5:5498.
25. Keenan SW, Engel AS, Elsey RM. The alligator gut microbiome and implications for archosaur symbioses. Sci Rep. 2013;3:2877.
26. Spor A, Koren O, Ley R. Unravelling the effects of the environment and host genotype on the gut microbiome. Nat Rev Microbiol. 2011; 9(4):279–90.
27. Larsson MHMA, Flores AS, Fedullo JDL, Mirandola RMS, Ito FH, Pessoa RB, Itikawa PH. Biochemical parameters of wild felids (Panthera leo and Panthera tigris altaica) kept in captivity. Semin Cienc Agrar. 2017;38(2):791.
28. Shrivatav AB, Singh KP, Mittal SK, Malik PK. Haematological and biochemical studies in tigers (Panthera tigris tigris). Eur J Wildl Res. 2012;58(1):365–7.
29. Junginger J, Hansmann F, Herder V, Lehmbecker A, Peters M, Beyerbach M, Wohlsein P, Baumgärtner W. Pathology in captive wild felids at German zoological gardens. PLoS One. 2015;10(6):e0130573.
30. Mohapatra RK, Panda S, Acharya UR. Study on activity pattern and incidence of stereotypic behavior in captive tigers. J Vet Behav. 2014;9(4):172–6.
31. Bashaw MJ, Kelling AS, Bloomsmith MA, Maple TL. Environmental effects on the behavior of zoo-housed lions and tigers, with a case study of the effects of a visual barrier on pacing. J Appl Anim Welf Sci. 2007;10(2):95–109.

Permissions

All chapters in this book were first published in VR, by BioMed Central; hereby published with permission under the Creative Commons Attribution License or equivalent. Every chapter published in this book has been scrutinized by our experts. Their significance has been extensively debated. The topics covered herein carry significant findings which will fuel the growth of the discipline. They may even be implemented as practical applications or may be referred to as a beginning point for another development.

The contributors of this book come from diverse backgrounds, making this book a truly international effort. This book will bring forth new frontiers with its revolutionizing research information and detailed analysis of the nascent developments around the world.

We would like to thank all the contributing authors for lending their expertise to make the book truly unique. They have played a crucial role in the development of this book. Without their invaluable contributions this book wouldn't have been possible. They have made vital efforts to compile up to date information on the varied aspects of this subject to make this book a valuable addition to the collection of many professionals and students.

This book was conceptualized with the vision of imparting up-to-date information and advanced data in this field. To ensure the same, a matchless editorial board was set up. Every individual on the board went through rigorous rounds of assessment to prove their worth. After which they invested a large part of their time researching and compiling the most relevant data for our readers.

The editorial board has been involved in producing this book since its inception. They have spent rigorous hours researching and exploring the diverse topics which have resulted in the successful publishing of this book. They have passed on their knowledge of decades through this book. To expedite this challenging task, the publisher supported the team at every step. A small team of assistant editors was also appointed to further simplify the editing procedure and attain best results for the readers.

Apart from the editorial board, the designing team has also invested a significant amount of their time in understanding the subject and creating the most relevant covers. They scrutinized every image to scout for the most suitable representation of the subject and create an appropriate cover for the book.

The publishing team has been an ardent support to the editorial, designing and production team. Their endless efforts to recruit the best for this project, has resulted in the accomplishment of this book. They are a veteran in the field of academics and their pool of knowledge is as vast as their experience in printing. Their expertise and guidance has proved useful at every step. Their uncompromising quality standards have made this book an exceptional effort. Their encouragement from time to time has been an inspiration for everyone.

The publisher and the editorial board hope that this book will prove to be a valuable piece of knowledge for researchers, students, practitioners and scholars across the globe.

List of Contributors

Izabela Janus, Marcin Nowak, Rafał Ciaputa and Małgorzata Kandefer-Gola
Division of Pathomorphology and Veterinary Forensics, Department of Pathology, Wroclaw University of Environmental and Life Sciences, Wroclaw 50375, Poland

Agnieszka Noszczyk-Nowak and Urszula Pasławska
Department of Internal Medicine and Clinic of Diseases of Horses, Dogs and Cats Wroclaw University of Environmental and Life Sciences, Wroclaw 50366, Poland

Ronaldo Casimiro da Costa and Carolina Gonçalves Dias Lima
The Ohio State University, 601 Vernon Tharp St., Columbus, OH 43210, USA

Marília de Albuquerque Bonelli
The Ohio State University, 601 Vernon Tharp St., Columbus, OH 43210, USA
Department of Veterinary Medicine, Federal Rural University of Pernambuco, R. Dom Manoel de Medeiros s/n, Recife, PE 52171-900, Brazil

Paula Martin-Vaquero
The Ohio State University, 601 Vernon Tharp St., Columbus, OH 43210, USA
Ogilvy Healthworld, Avda. de Burgos 21, C. P. 28036 Madrid, Spain

Camila Peres Rubio, Silvia Martinez-Subiela and José Joaquin Cerón
Interdisciplinary Laboratory of Clinical Analysis Interlab-UMU, Faculty of Veterinary Medicine, Regional Campus of International Excellence 'Campus Mare Nostrum', University of Murcia, Espinardo, Murcia 30100, Spain

Asta Tvarijonaviciute
Interdisciplinary Laboratory of Clinical Analysis Interlab-UMU, Faculty of Veterinary Medicine, Regional Campus of International Excellence 'Campus Mare Nostrum', University of Murcia, Espinardo, Murcia 30100, Spain
Department of Animal Medicine and Surgery, Veterinary School, University Autonoma of Barcelona, Barcelona, Spain

Josefa Hernández-Ruiz
Department of Plant Biology (Plant Physiology), Faculty of Biology, University of Murcia, Murcia, Spain

Anna Szabelska
Department of Prosthetic Dentistry, Medical University in Lublin, ul. Karmelicka 7, 20-081 Lublin, Poland

Marcin R. Tatara
Department of Animal Physiology, Faculty of Veterinary Medicine, University of Life Sciences in Lublin, ul. Akademicka 12, 20-950 Lublin, Poland

Witold Krupski
II Department of Radiology, Medical University in Lublin, ul. Staszica 16, 20-081 Lublin, Poland

W. Dingemanse, H. van Bree and I. Gielen
Department of Medical Imaging of Domestic Animals and Orthopaedics of Small Animals Faculty of Veterinary Medicine, Ghent University, Merelbeke, Belgium

M. Müller-Gerbl
Institute of Anatomy, Basel University, Basel, Switzerland

I. Jonkers
Human Movement Biomechanics Research Group, Faculty of Kinesiology and Rehabilitation Sciences, KU Leuven, Leuven, Belgium

J. Vander Sloten
Biomechanics Section, Faculty of Engineering Science, KU Leuven, Leuven, Belgium

W. Dingemanse, H. van Bree and I. Gielen
Department of Medical Imaging of Domestic Animals and Orthopaedics of Small Animals Faculty of Veterinary Medicine, Ghent University, Merelbeke, Belgium

M. Müller-Gerbl
Institute of Anatomy, Basel University, Basel, Switzerland

I. Jonkers
Human Movement Biomechanics Research Group, Kinesiology Department, KU Leuven, Leuven, Belgium

J. Vander Sloten
Biomechanics Section, Faculty of Engineering Science, KU Leuven, Leuven, Belgium

Frine Eleonora Scaglione, Andrea Peano, Enrico Bollo, Francesca Tiziana Cannizzo and Mario Pasquetti
Dipartimento di Scienze Veterinarie, Università degli Studi di Torino, Largo Paolo Braccini 2, 1s0095 Grugliasco (To), Italy

Sara Piga and Stefano Meda
Zoom Torino, Strada Piscina 36, 10040 Cumiana, Italy

Henrik Elvang Jensen
Department of Veterinary Disease Biology, University of Copenhagen, Ridebanevej 3, DK-1870 Frederiksberg C, Copenhagen, Denmark

Chiara Locatelli, Cristian Piras, Giulia Riscazzi, Isabella Alloggio, Ilaria Spalla, Alessio Soggiu, Luigi Bonizzi and Paola G. Brambilla
DIMEVET, Department of Veterinary Medicine, University of Milan, Milan, Italy

Viviana Greco
Fondazione Santa Lucia -IRCCS, Rome, Italy

Paola Roncada
Istituto Sperimentale Italiano L. Spallanzani, Milan, Italy

Sarah Hindenberg, Sabine Zielinsky, Natali Bauer and Andreas Moritz
Department of Veterinary Clinical Sciences, Clinical Pathology and Clinical Pathophysiology, Justus-Liebig-University Giessen, 35392 Giessen, Germany

Stefanie Klenner-Gastreich and Nicole Kneier
Scil animal care company GmbH, 68519 Viernheim, Germany

Kris Gommeren
Department of Clinical Sciences, School of Veterinary Medicine, University of Liège, 4000 Liège, Belgium

Meredith J. Bashaw
Wildlife Reproductive Centre, Taronga Conservation Society of Australia, Dubbo, NSW, Australia
Department of Psychology, Franklin & Marshall College, Lancaster, PA, USA

Florian Sicks
Tierpark Berlin, Berlin, Germany

Rupert Palme and Franz Schwarzenberger
Department of Biomedical Sciences, University of Veterinary Medicine, Vienna, Austria

Adrian S. W. Tordiffe
Department of Paraclinical Sciences, Faculty of Veterinary Science, University of Pretoria, Onderstepoort, Pretoria, South Africa
National Zoological Gardens of South Africa, Pretoria, South Africa

Andre Ganswindt
National Zoological Gardens of South Africa, Pretoria, South Africa
Department of Anatomy and Physiology, Endocrine Research Laboratory, Faculty of Veterinary Science, University of Pretoria, Onderstepoort, Pretoria, South Africa

Ulrike Kordass, Regina Carlson, Veronika Maria Stein and Andrea Tipold
Department of Small Animal Medicine and Surgery, University of Veterinary
Medicine Hannover, Hannover, Germany

Björn G.M. Eussen, Jaap Schaveling, Maria J. Dragt and Robert Jan Blomme
Center for Leadership and Management Development, Nyenrode Business University, AC Breukelen, Netherlands

Erica J. Moore, Stanley E. Kim, Scott A. Banks, Antonio Pozzi, Jason D. Coggeshall and Stephen C. Jones
Comparative Orthopaedics Biomechanics Laboratory, College of Veterinary Medicine, University of Florida, SW 16th Ave, Gainesville, FL 32610-0126, USA

Alexander Otterlei, Daniel Jensen and Are Nylund
Fish Diseases Research Group, Department of Biology, University of Bergen, Bergen, Norway

Patricia Apablaza, Henrik Duesund and Øyvind J. Brevik
Cermaq Group AS, Dronning Eufemias gate 16, SentrumN-0102 Oslo, Norway

Petter Frost and Ingunn Sommerset
MSD Animal Health, Thormølensgt. 55, 5008 Bergen, Norway

Julio Mendoza
Cermaq Chile, Diego Portales 2000, piso 10, Puerto Montt, Chile

Peter McKenzie
Cermaq Canada, 203 - 919 Island Highway, Campbell River, BC V9W 2C2, Canada

Dora Pinheiro
University of Trás-os-Montes e Alto-Douro (UTAD), Vila Real, Portugal

João Machado
Veterinary Teaching Hospital, UTAD, Vila Real, Portugal

Luís Cardoso and Ana Martins-Bessa
Veterinary Teaching Hospital, UTAD, Vila Real, Portugal
Department of Veterinary Sciences, School of Agrarian and Veterinary Sciences, UTAD, Vila Real, Portugal

Carlos Viegas
Department of Veterinary Sciences, School of Agrarian and Veterinary Sciences, UTAD, Vila Real, Portugal
Centre for the Research and Technology of Agro-Environmental and Biological Sciences (CITAB), UTAD, Vila Real, Portugal

Maria A. Pires
Department of Veterinary Sciences, School of Agrarian and Veterinary Sciences, UTAD, Vila Real, Portugal
Animal and Veterinary Research Centre (CECAV), UTAD, Vila Real, Portugal

Cláudia Baptista
Department of Veterinary Clinics, UPVet, Instituto de Ciências Biomédicas Abel Salazar, Universidade do Porto, Oporto, Portugal

Estela Bastos
Department of Genetics and Biotechnology, School of Life and Environment Sciences, UTAD, Vila Real, Portugal

Joana Magalhães
UCIBIO, REQUIMTE, Department of Chemical Sciences, Faculdade de Farmácia, Universidade do Porto, Oporto, Portugal

Marjolein L. den Toom, Agnes E. Meiling and Peter A. J. Leegwater
Department of Clinical Sciences of Companion Animals, Faculty of Veterinary Medicine, Utrecht University, Yalelaan 108, 3508, TD, Utrecht, The Netherlands

Henri C. M. Heuven
Department of Clinical Sciences of Companion Animals, Faculty of Veterinary Medicine, Utrecht University, Yalelaan 108, 3508, TD, Utrecht, The Netherlands
Animal Breeding and Genomics Centre, Wageningen University, 6700, AH, Wageningen, The Netherlands

Rachel E. Thomas
Department of Pathobiology, Faculty of Veterinary Medicine, Utrecht University, Yalelaan 1, 3485, CL, Utrecht, The Netherlands

Asta Tvarijonaviciute, Tomas Barranco, Silvia Martinez-Subiela, Fernando Tecles, Juana Dolores Carrillo and José J. Cerón
Animal Medicine and Surgery Department, School of Veterinary Medicine, University of Murcia, Campus of Espinardo s/n, 30100 Murcia, Spain

Monica Rubio and Jose Maria Carrillo
Animal Medicine and Surgery Department, School of Veterinary Medicine, Universidad CEU Cardenal Herrera of Valencia, Valencia, Spain
Garcia Cugat Foundation CEU-UCH Chair of Medicine and Regenerative 3 Surgery, Barcelona, Spain

Lionel Sebbag
Department of Veterinary Clinical Sciences, Iowa State University, College of Veterinary Medicine, Ames, IA 50011, USA

Emily M. McDowell and Patrick M. Hepner
Lloyd Veterinary Medical Center, Iowa State University, College of Veterinary Medicine, Ames, IA 50011, USA

Jonathan P. Mochel
Department of Biomedical sciences, Iowa State University, College of Veterinary Medicine, Ames, IA 50011, USA

José A. Camassa, Camila C. Diogo and João P. A. Bordelo
Department of Veterinary Sciences, Agricultural and Veterinary Sciences School (ECAV), University of Trás-os-Montes and Alto Douro (UTAD), Quinta de Prados, 5001-801 Vila Real, Portugal

Isabel R. Dias and Carlos A. Viegas
Department of Veterinary Sciences, Agricultural and Veterinary Sciences School (ECAV), University of Trás-os-Montes and Alto Douro (UTAD), Quinta de Prados, 5001-801 Vila Real, Portugal
CITAB - Centre for the Research and Technology of Agro-Environmental and Biological Sciences, UTAD, Vila Real, Portugal

Marília de A. Bonelli
Federal Rural University of Pernambuco (UFRPE), R. Dom Manoel de Medeiros, s/n, Dois Irmãos, Recife, PE 52171-900, Brazil

Jorge T. Azevedo
Department of Animal Sciences, ECAV, UTAD, Vila Real, Portugal
CECAV - Centre for Animal Sciences and Veterinary Studies, UTAD, Vila Real, Portugal

Nuno Dourado
CMEMS-UMinho, Department of Mechanical Engineering, University of Minho, Campus de Azurém, 4804-533 Guimarães, Portugal

Moran Tal, Adronie Verbrugghe and Charlotte Chau
Department of Clinical Studies, Ontario Veterinary College, University of Guelph, Guelph, ON N1G 2W1, Canada

J. Scott Weese
Department of Pathobiology, Ontario Veterinary College, University of Guelph, Guelph, ON N1G 2W1, Canada

Diego E. Gomez
Department of Pathobiology, Ontario Veterinary College, University of Guelph, Guelph, ON N1G 2W1, Canada
College of Veterinary Medicine, University of Florida, Gainesville, Florida, USA

María J. García-Iglesias and Claudia Pérez-Martínez
Department of Animal Health, Faculty of Veterinary Science, Institute of Biomedicine (IBIOMED), University of León, Campus de Vegazana, s/n, 24071 León, Spain

César B. Gutiérrez-Martín
Department of Animal Health, Faculty of Veterinary Science, University of León, Campus de Vegazana, s/n, 24071 León, Spain

Ana M. Sahagún-Prieto and Raquel Díez-Laiz
Department of Biomedical Sciences, Faculty of Veterinary Science, Institute of Biomedicine (IBIOMED), University of León, Campus de Vegazana, s/n, 24071 León, Spain

Lieven Van Meulebroek, Nathalie De Clercq, Julie Vanden Bussche and Lynn Vanhaecke
Faculty of Veterinary Medicine, Department of Veterinary Public Health & Food Safety, Laboratory of Chemical Analysis, Ghent University, Salisburylaan 133, 9820 Merelbeke, Belgium

Mathias Devreese and Siska Croubels
Faculty of Veterinary Medicine, Department of Pharmacology, Toxicology and Biochemistry, Laboratory of Pharmacology and Toxicology, Ghent University, Salisburylaan 133, 9820 Merelbeke, Belgium

Eric Fichant and Philippe Delahaut
Département Santé, CER Groupe, Rue du Point du Jour 8, Marloie 6900, Belgium

Jennifer Kylie, J. Scott Weese and Patricia V. Turner
Department of Pathobiology, University of Guelph, Guelph, ON N1G 2W1, Canada

Yoshihiko Yu, Daisuke Hasegawa, Aki Fujiwara-Igarashi, Yuji Hamamoto, Shunta Mizoguchi, Takayuki Kuwabara and Michio Fujita
Department of Clinical Veterinary Medicine, Nippon Veterinary and Life Science University, 1-7 1 Kyonan-cho, Musashino-shi, Tokyo 180-8602, Japan

Fengping He, Le Zhang and Jiancheng Zhai
College of Wildlife Resources, Northeast Forestry University, Harbin 150040, China

Dan Liu
Heilongjiang Siberian Tiger Park, Harbin 150040, China

Yue Ma and Yanchun Xu
College of Wildlife Resources, Northeast Forestry University, Harbin 150040, China
State Forestry Administration Detecting Center of Wildlife, Harbin 150040, China

Ke Rong, Jianzhang Ma and Guangshun Jiang
College of Wildlife Resources, Northeast Forestry University, Harbin 150040, China
China Feline Research Center of Chinese State Forestry Administration, Harbin 150040, China

Index